JUSTINE BASSANI

EATING LESSONS
FOR THE BODY AND MIND

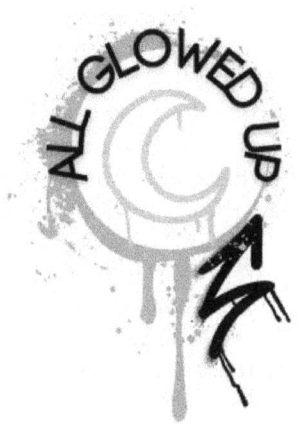

First published by ALL GLOWED UP LLC.

Copyright 2024 by Justine Bassani

All rights reserved. No part of this publication may be reproduced, stored or transmitted in any form or by any means, electronic, mechanical, photocopying, recording, scanning, or otherwise without written permission from the publisher. It is illegal to copy this book, post it to a website, or distribute it by any other means without permission. Justine Bassani has no responsibility for the persistence or accuracy of URLs for external or third-party Internet Websites referred to in this publication and does not guarantee any content on such Websites is, or will remain, accurate or appropriate.

Justine Bassani has no responsibility for the persistence or accuracy of URLs for external or third-party Internet Websites referred to in this publication and does not guarantee that any content on such Websites is, or will remain, accurate or appropriate.

Designations used by companies to distinguish their products are often claimed as trademarks. All brand names and product names used in this book and on its cover are trade names, service marks, trademarks and registered trademarks of their respective owners. The publishers and the book are not associated with any product or vendor mentioned in this book. None of the companies referenced within the book have endorsed the book.

The information provided in this book is for educational and informational purposes only and is not a substitute for professional medical advice, diagnosis, or treatment. Always consult with a physician or qualified healthcare provider before making significant changes to your diet, exercise routine, or using any supplements, especially if you have pre-existing medical conditions or concerns. The author and publisher disclaim any liability for adverse effects or consequences resulting from the use of any suggestions, products, or procedures discussed in this book. Individual nutritional and health needs vary, so use this information as a general guide and seek personalized advice from a registered dietitian, nutritionist, or healthcare professional. If you are experiencing psychological or emotional distress, please seek help from a licensed mental health professional. By reading this book, you acknowledge that you are responsible for your own health decisions.

Second edition 2024
EPUB 979-8-9897915-0-7 / Paperback 979-8-9897915-1-4
Hardcover 979-8-9897915-2-1

To my mom, who taught me the value of perseverance and compassion.

To Sese, for always believing in me and encouraging me to follow my dreams. And to my loyal customers, whose curiosity and conversations sparked the inspiration for this book. This journey wouldn't have been possible without your trust and support.

Thank you for being a part of my world.

CONTENTS

PREFACE	v
WHY DIETS ARE BAD	1
WATER YOU DRINKING?	15
RECOVERING FOODIE	33
MACROS & DON'T FORGET THE MICROS	47
THE HYPE ABOUT FASTING	60
WHAT'S WITH FIBER, THO?	73
THROWING SHADE AT CARBS	89
THE LIES THEY TOLD YOU ABOUT PROTEIN	111
OMEGA WARS	128
EAT BEFORE YOU'RE HUNGRY DRINK BEFORE YOU'RE THIRSTY	150
KNOW YOUR CRAVINGS	165
MUSCLE, MOOD, & THE HOPE MOLECULE: HORMONE HEALTH	188
TRUST YOUR GUT	200
SODIUM SUCKS. NAVIGATING FOOD LABELS	217
ORGANIC VS. EVERYTHING ELSE	234
DON'T EAT YOUR WHEATIEZ	251
SOMETHING'S FISHY	269
SOY NICE TO MEET YOU!	282
NOT MYLK!	295
EAT THE RAINBOW, WHY RAW IS BETTER	311
BOOZE IS MAKING YOU FAT	337
SUPP WITH YOU?	352
WORKBOOK	367

PREFACE

In a world filled with conflicting nutritional advice and relentless pressure to conform to societal beauty standards, I wrote this book to offer a beacon of clarity and empowerment. It is not just another diet book; it's a guide to transforming your relationship with food, your body, and your overall well-being.

The promise of this book is simple yet profound: to help you break free from the cycle of restrictive diets and unhealthy habits and to lead you towards a balanced, nourishing approach to health that honors your body's natural wisdom.

Throughout my life, I struggled with dieting, often feeling lost and overwhelmed by the flood of advice and the latest trends that promised quick fixes. I, like many others, was caught in the trap of believing that achieving the ideal body meant adhering to strict, often unsustainable diets. But over time, I realized that good health and a fit body do not require a deprivation diet to achieve. It's about learning and allowing ourselves to seek physical and emotional nourishment. This book is born from that realization and my desire to help others navigate the confusing landscape of modern nutrition.

The journey to writing this book began in childhood when my family's traditions profoundly influenced my perspectives on food. My mother, a woman of strength and conviction, always took me to the health food store instead of the traditional grocery store and was the first to instill in me the importance of choosing foods as close to nature as possible.

EATING LESSONS

Her journey began at the tender age of seven when she consciously decided to become a pescatarian after witnessing the harsh realities of animal farming. This decision, rooted in compassion and a deep respect for life, was a defining moment for me as I learned to understand the meaning of food and where it came from.

Our family's roots run deep in the soil of Italy, where my grandparents lived as farmers before immigrating to the United States in the 1950s. Their stories of life in Ripi, a small town where self-sufficiency was not just a choice but a necessity, have always resonated with me. My grandparents brought their farming traditions with them to America, transforming our family's small plots of land into abundant gardens that provided us with fresh produce year-round.

My earliest memories are of summers spent helping in the garden, my tiny hands eagerly shucking peas, snapping beans, and harvesting tomatoes under the warm sun.

These experiences were more than just chores. They were lessons in patience, hard work, and the value of what I put into my body.

Watching my Grandparents tend to the earth and reap its rewards taught me that food is more than sustenance; it is a connection to our heritage, a source of pride, and a foundation for health. The rows of tomatoes, beans, and lettuces in my grandparents' garden were more than just plants; they were a testament to the life-giving power of the earth and the dedication of those who worked it.

My mother's unwavering commitment to feeding me the cleanest, most nourishing foods shaped my early years in ways I didn't fully appreciate until much later. She raised me on meals prepared with fresh, homegrown ingredients and foods as close to nature as possible. We lived by the principles of the Moosewood Cookbook, eschewing processed foods and refined sugars in favor of

Preface

whole grains, legumes, and vegetables. The kitchen was our sanctuary, and I learned from an early age that the best meals came from our hands, cultivated from the earth with care and respect.

My grandparents, now in their 90s, continue to work in their garden with the same vigor and passion they had in their youth. Their lifestyle, characterized by physical labor and a diet rich in homegrown produce, is a testament to the life-giving power of organic, whole foods. My grandmother, often seen climbing ladders to pick the highest beans, and my grandfather, tirelessly tending to the soil, are living proof that how we nourish our bodies profoundly impacts our longevity and vitality.

The garden has always been more than just a food source for our family. It symbolizes resilience, the strength that comes from working with nature rather than against it. The wild peppermint that chased the sun up the garden gate, the rows of vibrant green and purple lettuces, the squash and cucumbers that seemed to multiply overnight, these were the gifts of the earth, nurtured by hands that respected and understood the cycles of nature. The bounty of our garden sustained us, not just physically but emotionally, grounding us in the rhythms of the seasons and the simple joys of a life lived in harmony with the land.

However, as I grew older, the simplicity of my upbringing was overshadowed by the complexities of modern life. Like many young women, I became increasingly aware of societal beauty standards and the pressures to conform. The media bombarded me with images of perfection, and I began to believe that achieving a specific body type was the ultimate goal. I strayed from the nourishing principles I had been raised with, experimenting with every restrictive diet that promised quick results. Yet, despite my best efforts, these diets only left me feeling depleted, both physically and emotionally.

It took years of trial and error to realize that my worth was not tied to a number on the scale or the size of my clothes. The turning point came when I understood that the key to true health was not starvation or deprivation but balance and nourishment. My body was not the enemy; it was my greatest ally, capable of amazing things when given the right fuel. Instead of viewing hunger as something to be suppressed, I began to see it as a signal and an opportunity to nourish myself with foods that would support my energy, strength, and overall well-being.

The realization that naturally maintaining one's weight wasn't a myth reserved for those with perfect genetics was liberating. I began embracing the values my mother had instilled in me, eating whole natural foods and listening to my body. I knew this was the most basic concept yet often overlooked, but I knew in my heart if I gave it the consistency I gave all of the diets I tried, I could achieve the wellness I had always sought. This shift in perspective led me to pursue further education in personal training and nutrition to deepen my understanding and help others struggling with similar issues.

My mother's influence continued to guide me as I immersed myself in the study of nutrition. Her resilience and dedication inspired me to dig deeper, question the mainstream narratives, and seek the truth. I wanted to empower myself and others with the knowledge necessary to make informed decisions about our health. Through my studies and professional training, I learned the science behind what I had always intuitively known: that the best way to care for our bodies is to return to the basics, to the foods that nourish us on every level.

This book is the result of my journey, influenced by my family's wisdom, my personal struggles, and the knowledge I've gained. It is intended for those tired of the endless cycle of diets that promise results but fail to deliver. It is for those who feel overwhelmed by the conflicting advice that bombards us from every media outlet. It is for

Preface

those who want to break free from the patterns of restriction and deprivation and find a path to their individual best health and untapped vitality.

In these pages, you will learn the steps to change and how to understand the true impact of your food choices and how they impact not just your weight but your energy levels, mood, skin health, hormones, and overall well-being. You will discover why diets often fail and how to adopt a more sustainable approach to eating.

You will gain insights into how to listen to your body's hunger and fullness cues, using these signals to guide your food choices. You will empower yourself with the knowledge necessary to make informed decisions about what you eat based on science and not celebrity trends. In these pages, you will learn the steps to change and understand the true impact of your food choices. Discover how they affect not just your weight but also your energy levels, mood, skin health, hormones, and overall well-being.

This book will help you develop a balanced, nourishing approach to food that allows you to create satisfying and health-promoting meals without feeling deprived or restricted. You will move away from viewing food as the enemy and begin to see it as a powerful tool for enhancing your health and quality of life. You will understand how to achieve and maintain your ideal weight naturally without resorting to extreme measures or diets.

My grandparents' garden strengthened my relationship to food and taught me that how we nourish our bodies has a profound impact on our health and longevity. This book is a testament to that lesson, and I hope that it will inspire you to cultivate your relationship with food, one that is based on respect, understanding, and a deep appreciation for the nourishment that the earth provides.

If you've ever felt overwhelmed by the endless stream of nutritional advice or disheartened by diets that don't deliver on their promises, you're not alone. I've come out the other side with a renewed understanding of what it means to be truly healthy. The core message of this book is that your body already has the wisdom to guide you; you need to learn how to listen to it.

True transformation begins with the decision to prioritize your health, and by picking up this book, you've already taken the first step. I invite you to join me on this journey to explore the power of nourishing your body with intention and to discover the joy of living in alignment with your natural rhythms. Your body is capable of incredible things; together, we can unlock its full potential.

Let this book be your guide to a healthier, more vibrant life. The path may not always be easy, but it is always worth it. And remember, the most important relationship you will ever have is the one with yourself, so nourish it well!

1
WHY DIETS ARE BAD

A journey through the olfactory memory lane is more than a simple recollection of past tastes and smells. It's a deep dive into the sensory experiences that have shaped our food habits, from our holiday menu traditions to what we crave for comfort and our go-to grocery items. The aroma and flavor of our past meals linger in us from the earliest days of childhood. These memories form the foundation of our relationship with food, intertwining with our emotions, traditions, and identities. Understanding how these sensory memories influence our present-day eating habits is crucial for developing a healthier, more balanced approach to food.

The olfactory system, with its intricate network of scent receptors, acts as a powerful gateway to our memories. A simple whiff of a familiar aroma can transport us back to a cherished moment, whether the comforting scent of freshly baked bread filling the kitchen or the nostalgic sweetness of Grandma's apple pie cooling on the windowsill. These scents do more than remind us of past pleasures. They trigger emotions and memories that influence our cravings and shape our culinary preferences. They are the silent architects of our food-related experiences, connecting us to the past with each inhalation.

Taste, like our sense of smell, is closely connected to memory. Our taste buds provide direct feedback, translating the flavors we consume into immediate sensations. The delicate dance of sweetness on our tongues, the bold bite of bitterness, and the tang of something sour all leave their mark on our palates, etching themselves into our minds and guiding our future culinary choices. As we grow older, these taste preferences, often rooted in childhood, evolve under the influence of various external factors.

However, as we mature, our palates often become misguided by a host of external influences. Cultural traditions, dietary trends, adolescent school lunches, and annual holiday feasts shape our eating habits. From the once authoritative food pyramid to today's media incessantly promoting the latest food trends, these influences shape our views on food and, consequently, our eating habits. When bombarded with conflicting advice and unhealthy food options, it's easy to become disconnected from our natural instincts about what our bodies truly need.

Entering adulthood presents its own set of challenges. The notorious "freshman 15," post-pregnancy weight changes, or the struggle to bounce back from an injury, push us toward various diets, each one promising that elusive ideal physique. Despite our best efforts, we have all questioned whether our nutritional understanding is as solid as it should be. Are we merely skimming the surface with a multivitamin, hoping it will counterbalance the lack of leafy greens on our plates? Do we grapple with the confusion surrounding daily fiber intake, hydration mistakes, or the persistent feeling of being simultaneously parched and bloated, even after downing an entire bottle of water?

These questions reflect a common struggle in our modern relationship with food. We yearn to return to simpler times when food was just food, an experience of pure joy and nourishment, free from the complexities of dietary trends and nutritional confusion. Yet, as we navigate the maze of adult eating habits, we often find ourselves longing for childhood's uncomplicated flavors and aromas, the very scents and tastes that first shaped our love for food and continue to influence us today.

However, this nostalgia can also be misleading. While the

foods of our past may bring comfort, they are not always aligned with our current health needs. The combination of neurobiological, hormonal, gut-related, psychological, and environmental factors can create a physical dependency on detrimental foods, making it challenging for individuals to break free from unhealthy eating patterns. In the intricate dance of our day-to-day lives, these unhealthy foods insinuate themselves into our habits, making it feel almost impossible to break the cycle.

This ghostly dependence is not merely a matter of willpower but is deeply rooted in the complex interplay of biological, psychological, and environmental factors. It's time to confront the truth. We have been led astray, albeit unintentionally in some cases, but misled nonetheless. From diet fads and celebrity diets to misinformation in magazines, we have been bombarded with conflicting advice that has only added to our confusion.

Many "diets" notably forbid long-term success, enforce severe calorie restrictions, promote various supplements, or even exclude entire whole foods necessary for adequate fiber, which can lead to deficiencies in essential micronutrients at the minimum. Fad diets, hyped by the media, may offer too-good-to-be-true promises of miraculous weight loss but typically fail. Their short-term effectiveness is due to water weight loss and the practical difficulties of maintaining strict rules amidst a busy lifestyle and on-the-go eating habits.

Dietary plans like keto, paleo, South Beach, Whole 30, and FODMAP have become media sensations, attracting those pursuing a quick weight-loss solution. Some diets yield temporary benefits, while others are unsuccessful, possibly due to inconsistent adherence, self-sabotage, or biological factors. These complex and often costly diets require significant focus and planning, raising questions about their long-term practicability. Meanwhile, the high fat and protein intake required in the Keto or Atkins diet can harbor long-term micronutrient imbalances. This type of diet, if done consistently enough to be considered successful for the goal of weight loss, has so many detrimental effects in the long term that any weight loss would pale in comparison.

In contemporary dietary trends, popular regimes such as the ketogenic or Atkins diets, with their pronounced predilection for fats and proteins, present potential risks for long-term nutritional deficits. This is primarily due to their exclusion of carbohydrates commonly obtained from fruits and vegetables, vital sources of essential nutrients. While these diets can lead to rapid weight loss and improved metabolic markers in the short term, the restriction of carbohydrates often results in a limited intake of vitamins, minerals, and fiber abundant in plant-based foods.

Fruits and vegetables are rich in vitamin C, potassium, folate, and dietary fiber. These nutrients play critical roles in maintaining health. For instance, vitamin C is essential for immune function and skin health, potassium helps regulate blood pressure, and dietary fiber is crucial for digestive health and maintaining stable blood sugar levels. The absence or severe limitation of these nutrients can lead to deficiencies that might not be immediately apparent but can have significant health implications over time. For example, diets that severely limit fruits and vegetables may increase the risk of vitamin deficiencies like vitamin C, leading to symptoms such as weakened immunity and fatigue. Similarly, the lack of dietary fiber from whole grains, fruits, and vegetables can lead to digestive issues such as constipation and may increase the risk of colon cancer.

Potassium, naturally found in many fruits and vegetables, can lead to imbalances that affect heart and muscle function. In addition to micronutrient deficiencies, the high intake of saturated fats and animal proteins promoted by ketogenic and Atkins diets has raised concerns about cardiovascular health. While some studies suggest that these diets can improve specific markers of heart health, such as triglyceride levels and HDL cholesterol, the long-term effects on cardiovascular health remain uncertain.

Many observational studies have associated high consumption of saturated fats, particularly from animal sources, with an increased risk of heart disease. Moreover, the focus on high-fat foods may lead to an overconsumption of calories, potentially offsetting any weight loss benefits over the long term.

The exclusion of whole grains, legumes, fruits, and many vegetables in these diets also reduces the intake of phytonutrients—compounds that have been shown to protect against chronic diseases such as cancer and heart disease. Phytonutrients, such as flavonoids, carotenoids, and polyphenols, have antioxidant and anti-inflammatory properties that help protect cells from damage and support overall health. By limiting the intake of a wide variety of plant foods, individuals on low-carb diets may miss out on these important health benefits.

While ketogenic and Atkins diets can be effective for short-term weight loss and managing specific health conditions such as epilepsy or type 2 diabetes, it is important to consider their long-term sustainability and nutritional adequacy. A balanced approach that includes a wide range of nutrient-dense foods is essential for maintaining overall health and preventing chronic diseases. Incorporating moderate amounts of healthy carbohydrates, such as those found in fruits, vegetables, and whole grains, can provide the necessary nutrients to support long-term health while allowing for weight management and metabolic benefits.

Diets rich in high-fat and animal protein content bear a significant load of cholesterol and sodium and fall short of providing the dietary fiber vital for a balanced intestinal microbiome, placing undue strain on the body's hepatic and renal systems. The detrimental effects of adhering to such diets far exceed the benefits of any weight loss achieved in the interim. The consumption of saturated animal fats in excessive quantities is associated with a wide array of health risks, including heart disease, high cholesterol, and other cardiovascular issues. These fats can contribute to the buildup of plaque in arteries, leading to atherosclerosis and an increased risk of heart attacks and strokes. Additionally, excessive intake of saturated fats has been linked to obesity and type 2 diabetes, further compounding the risk of chronic illnesses.

On the other hand, carbohydrates are essential for the optimal functioning of the brain and muscles, providing the primary energy source, glucose. Ketogenic diets drastically reduce carbohydrate intake, which can have long-term health implications. By shifting the body's energy source to fats through ketosis, these diets may increase the risk of nutrient deficiencies, liver problems, and cardiovascular diseases due to the high intake of saturated fats. Furthermore, the lack of dietary fiber in ketogenic diets can lead to digestive issues, such as constipation and an increased risk of colon cancer. Hence, while ketogenic diets can offer short-term benefits like weight loss and improved blood sugar control, they may pose significant long-term health risks if not carefully managed.

These unnatural dietary patterns invariably thrust the body's regulatory mechanisms into a state of heightened activity or "survival mode" as it attempts to maintain equilibrium while facing suboptimal nutrient absorption. The single-minded pursuit of weight loss through dieting often results in meals that are, at best, unsatisfying and, at worst, severely lacking in essential nutrients. Focusing solely on reducing calorie intake or eliminating certain food groups can lead to unbalanced diets that fail to provide the body with the vitamins, minerals, and macronutrients it needs to function optimally. This approach diminishes the enjoyment and satisfaction that should come from eating and increases the risk of nutrient deficiencies, fatigue, and other health issues.

Restrictive dieting is inherently unsustainable as a long-term lifestyle practice. Constant deprivation and a focus on weight loss can lead to a cycle of yo-yo dieting, where any weight loss is quickly regained once normal eating patterns resume. This can result in frustration, a negative relationship with food, and a diminished quality of life. Sustainable health and well-being require a balanced approach that nourishes the body while allowing for enjoyment and flexibility in eating habits.

When individuals embark on a diet, they typically focus on eating fewer calories to achieve a slimmer figure. This frequently leads them to forgo entire meals or bypass flavorful additions like sauces and dressings. Instead, they attempt to make more health-conscious meals tasty using low-calorie substitutes and artificial sweeteners. However, such eating habits leave them hungry soon after eating, an approach that is hardly maintainable in the long haul.

The abundance of processed meats, cheese, refined carbohydrates, sugar-free drinks, and alcoholic drink consumption in many diets sends confusing signals to the body, influencing cravings and disrupting the gut microbiome. When following a low-carb diet, this overload on the digestive and endocrine systems, combined with calorie-dense but nutrient-poor foods, forces the body's metabolic processes to focus on burning stored fat rather than utilizing energy from consumed food. While this strategy may be theoretically viable as long as excess fat is utilized, it comes with significant caveats.

Low-carb diets rely on the assumption that one can adhere strictly to a regimen that severely restricts carbohydrate intake, altering the body's entire metabolic operation. However, these diets often neglect many foods that are essential for the optimal functioning of our cells and bodily systems. The exclusion of nutrient-rich, carbohydrate-containing foods can lead to imbalances that affect overall health and well-being. To counteract the imbalances caused by a low-carb diet, it is crucial to restore gut microbiome health by incorporating fiber-rich, nutrient-abundant foods into your meals.

These foods enhance cellular vitality and support a flourishing microbiome, which is essential for digestion, immunity, and overall metabolic health. By prioritizing a balanced and diverse diet, you can achieve a more sustainable and healthy way of eating that better aligns with the body's natural needs. Whole foods such as fruits, vegetables, legumes, and whole grains provide carbohydrates, essential vitamins, minerals, and fiber. These nutrient-dense carbs are digested more slowly, leading to a steady release of energy that helps maintain blood sugar levels and keeps cravings in check. Unlike refined carbohydrates, which can spike insulin and contribute to metabolic issues, whole-food carb sources nourish the body to support long-term health, gut microbiome balance, and overall well-being. Incorporating these foods into your diet can help you enjoy the benefits of carbohydrates without compromising your low-carb goals.

Understanding what truly fuels your body and embracing the personal balance of nutrients that make you feel your best naturally crafts a body that reflects your body's ideal shape while enhancing the vitality of your hair, skin, and nails. It's about fine-tuning your body's intricate biochemical symphony to feel your best. It's time to take control, nourish intelligently, and rewrite your story with food. With awareness, support, and a concerted effort to adopt healthier habits, overcoming food dependencies and establishing a balanced and nourishing relationship with food is entirely possible.

Modifying our diet can sometimes feel daunting, causing us to fear missing out at food-centric gatherings, on dates, and at work. The topic of a diet change can become the start of a conflict for many.

Why Diets Are Bad

Having to explain oneself when dining with others or at family meals because you are eating differently may raise questions. Routines at mealtime are silently cherished and emotionally charged; the people you share them with will initially want to protect the traditions you've created together; whether it be Taco Tuesday or Superbowl Sunday, it's about more than food; it is a comforting habit. While it may feel challenging to start altering our eating habits, we can develop a positive connection with our bodies. At the same time, we positively impact those around us.

The main hurdle is knowing where to begin, what foods to cut out, and which to start consistently integrating into your diet. People who have a yo-yo diet often stick to repetitive "safe" foods when dieting, worrying that trying new things will set them back. They usually choose foods containing lots of water that are low in calories, like celery, lettuce, low-fat dairy products, or reduced-fat sweets, which generally have little nutritional value outside hydration. Our bodies continually seek essential nutrients from our food to sustain us. This is why extreme diets that don't provide a variety of nutrients will fail consistently on a timeline. Disrupting how we feel about the food we repeatedly choose and questioning them is essential to achieving real and lasting dietary changes.

Introducing a more comprehensive range of nutritious foods into your daily meals is an excellent way to explore the many fruits, nuts, legumes, roots, leaves, gourds, berries, and vegetables available beyond your usual inclinations. Expanding your diet to include these whole foods provides a wide variety of nutrients essential for maintaining good health. It encourages a deeper connection to the natural flavors and textures of food. If you struggle to enjoy eating these whole foods, it might be valuable to consider whether they aren't satisfying the need for a hit of endorphins, which comfort foods often provide. This is a common experience, as many comfort foods are designed to be highly palatable, usually loaded with sugars, fats, and salts that trigger the brain's pleasure centers.

Understanding the difference between true hunger and eating for psychological or emotional reasons is crucial in making healthier food choices. True hunger is a physical need for nutrients and energy, while emotional eating often seeks to fill a void or cope with stress, boredom, or other emotions. Asking yourself at every meal, "Am I eating because I'm truly hungry, or am I eating to satisfy an emotional need?" can be a powerful tool for mindful eating. This self-awareness allows you to make more conscious choices, selecting foods that nourish your body rather than simply providing temporary comfort.

Instead of resorting to low-calorie meal replacements to keep your calorie count low, expanding your diet to include nutrient-dense foods can help your mind and taste buds acclimate to the variety of flavors and textures that whole foods offer. These nutrient-dense foods, such as avocados, beans, nuts, seeds, whole grains, and leafy greens, provide essential vitamins, minerals, and healthy fats that support overall well-being. They also promote satiety, helping you feel full and satisfied after meals, which can reduce the urge to overeat or snack on less healthy options.

By incorporating a diverse range of whole foods into your diet, you can create a more sustainable and enjoyable way to manage your diet and maintain a healthy lifestyle. Over time, your taste preferences will shift, and you naturally gravitate toward more nutritious choices that support your physical and emotional well-being. This holistic approach to eating can lead to lasting changes in your relationship with food, making it easier to maintain a balanced and nourishing diet that supports your overall health and happiness.

Why Diets Are Bad

While consuming hydrating foods like watermelon and celery is beneficial due to their high water content and ability to keep you hydrated, it's equally important to include calorie-rich, nutritious foods in a balanced diet. These foods provide the energy needed to support bodily functions and maintain overall health. Calorie-rich foods such as avocados, nuts, seeds, and whole grains are packed with essential nutrients, healthy fats, and fiber, crucial for maintaining energy levels, supporting metabolic functions, and promoting satiety.

By broadening your dietary horizons and trying new foods, you can reset your body and mind, making it easier to gravitate toward healthier food choices naturally.

When you expose yourself to a variety of flavors and textures from newly introduced whole foods, your brain begins to associate those flavors with the nutritional benefits they provide. This association helps your body recognize and crave the nutrients it needs rather than just the flavor. Over time, this shift in mindset can lead to more intuitive eating, where you can better listen to your body's hunger cues and make choices that nourish and satisfy you. This process allows you to distinguish between true physiological hunger and cravings driven by habit or emotional needs.

As your body receives the nutrients from whole foods, the urge to continue snacking diminishes because your body's nutritional needs are being met. Processed foods, on the other hand, are often high in empty calories but low in essential nutrients, leaving your body craving more in an attempt to fulfill its nutritional requirements. By choosing whole foods, you provide your body with a wealth of vitamins, minerals, fiber, and antioxidants, all of which help to regulate hunger and maintain energy levels.

Training your brain to recognize and appreciate the nutritional benefits of whole foods is a critical step in developing healthier eating habits. When you consistently choose nutrient-rich options, your taste preferences shift, and you crave the natural flavors of whole foods rather than the artificial flavors of processed snacks. This shift is not just about changing what you eat but also about changing how you think about food. Instead of viewing food as merely a source of pleasure or a way to cope with emotions, you start to see it as a source of nourishment and well-being.

Over time, this practice can transform your relationship with food, making it easier to make choices aligned with your body's actual needs. By focusing on the quality of the food you consume, you promote a more balanced and satisfying diet. This approach helps you maintain a healthy weight, supports your immune system, and enhances your overall physical and mental health. Moreover, it reduces the likelihood of developing chronic diseases such as obesity, diabetes, and heart disease, which are often linked to poor dietary choices.

By choosing whole foods rich in nutrients, such as fruits, vegetables, whole grains, amino acid-rich foods, and healthy fats, you provide your body with the essential vitamins and minerals it needs to function optimally. These nutrients play crucial roles in maintaining cellular health, supporting metabolic processes, and protecting against oxidative stress and inflammation. For example, antioxidants found in colorful fruits and vegetables help to neutralize free radicals, reducing the risk of chronic diseases and promoting longevity. Fiber from whole grains and legumes supports digestive health, helps regulate blood sugar levels, and lowers cholesterol, further protecting against heart disease and diabetes.

To start this journey toward healthier eating, it's important to set clear and achievable goals. Ask yourself, "What is the best choice for me?" This simple question encourages mindful eating and helps you focus on making food choices that align with your health and wellness objectives. Mindful eating involves paying attention to the taste, texture, and nutritional value of the food you eat, as well as how it makes you feel. By being present and conscious of your eating habits, you can identify emotional eating patterns and make more informed choices.

A fundamental shift in mindset is essential for achieving long-term health and well-being, not a diet. Rather than obsessing over reducing the number on the scale, the focus should be on nourishing the body with a diverse array of vitamins, minerals, fibers, and phytonutrients. This shift in thinking requires a thorough reevaluation of one's relationship with food.

Food should be seen as a means to control weight and a source of nourishment and pleasure supporting physical and mental well-being. Embracing a diet rich in whole foods, such as fruits, vegetables, whole grains, legumes, nuts, seeds, and healthy fats, can lead to more satisfying meals that provide the body with everything it needs to thrive. In turn, this mindset fosters a healthier, more sustainable approach to eating that supports long-term health goals without the need for restrictive or unsatisfying diets. Conscious engagement with the choices made at the table creates daily habits.

Learning to navigate your dietary choices independently, utilizing your natural faculties. Your vision, cognitive function, and hunger cues are instrumental in identifying nourishing foods that promote a healthy weight for your body. There's no necessity for perpetual adherence to a stringent diet plan. Instead, you'll develop the skill of intuitive eating. Although plentiful resources catering to those who favor structured meal guides and culinary inspiration are readily accessible in our digital landscape, I advocate for an adaptable eating framework over rigid regimens, which often prove challenging for many individuals.

Conventional approaches to diet and physical activity often

concentrate on cardiovascular workouts and diets characterized by low fat, elevated protein, and reduced carbohydrates. The concept of intermittent fasting also garners widespread attention. Countless individuals are experimenting with various methods to shed pounds, yet the purpose and rationale behind these techniques remain misunderstood.

To lose weight effectively, one must ingest fewer calories than one expends daily. Therefore, it's critical to view each calorie consumed as energy and a potential vessel for nutrition that enriches one's bloodstream and provides diverse fiber to one's gut microbiota. Adopt the mindset of a judicious consumer operating within a budget, striving to obtain maximal nutritional value from each calorie while ensuring one's sense of satiety.

2
WATER YOU DRINK-ING?

Water is essential to life. We drink it, cook with it, bathe in it, and rely on it every single day. Yet, despite its fundamental role in our lives, many of us don't fully understand the journey water takes before it flows from our taps. We know tap water isn't always ideal—after all, a significant number of Americans use water filters. But what's the real story behind our water? Let's dive into the history of water treatment, the pipes that transport it, and the contaminants that are often introduced along the way.

The treatment of drinking water dates back thousands of years. Ancient civilizations used rudimentary methods to clean their water, such as boiling and filtering through sand. The Greeks and Romans developed aqueducts and other sophisticated systems to transport and filter water, recognizing early on the importance of clean water for public health.

Fast forward to the 19th century, when the Industrial Revolution brought rapid urbanization. Cities grew exponentially, and with them, the demand for clean, safe water. This urban explosion highlighted the inadequacies of existing water systems and the dire need for more systematic approaches to water treatment. In the mid-1800s, London faced a series of cholera outbreaks linked to contaminated water. This led to significant advancements, including the construction of large-scale sewer systems and the adoption of sand filtration.

The turning point came with the introduction of chlorine as a disinfectant. In 1908, Jersey City, New Jersey, became the first city in the United States to chlorinate its drinking water, significantly reducing the incidence of waterborne diseases like cholera and typhoid. This practice quickly spread, and by the mid-20th century, chlorination had become a standard practice in water treatment facilities worldwide.

Once water is treated, it travels through an extensive network of pipes to reach our homes. Many of these pipes are old, some even dating back to the early 20th century. Aging infrastructure can pose significant risks, including leaks, breaks, and the potential for contaminants to enter the water supply. Corrosion in old pipes can introduce metals such as lead and copper into the water, posing serious health risks.

Treatment facilities add various chemicals to ensure water is safe to drink because it began as polluted water full of potentially dangerous microbes, bacteria, pesticide runoff, and errant medications that are passed through into our water supply through the septic system. Chlorine is the most common disinfectant used to kill harmful bacteria and viruses. However, while chlorine effectively purifies water, it can react with natural organic matter to form disinfection byproducts (DBPs), some of which are potentially harmful if consumed over long periods. Fluoride is another additive that was introduced to help reduce dental cavities, but its inclusion remains a topic of debate among health professionals and the public.

Despite rigorous treatment processes, several contaminants can still find their way into our tap water. Heavy metals like lead and copper can leach from old pipes and fixtures, posing significant health risks, largely to children and pregnant women. Pesticides and herbicides from agricultural runoff can introduce these chemicals into water sources. Industrial pollutants from factories and industrial plants can release various chemicals into nearby water bodies, which may eventually end up in our drinking water. Microplastics, tiny plastic particles from various sources, have been detected in tap water, raising concerns about their long-term health impacts.

Given these potential contaminants, it's no surprise that many people turn to water filters to improve the quality of their drinking water. Filters can reduce or eliminate many of these harmful substances, providing an extra layer of protection. However, not all filters are created equal, and it's crucial to choose one that's suitable for the specific contaminants present in your water supply.

Choosing to drink pure water means recognizing that the water you use for washing dishes shouldn't be the same as the water you use to hydrate your cells. Tap water contains a range of contaminants, with chlorine being one of the most noticeable due to its distinct smell. After I stopped drinking tap water, I began to notice a bleach-like odor every time I turned on the tap. This led me to investigate further, and I quickly discovered information that made me reluctant to even wash my hair with tap water without an additional filter.

I prefer to keep my home drinking water in a glass 5-gallon decanter, which I purchase through Alive Waters, a premium water delivery service. They utilize two springs that have zero industrial contaminations, including no radioactive isotopes, which are often found in other springs. Their water also boasts the perfect mineral balance, making it ideal for health and great-tasting water. Even if you don't want to subscribe to their delivery service—which arrives in glass containers—you can purchase their stunning decanter with a spout separately. You can explore their offerings at www.alive-waters.com, and using my personal discount code "EL" gives 15% off any purchase, whether you opt for premium water delivery or just the Italian Glass Water decanter.

Keeping your water out of plastic is ideal, and this decanter allows you the space to add energetically charged stones to the water as it sits. I like to add rose quartz stones to the base of the decanter to infuse the water with positive energy. Using gemstones to "Energetically Charge" water is a practice rooted in holistic and metaphysical traditions. However, not all gemstones are safe for this purpose, as some can leach toxic substances or dissolve in water. Still, several stones are commonly considered safe and are believed to impart positive energies or beneficial vibrations to water.

Clear quartz, known as a master healer, is believed to amplify energy and thought, enhancing the properties of other stones. It is safe for direct contact with water because it is hard and does not dissolve or leach toxic substances. Amethyst, associated with calmness, clarity, and spiritual awareness, is often used to promote relaxation and balance. Amethyst is a form of quartz that does not dissolve in water, making it safe for use. Rose quartz, linked to love, compassion, and emotional healing, is thought to open the heart chakra. It is another form of quartz and is durable in water, making it safe to use.

Citrine, associated with abundance, joy, and prosperity, is believed to attract positivity and success. It is safe for water use, though natural citrine can be rare. Heat-treated amethyst, sold as citrine, is also safe. Aventurine, known as the stone of opportunity, is thought to attract luck and improve prosperity. It is generally safe in water and does not leach harmful substances.

Carnelian, linked to creativity, motivation, and courage, is used to boost confidence and personal power. It is a hard stone and does not dissolve in water. Black obsidian is known for its protective properties and is thought to shield against negativity and aid in grounding. It is safe for short-term use in water; being volcanic glass, it should not be left in water for extended periods. Smoky quartz, associated with grounding and protection, is used to neutralize negative energies. It is similar to clear quartz in terms of durability and is safe to use in water.

When using gemstones to charge water, it is important to ensure the stones are clean. Always clean the gemstones thoroughly before placing them in water to remove any dirt, oil, or residue. Using polished (tumbled) stones can avoid sharp edges that could harbor bacteria or cause scratches. For those unsure about a stone's safety, placing it in water for only short periods and avoiding prolonged soaking can provide an extra level of caution. Alternatively, using the indirect method, where stones are placed around the water container or in a separate container placed inside the water vessel, can charge the water energetically without direct contact, reducing any risk of contamination. Using these gemstones to charge water can be a meaningful and enriching practice, combining the physical properties of water with the metaphysical properties of the stones.

Understanding the history and treatment of our tap water, the journey it takes through our aging infrastructure, and the potential contaminants it can carry helps us make informed decisions about our water consumption. In the chapters that follow, we'll delve deeper into the specifics of water quality, the types of filters available, and how to ensure you're drinking the best water possible for your health and well-being.

When I think back to chemistry class, I vividly remember learning about solvents. Rubbing alcohol was often cited as an example—a substance capable of dissolving and interacting with the molecules around it. But in reality, water is the most effective solvent we know. Just imagine those majestic rock formations with lines intricately carved out over centuries by trickling water. That's the true power of water as a solvent.

This incredible property of water is why the importance of

carrying it in glass containers has gained so much popularity. Media outlets have been buzzing with warnings about contaminants leaching from plastic bottles, especially when they are reused. While everyone knows they should drink water, not everyone makes it a priority. And even for those who do, the variety of options can be overwhelming. Water is not just water.

From tap water to spring water, from fruit-infused water to energy drinks, water is ubiquitous. But what is the best type of water, and how much should you drink? Water's extensive ability to dissolve a wide variety of molecules has earned it the designation of "universal solvent." This capability makes water an invaluable life-sustaining force. On a biological level, water's role as a solvent is crucial—it helps cells transport and utilize essential substances like oxygen and nutrients.

The idea that speaking to water or exposing it to external factors can change its properties dynamically has intrigued both scientists and metaphysical enthusiasts for decades. The most notable exploration of this concept comes from the work of Dr. Masaru Emoto, a Japanese researcher who claimed that human consciousness could affect the molecular structure of water.

Emoto's experiments involved exposing water to different types of stimuli, such as spoken words, music, and written phrases, then freezing the water and examining the resulting ice crystals under a microscope. According to Emoto, positive words and pleasant music produced beautiful, well-formed crystals, while negative words and harsh music led to disordered, asymmetrical crystals. His work suggested that water could hold memory or be influenced by vibrations, reflecting the intent or energy directed at it.

While Emoto's work is widely discussed in alternative and holistic health circles, it has faced criticism and skepticism from the scientific community. Critics argue that his experiments lacked rigorous scientific controls and that his findings were not reproducible in other studies. The main contention is the subjective nature of determining the "beauty" of the ice crystals, as well as the potential for observer bias—where expectations of the outcomes could influence the results. Despite the lack of scientific consensus, the idea has sparked considerable interest in the potential of water to interact with its environment in ways that go beyond traditional chemistry.

From a scientific perspective, water is a highly sensitive substance with unique properties. Its molecular structure allows it to form hydrogen bonds, making it an excellent solvent capable of interacting with various substances and energies. While conventional science does not yet support the notion that thoughts or spoken words can alter water's structure in the way Emoto described, it acknowledges that water is sensitive to temperature, pressure, and impurities, which can affect its behavior. For instance, external factors like electromagnetic fields, sound waves, or physical motion can influence the state of water at a molecular level, impacting its solubility, freezing point, and evaporation rate. This sensitivity underlines water's capacity to respond to its environment, though not necessarily in the dramatic fashion of Emoto's interpretations.

The study of cymatics, which explores how sound waves affect physical mediums like sand, water, and air, provides a more scientific basis for understanding how vibrations can influence water. Cymatics demonstrates that sound frequencies can cause water to form distinct patterns, suggesting that sound waves indeed affect the physical state of water. These observations align with the basic principles of physics, where vibration and resonance can lead to changes in matter. However, the leap from sound-induced patterns to emotional or intention-driven changes in water is still a significant one, requiring further scientific validation.

While the idea that thoughts, words, or intentions can dynamically change water remains controversial and largely unsupported by rigorous scientific evidence, the broader concept of water's sensitivity to external factors is well-documented. Water's ability to respond to physical vibrations and environmental changes opens the door to further exploration into how subtle energies might influence its state. The field remains ripe for inquiry, blending the boundaries between science, consciousness, and the intrinsic properties of one of life's most essential elements.

Water is involved in every aspect of our health. It aids in colon health and digestion, facilitates toxin removal through sweat, regulates blood pressure, and sustains our energy levels. Quite literally, water is flowing through us at all times. To maintain optimal health, it's essential to ensure you're consuming the best quality water available.

Surface water is collected from rivers, lakes, reservoirs, and other above-ground water sources. It is commonly used as a source of tap water in urban areas. Surface water undergoes treatment processes to remove impurities and ensure it meets the required quality standards for safe consumption. Treatment may involve processes such as coagulation, sedimentation, filtration, disinfection, and pH adjustment.

Groundwater is water that is stored beneath the Earth's surface in aquifers, which are layers of permeable rock, gravel, or sand that contain water. Groundwater is accessed by drilling wells into the aquifers. It is typically extracted using pumps and brought to the surface for treatment. Groundwater is often used as a source of tap water in both urban and rural areas. Similar to surface water, groundwater also undergoes treatment processes to ensure its safety and quality.

The specific sources of tap water can vary depending on the

location and local water supply infrastructure. Municipal water treatment facilities are responsible for treating and distributing tap water to homes and businesses in accordance with regulatory standards to ensure it is safe for drinking, cooking, and other domestic uses. If your tap water contains high levels of nitrates, boiling can increase their concentration rather than removing them. This is because boiling causes water to evaporate, leaving behind the nitrates in a more concentrated form.

Distilled water is water that has been purified through the process of distillation, which involves boiling the water and then collecting the steam and condensing it back into a liquid form.

Distillation removes most impurities, including minerals, bacteria, viruses, and contaminants with higher boiling points, resulting in water that is essentially pure H2O.

Distilled water is commonly used in medical and laboratory settings where the absence of impurities is crucial, such as in medical procedures, pharmaceutical preparations, and scientific experiments. Its properties are recommended for use in humidifiers and steam irons to prevent the buildup of mineral deposits that can occur with tap water.

Distilled water is preferred for topping up automotive cooling systems and filling lead-acid batteries to prevent mineral buildup and corrosion. While distilled water is safe to drink, it lacks minerals that are naturally present in other water sources. Drinking solely distilled water over an extended period may not provide necessary minerals that contribute to overall health. It's generally recommended to obtain minerals through a balanced diet rather than relying solely on water.

Distilled water does not contain electrolytes, which are essential for rehydration during intense physical activity or in cases of dehydration.

Some people find that distilled water can give a flat or bland taste to certain foods and beverages compared to water with naturally occurring minerals. Other types of water, such as filtered water or mineral water, may be preferred for cooking, brewing coffee or tea, and enhancing the flavor of certain dishes. While this side effect may not necessarily make the water toxic, it can affect the taste, odor, and overall quality of the water.

Some of my plants have unexpectedly died when given tap water, and I noticed a white, flaky coating on the soil. My orchids only thrive with well or spring water misted on them regularly. The delicate roots of these plants literally dissolve under constant tap water. Personally, if my plant can't tolerate it, then neither can I. It's important to treat yourself with the same care you give to something you cherish.

Often, we go through our routines without considering how these small actions can accumulate into an overall feeling of unwellness. There are many people who rent and others who own, all with different budgets, making it difficult to recommend just one type of filter for everyone. Depending on the contaminants in your local water supply, different types of filtration may be necessary for each situation. From high-end household water filters that clean all the water entering your home to handheld pitcher filters, countertop filters, advanced technology that creates water from the air, shower head filters, and sink tap filters, the options can be overwhelming at first, but start with changing the water you drink first.

One fascinating alternative to tap water is the water found in fruits. The molecular structure of water within fruits is unique and highly beneficial. Fruit water is not only absorbed more efficiently by the body but also comes with a host of natural nutrients and antioxidants. This superior absorbency can aid in more effective hydration, as the water in fruits is often accompanied by electrolytes and minerals that enhance their hydrating properties.

Considering fruit juices as a hydration source raises important points about balance and sugar content. Freshly squeezed fruit juices can indeed contribute to hydration and offer essential vitamins and minerals. However, it's crucial to be mindful of their natural sugar content. While fruit juices provide hydration and nutrients, consuming them in moderation is key to managing sugar intake and avoiding excessive calorie consumption.

Ultimately, while fresh pressed fruit juices can be beneficial in a balanced diet, they should complement, not replace, plain water. A diverse approach to hydration, combining clean water with nutrient-rich fruit juices, can support overall health and ensure you meet your hydration needs effectively.

Watermelon juice stands out due to its high water content and relatively low natural sugar levels compared to other fruit juices. Comprising about 90% water, watermelon juice is exceptionally hydrating, making it an excellent option for quenching thirst and maintaining hydration. This high water content, combined with watermelon's natural electrolytes like potassium, helps in efficient fluid balance and replenishment.

Additionally, watermelon juice contains antioxidants such as lycopene and citrulline, which contribute to overall health. Lycopene has been linked to various health benefits, including reduced inflammation and improved cardiovascular health, while citrulline may help improve blood flow and reduce muscle soreness. While watermelon juice is lower in sugar compared to some other fruit juices, it's still wise to consume it in moderation if you are eating other sources of commercial sugar. However, its hydrating properties and nutritional benefits make it a favorable choice for hydration, particularly in hot weather or after physical activity.

Ordering 5-gallon spring water delivery is the best option for many offices, but it can also be a very affordable option for at home.

Check your membership club stores for even bigger discounts on at-home water delivery. Spring water carries minerals sourced from natural underground springs that often pass through mineral-rich rock formations. The composition of minerals in spring water can vary depending on the specific geology of the area where the spring is located. Common minerals found in spring water include calcium, magnesium, potassium, and trace elements like iron, zinc, and manganese.

It's important to note that the mineral content of spring water can vary from one source to another. Some springs may have higher mineral concentrations, while others may have lower levels. The mineral composition of spring water is influenced by factors such as the surrounding soil, the depth and location of the aquifer, and the natural geological processes.

The presence of minerals in spring water can contribute to its taste and potential health benefits. Some people prefer the taste of spring water due to its natural mineral content. Additionally, minerals in water can provide a small contribution to the daily intake of essential minerals in the diet.

The types of water filters available work differently: carbon filters, such as activated carbon or charcoal filters, are widely used for water filtration. They work through a process called adsorption, where impurities in the water stick to the surface of the carbon filter media. Carbon filters can effectively remove chlorine, volatile organic compounds (VOCs), certain pesticides, and some taste and odor compounds.

Reverse osmosis systems use a semipermeable membrane to remove a wide range of impurities from water. Water is forced through the membrane under pressure, effectively filtering out contaminants such as dissolved minerals, heavy metals, bacteria, viruses, and certain chemicals. RO systems are highly efficient at removing a variety of impurities but may produce wastewater in the process.

Ceramic filters consist of porous ceramic material that traps sediment, bacteria, and larger particles as water passes through. Some ceramic filters are impregnated with silver, which can help inhibit bacterial growth. These filters are often used in conjunction with other filtration methods to provide additional purification.

UV (Ultraviolet) filters disinfect water by inactivating bacteria, viruses, and other microorganisms. UV light damages microorganisms' DNA, preventing them from reproducing. UV filters are typically used in combination with other filtration methods to ensure both disinfection and removal of particulate matter.

Ion exchange filters work by replacing undesirable ions in the water with more desirable ions. These filters are commonly used for water softening to remove minerals like calcium and magnesium that cause hardness. Ion exchange filters are not designed to remove all types of contaminants but can improve water taste and address specific concerns related to water hardness.

The term "15-stage water filter" is often used in marketing to describe a multi-stage filtration system that incorporates various filtration media and technologies. While these filters may offer multiple stages of filtration, it's important to note that the number of stages alone does not necessarily indicate superior performance or effectiveness. The performance of a water filter depends on several factors, including the specific filtration technologies used, the quality of the filter media, and the contaminants being targeted.

The effectiveness of a water filter is typically determined by its ability to remove specific contaminants of concern, such as chlorine, sediment, heavy metals, bacteria, or other impurities. Different filtration stages or media can address specific types of contaminants. For example, activated carbon is effective at removing chlorine and certain organic compounds, while a membrane filter like reverse osmosis can remove dissolved minerals and other substances.

When considering a water filter, it's important to evaluate its performance based on independent third-party certifications or testing results, such as NSF/ANSI standards. These certifications can provide assurance that the filter meets specific criteria for contaminant removal. While multi-stage filters may offer the advantage of combining different filtration technologies, it's crucial to choose a filter that targets the specific contaminants present in your water supply. Additionally, factors such as filter maintenance, replacement frequency, and overall cost should also be considered.

Ultimately, the effectiveness of a water filter depends on the combination of filtration technologies, the quality of the filter media, and its ability to address the specific contaminants of concern. It's recommended that you review product specifications, performance data, and independent testing to make an informed decision about the best water filter for your needs. https://www.ewg.org is a free website where you can enter your zip code, see for yourself the contaminants present in your municipality's water supply, and determine what is best for you. A shower and hand sink filter is also recommended, as our skin is our largest organ, and our hair, nails, and skin can suffer from the daily onslaught of pollutants in our water.

Water itself does not have a fixed pH. Its pH can vary based on factors like its source, mineral content, or treatment process. However, a neutral or slightly alkaline pH is generally considered ideal for drinking purposes. The body's pH is usually maintained in a narrow range of 7.35 to 7.45, which is somewhat alkaline. Maintaining this pH balance is essential for various physiological functions. The body's pH influences enzyme activity, cellular operations, and the overall balance of bodily fluids. Any deviation from this optimal range can disrupt normal functions and potentially lead to health issues.

Water You Drinking?

When consuming acidic substances such as sodas or alcohol, the body has natural buffering systems to maintain its pH balance. These involve various organs, including the kidneys and lungs. Upon consuming acidic substances, the body neutralizes the acidity to keep its pH within the normal range. For instance, the kidneys help regulate pH by excreting excess acids or retaining bicarbonate ions to counterbalance acidity. The respiratory system can also adjust pH by changing breathing rates.

However, consistently consuming acidic substances, such as excessive amounts of soda or alcohol, can challenge the body's buffering systems and potentially disrupt pH balance. Over time, this can adversely affect health, including potential organ damage or increased susceptibility to certain health conditions.

The body has its own mechanisms to regulate PH balance, and the impact of specific drinks on overall pH can be minimal. However, some beverages are often associated with alkalizing properties or potential health benefits. Plain water is generally neutral and does not significantly affect the body's PH. Staying well-hydrated with water is vital for overall health and maintaining proper bodily functions. Although acidic, lemon and lime water can have an alkalizing effect on the body when consumed. This is due to their potential to stimulate bicarbonate production in the body, which helps buffer acidity.

Alkaline water has a higher pH than regular water, often achieved through the addition of minerals or electrolytes. While it may have a slightly alkalizing effect when consumed, the long-term health benefits and significant impact on the body's pH are still subjects of scientific debate.

Deuterium-depleted water is water with reduced deuterium levels, a heavy form of hydrogen. While there are claims about its potential health benefits, its impact on the body's pH is unclear, and more research is needed to establish its effectiveness.

Coconut water has become increasingly popular as a hydrating natural beverage, known for its refreshing taste and high electrolyte content, which makes it a favored choice for athletes and health enthusiasts alike. Rich in potassium, magnesium, and calcium, coconut water is celebrated for aiding in hydration and replenishing electrolytes lost through sweat. However, as its popularity has surged, so have concerns about the environmental impact and ethical practices associated with its production.

Coconut farming, particularly on a large scale, can pose significant environmental challenges. These include deforestation, biodiversity loss, and the depletion of natural resources. Additionally, the global demand for coconut water has raised questions about the fair treatment of farmers and the sustainability of farming practices. Ethical sourcing has become a critical factor for consumers who want to enjoy the benefits of coconut water without contributing to environmental degradation or social injustice.

Addressing these concerns, brands like Vita Coco have taken steps to ensure that their coconut water is ethically sourced. Vita Coco is committed to sustainable farming practices and works directly with smallholder farmers, supporting their communities and providing fair wages. They emphasize transparency in their supply chain, aiming to reduce their environmental footprint and contribute positively to the local economies where their coconuts are grown. This commitment helps preserve the environment and ensures that the people who grow and harvest the coconuts are treated fairly and ethically.

Vita Coco is a responsible choice for those who enjoy healthy and ethically sourced coconut water. You can enjoy the benefits of their coconut water with the assurance that it supports sustainable practices and the well-being of farmers. To get 25% off your purchase of Vita Coco, you can use this link: https://vitacoco.com/JUS-TINEBASSANI. This 25% discount gives you an alternative to water while you stay hydrated with a clean conscience, knowing that you support ethical sourcing and sustainable agriculture. I love to freeze the Vita Coco Original and use them as ice cubes for everything from mock-tails to iced lattes.

Reverse osmosis water is the best-rated home filtration option because of its thoroughness, but the price points vary tremendously. Reverse osmosis (RO) is a water purification process that removes impurities and contaminants from water by using pressure to force the pure water through a semipermeable membrane, leaving impurities behind. The process involves several stages.

The water passes through a series of pre-filters to remove larger particles, sediment, and chlorine. These pre-filters help protect the RO membrane from damage. The pre-filtered water is then forced through a semipermeable membrane with tiny pores. This membrane allows water molecules to pass through while blocking larger molecules, ions, and contaminants such as bacteria, viruses, heavy metals, and some dissolved solids.

Post-filtration: After passing through the RO membrane, the purified water goes through additional post-filters to further improve its taste and remove any remaining odors or residual impurities.

The reverse osmosis process results in purified water that is typically free from a wide range of impurities. The efficiency of an RO system in removing contaminants depends on factors such as the quality of the membrane and the system's design.

The cost of an at-home reverse osmosis system can vary depending on the brand, model, features, and where you purchase it. Basic under-sink RO systems can range from around $150 to $500, while more advanced models with additional features may cost upwards of $1,000 or more. Additionally, ongoing costs are associated with replacing filters and membranes periodically, usually every 6-12 months, depending on water usage and quality.

Although reverse osmosis water is the best way to clean large volumes of water processed at a municipality, it is still just a filtered version of water and inferior to water originating in a natural, untainted source.

The journey of tap water from treatment facilities through aging pipes to our homes reveals the complexities and potential pitfalls of relying on municipal water systems for drinking and daily use. Understanding the extensive treatment processes, the chemicals added, and the possible contaminants helps underscore why many people turn to alternative solutions for purer water.

By investing in high-quality water and being mindful of the sources of our water, we can make more informed decisions about our health and well-being. Drinking pure water is not just about preference it's a commitment to ensuring that the water we consume supports our health rather than potentially undermines it.

3
RECOVERING FOODIE

A "foodie," as defined by the Urban Dictionary, is someone with a deep passion for discovering, experiencing, and appreciating various types of cuisine and culinary experiences. For many, this passion extends beyond mere sustenance; it's an exploration of food culture, history, and gastronomic creativity. Foodies often delight in exploring new restaurants, experimenting with cooking techniques, trying unique ingredients, and staying abreast of the latest food trends. They revel in sharing their culinary adventures on social media, engaging in spirited discussions about food, and participating in food-related events.

For most, this interest stems from a genuine love of culinary artistry and gastronomic exploration, where the joy of food lies in its ability to connect people, evoke emotions, and tell stories. However, for some individuals, particularly those prone to addictive behaviors or struggling with emotional eating, the foodie culture can become a way to justify or rationalize their complicated relationship with food. In these cases, what begins as an innocent indulgence in culinary pleasures can spiral into patterns of compulsive overeating or unhealthy behaviors. These individuals must recognize when their passion for food crosses the line into a detrimental relationship and take steps to cultivate healthier eating habits.

While being a foodie is often about celebrating the joys of food in a balanced and mindful way, it's important to ensure that this appreciation doesn't slip into patterns of overconsumption or emotional reliance on food. The concept of addiction is often associated with a reliance on substances or behaviors that individuals feel they cannot do without. This is why the idea of food addiction can be overlooked; eating is essential to survival, making it a fundamental need rather than an addiction in the traditional sense. However, the focus should be less on the act of eating itself and more on the choices we make about what we eat and how we care for ourselves.

Food addiction, unlike a simple passion for culinary experiences, involves compulsive overeating or binge eating driven by emotional or psychological factors rather than genuine enjoyment of food. This type of addiction is not about the pleasure of eating; it's about a compulsive drive to eat, often in the absence of hunger, which is linked to deeper emotional or psychological triggers.

Scientific studies have shown that highly palatable foods, significantly those high in sugar, fat, and salt, can stimulate the brain's reward system, like addictive drugs like cocaine or nicotine. These foods trigger the release of dopamine, a neurotransmitter associated with pleasure and reward, in the brain's reward center. This dopamine release creates feelings of pleasure and reinforces the behavior, leading to repeated consumption of these foods even when not hungry.

Over time, the brain's reward system can become desensitized, requiring more of the addictive substance (in this case, food) to achieve the same level of pleasure. This leads to a cycle of overeating and intense cravings, which can be challenging to break. Brain imaging studies have shown that individuals with food addiction exhibit similar brain activity to those with drug addiction when exposed to their trigger foods. This evidence underscores the profound impact that certain foods can have on the brain, making it clear that food addiction is not merely a matter of willpower but involves a complex interplay of biological, psychological, and environmental factors.

Emotional eating, another critical aspect of the relationship between food and addiction, occurs when individuals use food as a way to cope with negative emotions such as stress, anxiety, depression, or boredom. Instead of addressing the underlying emotional issues, they may turn to food for comfort, temporarily alleviating their emotional distress. However, this relief is short-lived, and the negative emotions often return, leading to further emotional eating. This cycle can be particularly challenging because it is deeply rooted in the brain's reward and stress response systems.

When individuals eat in response to stress, the body releases cortisol, a hormone that increases appetite and encourages the consumption of high-calorie foods. Cortisol not only stimulates appetite but also promotes the storage of fat, particularly in the abdominal area, which can contribute to weight gain and increase the risk of chronic diseases such as type 2 diabetes and cardiovascular disease. The relationship between stress, cortisol, and eating behaviors highlights the importance of understanding the emotional and physiological triggers that drive unhealthy eating patterns.

Moreover, nutrition plays a significant role in mood regulation and mental health. The brain requires a steady supply of nutrients to function optimally, and deficiencies in certain nutrients can contribute to mood disorders such as depression and anxiety. For example, omega-3 fatty acids, flaxseeds, and walnuts are essential for brain health and have been shown to reduce symptoms of depression. Similarly, vitamins and minerals such as vitamin D, B vitamins, magnesium, and zinc are crucial for neurotransmitter production and regulation. A diet rich in these nutrients supports not only physical health but also mental and emotional well-being.

The gut-brain axis, a bidirectional communication system between the gastrointestinal tract and the brain, also plays a crucial role in mood regulation. The gut microbiome, which consists of trillions of microorganisms living in the digestive tract, has been shown to influence brain function and behavior. A healthy gut microbiome can produce neurotransmitters like serotonin, often called the "feel-good" hormone. Approximately 90% of the body's serotonin is made in the gut. A diet rich in fiber, prebiotics, and probiotics supports a healthy gut microbiome, promoting better mental health and emotional resilience.

Conversely, a diet high in processed foods, sugars, and unhealthy fats can disrupt the gut microbiome, leading to inflammation and an increased risk of mental health disorders. Chronic inflammation has been linked to a range of health issues, including depression, anxiety, and cognitive decline. This connection between diet, gut health, and mental health underscores the importance of mindful dietary choices supporting overall well-being.

Identifying a behavior as an addiction can sometimes make it more challenging to change.

One notable barrier is the stigma and shame often attached to addiction. This stigma can make people feel embarrassed or judged, discouraging them from acknowledging their struggles and seeking help. As a result, they may deny or downplay their issues, hindering any potential for improvement. Moreover, addiction labels can instill a sense of powerlessness and hopelessness. Individuals may perceive change as unattainable or beyond their control, creating a defeatist attitude that undermines efforts to initiate positive transformations. This defeatism can perpetuate cycles of relapse and demoralization, hindering progress and perpetuating the addiction cycle.

A more effective approach may involve reframing these issues as a series of ingrained habits rather than labeling them as addictions. For example, if you're struggling to stop eating junk food or find yourself overeating, the sense of helplessness you feel can be a significant barrier to adopting healthier habits. Negative habits are often established and settled into a routine, masking the actual addictive behaviors they represent. Focusing on the chronic nature of these behaviors makes it easier to develop strategies for change.

Habit formation is a well-studied area of psychology, and understanding how habits are formed and changed can provide valuable insights for those looking to improve their relationship with food. Habits are formed through a process called "context-dependent repetition," where a behavior is repeated in a specific context until it becomes automatic. For example, if you consistently eat a snack while watching TV in the evening, your brain begins to associate TV watching with eating, and eventually, the behavior becomes automatic.

Breaking a habit requires disrupting the context-behavior association and replacing the old behavior with a new one. This process is known as "habit replacement" and is a key strategy in behavior change. For example, if you want to break the habit of eating junk food while watching TV, you could replace the snack with a healthier option, such as a piece of fruit or a handful of nuts. Over time, your brain will associate the new behavior with the old context, and the new habit will become automatic.

Studies have shown that one of the most effective ways to break an addiction is to replace it with a new, healthier focus or activity. For instance, someone trying to quit drinking may find it easier if they start exercising regularly, replacing the habitual aspect of drinking with a new routine that is both consistent and positive. The goal is to find a new, reinforcing, and advantageous habit that furthers your goals rather than obstructing them. This concept, known as "habit replacement," is rooted in the understanding that habits are powerful and difficult to change. However, you can gradually replace negative habits with positive ones by introducing new behaviors that serve a similar function: stress relief, comfort, or social connection.

The role of self-worth in influencing our consumption choices cannot be overstated. The foods we choose to eat can reflect how we value ourselves and our bodies. For example, selecting organic products from independent producers and local sources demonstrates self-respect and a commitment to quality.

Conversely, choosing easily accessible fast food due to a lack of planning may reflect low self-worth. Prioritizing your needs and making deliberate, informed choices about your consumption is a sign of acknowledging your personal value. Understanding this is straightforward, yet it requires time to evaluate decisions and question whether you're making the best choices for your health multiple times a day. Consider asking yourself, "Is this the best decision for me now, and how could I improve my choices for my next meal?" "Am I eating this because it looks good?" "Do I know the ingredients in this dish?" "Would I eat them in a different setting, or is this convenient?"

Being mindful of your physical reactions to food before, during, and after meals is crucial. This awareness can help you distinguish between respecting your actual needs versus lazily submitting to convenience or familiarity. It's essential to be deliberate and not give in to impulsive or peer-pressured food consumption. For example, if you notice that certain foods make you feel sluggish or lead to cravings later in the day, this awareness can help you make different choices in the future. By paying attention to how food affects your body, you can make more informed decisions that support your long-term health and well-being.

Mindful eating involves paying full attention to the experience of eating and drinking, both inside and outside the body. It includes observing how the food makes you feel and the signals your body sends about taste, satisfaction, and fullness. Mindful eating can help you recognize the difference between physical and emotional hunger, reducing the tendency to eat in response to emotions.

Research shows that mindful eating can help people develop a healthier relationship with food, reduce overeating, and promote weight loss. A study published in the journal Obesity found that participants who practiced mindful eating were better able to control their eating habits, lost more weight, and maintained their weight loss more effectively than those who did not practice mindfulness.

Mindful eating can be practiced in many ways, such as eating slowly and savoring each bite, paying attention to your food's colors, smells, textures, and flavors, and listening to your body's hunger and fullness cues. Incorporating mindfulness into your eating habits can cultivate a more positive and balanced relationship with food.

Another common challenge is the tendency to view weekends as a time to indulge, often justifying it with the mindset that "the diet starts on Monday." This mentality creates a separation between the enjoyment of food and the weekly diet, making the latter feel like a chore rather than a pleasure. Instead, it's more effective to integrate enjoyable and healthy habits into a lifestyle that doesn't depend on the day of the week.

This approach emphasizes understanding and sustaining your needs, achieving a long-term goal rather than a temporary flavor fix. Food should be enjoyed, and healthy eating doesn't have to be restrictive or boring. By incorporating flavors and foods you love into a balanced diet, you can create a sustainable approach to eating that supports both pleasure and health.

Many people believe that significant changes, like starting a diet or adopting a new lifestyle, should begin at the start of a new year or week. However, time-enduring change is gradual. Real change looks like daily, weekly, and monthly progress, from crawling to walking or novice to expert.

Weekends often become a time of indulgence, where social events, dining out, and relaxation take precedence, leading to eating patterns that differ significantly from those during the week. When we allow indulgent weekends to pass without making any adjustments to our overall routine and then turn to a restrictive diet during the week to counterbalance these excesses, we find ourselves trapped in an unhealthy cycle. This pattern of indulgence followed by restriction can disrupt metabolism, lead to feelings of guilt or deprivation, and undermine long-term weight management efforts. These constant shifts between overeating and strict dieting can cause the body to store more fat during the periods of indulgence, anticipating future periods of restriction, thus making weight management even more challenging.

Effective change begins with the understanding that lasting habits are built gradually. You can steadily build momentum by focusing on making one positive change at a time, such as incorporating more whole foods into your diet, reducing portion sizes, or drinking more water. These small steps accumulate, laying a solid foundation for lasting habits that support your health. Each positive change reinforces the next, making it easier to continue progressing toward your goals. This steady, manageable approach is more sustainable. It minimizes the likelihood of reverting to old habits, as it doesn't rely solely on willpower but on gradually developing new routines.

Separating the enjoyment of food from the pleasure associated with social eating occasions is another critical component in establishing a solid foundation for healthier habits. Social events often revolve around food, and the pleasure derived from these occasions is as much about the company and experience as it is about the food itself. Building a healthy relationship with food doesn't mean giving up the foods you love; it means finding a balance that allows you to enjoy the taste and the benefits of what you eat. This can involve choosing nutrient-dense foods that satisfy both your body's needs and your taste preferences daily while allowing for occasional indulgences.

Most of the beliefs and information we hold as adults about food, diet, and nutrition, along with many of our core values, are shaped during adolescence. These "formative years" are so named because they are when we learn what our elders consider essential for survival. This age-old system of passing down knowledge has ensured the survival of all species, complemented by the unique genetic instincts encoded in our DNA. However, modern times present new challenges, especially concerning untainted, wholesome food availability. This shift means that each individual must actively seek out and uncover the truths about what is truly ideal for their body, mind, and spirit.

Metabolism, the process by which your body converts what you eat and drink into energy, plays a key role in this journey. Even at rest, your body needs energy for all its "hidden" functions, such as breathing, circulating blood, adjusting hormone levels, and growing and repairing cells. Your basal metabolic rate (BMR) accounts for about 60 to 75% of the calories you burn each day. Factors influencing BMR include age, sex, body composition, and genetics.

Understanding how metabolism works can help you set realistic expectations for weight loss. For example, as you lose weight, your BMR decreases because your body requires fewer calories to maintain a smaller body size. This is why weight loss can slow down over time and why focusing on building muscle mass through strength training becomes increasingly important. Muscle tissue burns more calories at rest than fat tissue, so increasing muscle mass can help offset the natural decline in BMR that occurs with weight loss.

It's also important to embrace that fat loss may not occur in one specific spot and that the body draws from fat stores all over the body. Spot reduction, or the idea of losing fat in one specific area by targeting that area with exercises, is a common myth. Fat loss occurs throughout the body based on overall energy expenditure and genetic factors.

If you are trying to lose weight in certain areas and focusing on those in the mirror, you may miss the small, less apparent milestones along the way. Celebrate the progress made daily throughout the journey. Relish your commitment to staying on your program, and remember that weight loss may not occur in one specific spot. Should you notice a deviation from your planned habits, examine the triggers and adjust these habits to reduce the likelihood of disappointment in your accountability.

Focusing on the overall goal of improved health and well-being can create a positive mindset and help us stay motivated on our journey to a healthier version of ourselves, one step at a time. As you simplify what you eat, you will gradually tune your brain and body into seamless communication. But flavors, like memories, stay in the frontal lobe.

Replacing the foods you've associated with pleasure with healthier, colorful food options will increase the number of foods you can choose from that will appeal to you because your body will crave the nutrients. This shift in cravings reflects the body's natural inclination towards balance and nourishment once it is no longer conditioned to seek out hyper-palatable, nutrient-poor foods.

Nutrient density refers to the amount of nutrients a food contains relative to the number of calories it provides. Nutrient-dense foods, such as vegetables, fruits, legumes, roots, and whole grains, provide essential vitamins, minerals, and other beneficial compounds with relatively few calories. These foods help you feel full and satisfied while supporting overall health.

Conversely, foods high in calories but low in nutrients, such as sugary snacks, fast food, and processed foods, can lead to overeating because they do not provide the nutrients your body needs to function properly. This can result in a cycle of overeating and cravings as your body continues to seek out the nutrients it lacks. For example, a salad with mixed greens, colorful vegetables, lean protein, and a healthy fat source like avocado or nuts can provide a balance of nutrients that keeps you full and energized. Incorporating various foods in different colors, textures, and flavors can make meals more enjoyable and reduce the desire for less healthy options.

The world of edible plants is vast and diverse, offering a wealth of flavors, textures, and nutritional benefits that can transform how we approach food. Despite there being over 20,000 known edible plant species on Earth, most diets rely on a small handful of staples like wheat, corn, and rice. This limited selection not only restricts our exposure to a broader range of nutrients but also narrows our culinary experiences. By exploring the wide variety of edible plants available, we can discover new tastes and expand our palates, leading to a more diverse and nourishing diet.

Leafy greens, root vegetables, legumes, nuts, seeds, fruits, and herbs provide an array of flavors that are both satisfying and healthful. For instance, the bitterness of arugula can add complexity to a dish, while the sweetness of beets or the earthiness of mushrooms can offer depth. Each plant has a unique flavor profile, and experimenting with different combinations can create meals that are both nutritious and delicious.

Changing our beliefs about what tastes good requires more than just exposure to new foods; it involves reconditioning the brain and palate to appreciate and crave healthier options. Genetic factors, early experiences, cultural influences, and repeated exposure to specific flavors shape our taste preferences. For many, the flavors of highly processed, sugar-laden foods have become the norm, leading to a preference for sweetness, saltiness, and rich, fatty textures. But this can be changed by gradually introducing healthier foods into our diet.

For those who consider themselves foodies, there is a common misconception that adopting a healthier or plant-based diet means sacrificing the enjoyment of food. However, being a foodie is about savoring flavors, appreciating culinary artistry, and exploring diverse tastes. With the vast array of plant-based ingredients available, it is possible to maintain a Foodie's identity while abstaining from unhealthy foods. Plant-based diets offer a canvas of vibrant, fresh, and wholesome ingredients that can be crafted into exquisite dishes. The possibilities are endless, from rich, creamy cashew sauces to hearty lentil stews, from vibrant fruit salads to spiced roasted vegetables. Exploring the culinary world of plant-based cooking allows one to remain a foodie, enjoying all the pleasures of gourmet dining without compromising health.

Research shows that the brain's reward system is highly responsive to hyper-palatable foods designed to be addictive. Over time, this can desensitize taste buds, making natural, whole foods seem less appealing. To shift these preferences, it's essential to gradually reintroduce the palate to the flavors of real, whole foods.

Incorporating small amounts of new, nutrient-dense foods into familiar dishes is a practical approach. For example, adding a handful of spinach to a smoothie or incorporating roasted vegetables into a pasta dish can begin to accustom the palate to different tastes without overwhelming it. Over time, as these flavors become more familiar, they may become more enjoyable, and the brain will start to associate them with positive feelings of satiety and well-being.

Beyond the physical aspects of nutrition, the psychological relationship with food plays a significant role in dietary habits and overall well-being. Many people use food as a coping mechanism, turning to it for comfort during times of stress, sadness, or boredom. This emotional eating can create a cycle where food is used to suppress or soothe uncomfortable feelings rather than to nourish the body. Understanding and addressing the emotional triggers that lead to unhealthy eating patterns is crucial for breaking this cycle and developing a healthier relationship with food.

Mindful eating plays a critical role in this process. By slowing down and fully experiencing each bite, we can retrain our taste buds to savor the natural sweetness of a ripe peach or the satisfying crunch of a fresh cucumber.It involves being fully present in the moment and paying attention to your thoughts, feelings, and bodily sensations while you eat. When applied to eating, mindfulness encourages you to savor each bite, notice the flavors and textures of your food, and pay attention to your body's hunger and satiety cues.

This practice can help you become more attuned to your body's needs and less likely to eat in response to emotional triggers. Over time, mindfulness can transform your relationship with food, making eating a more intentional and enjoyable experience. This awareness helps to break the cycle of mindless eating and re-establishes a connection with the sensory pleasures of whole foods.

Understanding the science behind taste and flavor can also help shift perceptions. Taste buds regenerate approximately every two weeks, meaning that with consistent exposure to healthier foods, our taste preferences can change relatively quickly. Studies suggest that reducing sugar and salt intake for even a short period can reset taste buds to be more sensitive to these flavors, making naturally sweet or savory foods more satisfying.

This gradual process requires patience, but the rewards are significant. As we begin to enjoy and crave nutrient-rich foods, we not only improve our overall health but also cultivate a deeper appreciation for nature's diverse flavors. This shift in perspective allows us to see food not just as fuel but as a source of nourishment, pleasure, and connection to the natural world.

Abstaining from unhealthy foods doesn't mean giving up the joy of eating or the pleasure derived from food. It means redefining what pleasure in food means. The world of plant-based cooking offers endless possibilities for creativity and satisfaction. Whether making a rich, creamy cashew Alfredo sauce or a decadent chocolate avocado mousse, plant-based ingredients can be transformed into indulgent dishes that are both healthful and satisfying. This approach allows you to remain a foodie, savoring the joys of culinary exploration while taking care of your body and health.

For many, emotional eating and food addictions stem from using food to cope with stress, boredom, or other negative emotions. Highly processed foods, rich in sugars, salts, and fats, trigger the release of dopamine, a neurotransmitter associated with pleasure and reward. This leads to a temporary feeling of relief or happiness but also reinforces the cycle of craving and consumption. Over time, this can develop into an addiction, where the brain begins to crave these foods, not for their taste or nutritional value, but for the dopamine hit they provide.

A plant-based diet can help break this cycle by reducing the intake of highly processed, addictive foods and replacing them with nutrient-dense, whole foods that support overall health and well-being. The variety of flavors, textures, and nutrients in plant-based foods can help satisfy cravings healthily, reducing the reliance on sugar-laden and fatty foods for emotional comfort. Moreover, the high fiber content of plant-based foods helps stabilize blood sugar levels, reducing the spikes and crashes that can trigger cravings.

By embracing a plant-based diet, individuals can begin to heal their relationship with food. They learn to appreciate whole foods' natural flavors and textures, finding joy and satisfaction in meals that nourish the body and soul. This shift in mindset allows for a more balanced approach to eating, where food is seen as a source of pleasure and a tool for health and well-being. Over time, this can help to heal emotional eating patterns and food addictions, leading to a healthier, more fulfilling relationship with food.

4
MACROS & DON'T FORGET THE MICROS

Modern discussions on diet and nutrition frequently focus on "Macros," with much of the attention centered on protein intake. This emphasis, often fueled by media trends, raises questions like, "Are you getting enough protein?" While protein is undeniably important, this narrow focus can lead to a misunderstanding of dietary needs, akin to refueling a car without attending to its other essential maintenance needs. A well-rounded diet must include a balanced intake of all macronutrients: carbohydrates, proteins, and fats. Each plays a distinct and vital role in the body, contributing to energy levels, cellular function, and overall metabolic processes.

Carbohydrates are often misunderstood, especially in modern dieting trends that sometimes vilify them. However, they are the body's primary energy source, particularly important for brain function and muscle activity during physical exertion. The key to including carbohydrates in a healthy diet is choosing the right kinds.

Complex carbohydrates, found in whole grains, fruits, vegetables, and legumes, break down slowly in the body, providing a steady release of energy. This slow release helps prevent spikes and crashes in blood sugar levels, which can lead to cravings and overeating. Fiber, a component of complex carbohydrates, plays a crucial role in digestion and satiety. It helps regulate the body's use of sugars, keeping hunger and blood sugar in check, supporting a healthy digestive system, and promoting feelings of fullness.

In contrast, simple carbohydrates common in sugary snacks, white bread, and many processed foods are quickly absorbed into the bloodstream. This rapid absorption causes sharp increases in blood sugar and insulin levels, often followed by sudden declines. These fluctuations can trigger hunger and a cycle of overeating as the body seeks to restore energy levels quickly. While carbohydrates are essential, the type and timing of carbohydrate intake are critical. Combining carbohydrates with fiber and protein can help moderate these effects, leading to more sustained energy and reduced hunger throughout the day.

Amino Acids, aka protein chains, are fundamental for tissue growth, repair, and maintenance, including muscle. They are also crucial for producing enzymes and hormones that regulate metabolism and other bodily functions. While the media often emphasizes animal-based protein sources, plant-based proteins such as beans, lentils, tofu, and quinoa are excellent alternatives, offering a host of additional nutrients, including fiber, vitamins, and minerals.

Fats have long been misunderstood and often demonized in diet culture, but they are essential for good health. Fats are necessary for absorbing fat-soluble vitamins (A, D, E, and K), providing essential fatty acids the body cannot produce, and serving as a long-term energy source. Healthy fats, such as those found in avocados, nuts, seeds, and oily fish, support brain health, reduce inflammation, and promote heart health. It's crucial to differentiate between healthy fats and unhealthy trans fats found in many processed foods. While fats are calorie-dense, incorporating healthy fats in moderation can help maintain satiety and reduce the likelihood of overeating or relying on unhealthy snacks.

Achieving a balanced intake of macronutrients is crucial in maintaining energy levels, supporting overall health, and managing weight. Each macronutrient contributes to the body's functioning in unique ways, and finding the right balance can help ensure that the body is well-nourished and operating efficiently.

Consider a daily intake of 2,000 calories, which is a common benchmark for nutritional guidelines. The recommended distribution for macronutrients is as follows:

- Carbohydrates: 45-65% of total calories (900-1,300 calories per day, or 225-325 grams)
- Proteins: 10-35% of total calories (200-700 calories per day, or 50-175 grams)
- Fats: 20-35% of total calories (400-700 calories per day, or 44-78 grams)

Balancing these macronutrients involves ensuring each category contributes appropriately to the total caloric intake. For example, a diet with 55% carbohydrates, 15% protein, and 30% fat translates to 1,100 calories (275 grams) from carbohydrates, 300 calories (75 grams) from proteins, and 600 calories (67 grams) from fats. A well-balanced diet includes a variety of foods from all food groups to meet both macronutrient and micronutrient needs. Whole grains, fruits, vegetables, legumes, nuts, and seeds provide a wide range of nutrients necessary for optimal health.

Many individuals struggle with balancing macronutrients and micronutrients. The media often emphasizes the importance of protein, sometimes overshadowing the need for a balanced intake of vitamins and minerals. Relying solely on high-protein diets without addressing other nutritional needs can lead to deficiencies and imbalances. It's essential to consider the complete nutritional profile of foods rather than focusing on just one aspect.

There is a common misconception that consuming animal products, such as meat and fish, provides all necessary nutrients.

While animal products offer certain nutrients, they lack phytonutrients and living enzymes beneficial for health. A varied diet that includes plant-based foods can provide comprehensive nutritional benefits and support overall well-being. Incorporating plant-based foods into the diet offers a range of nutrients and health benefits. Fruits, vegetables, legumes, nuts, and seeds are rich in vitamins, minerals, and antioxidants, providing essential nutrients without the added saturated fats and cholesterol found in all animal products.

Cravings can signal a need for specific nutrients. For example, craving citrus fruits may indicate a need for vitamin C, while a desire for leafy greens might suggest a lack of iron. Recognizing these signals can help individuals make informed dietary choices to meet their nutritional needs. Emotional and environmental factors, such as stress or past experiences, can also influence cravings. Cravings for processed foods, like sugary snacks or fried items, may indicate a need for more calories rather than specific nutrients. Ensuring a consistent intake of balanced meals can help stabilize hunger and reduce cravings for less healthy options. A varied diet that includes whole, nutrient-dense foods supports overall health and reduces the likelihood of unhealthy cravings.

Achieving a balance of macronutrients and micronutrients is essential for maintaining optimal health. While macronutrients provide the energy needed for daily activities, micronutrients support various physiological processes and prevent deficiencies. Incorporating a diverse range of plant-based foods into your diet can offer comprehensive nutritional benefits, enhance overall well-being, and support a healthy balance of bioelectricity in the body. By understanding and implementing these principles, individuals can improve their health and experience the benefits of a well-rounded diet.

The premise of a macrobiotic diet is rooted in the principles of balance, harmony, and natural foods. It originated from traditional

Eastern philosophies, primarily influenced by Zen Buddhism. The diet emphasizes the consumption of whole, unprocessed, and plant-based foods while promoting a mindful and balanced approach to eating.

This is a conscious shift to whole, non-harmful foods that are non-processed, have low environmental impact, and are thoughtfully grown. There is a belief that the less harm you do, the less negative karma will follow you. There are beliefs that when you ingest an animal, you are also ingesting all of the fear within it, and there is a counter belief that when you eat a raw living vegetable, you are increasing the joy because you are eating the wellness of a healthy plant that will become you.

The fundamental principles of a macrobiotic diet include many details and food pairings. These concepts are more advanced, as it does take some time to understand which foods they suggest pairing. Still, for someone looking to try a stable lifestyle plan that could encourage wellness, the macrobiotic template has been around for much longer than any of the diets trending today.

Eating with a positive spiritual mindset can only increase the positive momentum in your life. The macrobiotic diet aims to balance yin and yang energies in food. Yin represents cooling and expansive qualities, while yang represents warming and contracting qualities. The goal is to consume foods that create a harmonious balance between these energies. Foods are categorized as either "yin" or "yang" based on their perceived energetic qualities. The goal is to achieve a balance between these two opposing energies to promote overall well-being.

Yang Foods (Contractive, Warming): Whole grains like brown rice, barley, millet, quinoa, rye, and buckwheat; beans and legumes such as adzuki beans, lentils, chickpeas, black beans, and kidney beans; sea vegetables including nori, kombu, wakame, and hijiki; vegetables like root vegetables including carrots, daikon radish, onions, garlic, and winter squashes; and seeds and nuts like pumpkin seeds, sesame seeds, almonds, and walnuts.

Yin Foods (Expansive, Cooling): Vegetables such as leafy greens, cabbage, broccoli, cauliflower, celery, and lettuce; fruits including apples, pears, berries, melons, and citrus fruits; lightly processed foods like tofu, tempeh, miso, and soy milk; oils such as sesame oil, olive oil, and flaxseed oil; and beverages like herbal teas, green tea, and naturally fermented drinks such as kombucha.

The diet focuses on consuming whole grains, fresh vegetables, legumes, and sea vegetables. Processed foods, refined sugars, and artificial additives are generally avoided. Emphasis on the consumption of locally grown and seasonal foods, as they are believed to be in harmony with the environment and the individual's needs.

A macrobiotic diet encourages consuming a wide variety of foods to ensure nutritional balance. It emphasizes moderation in portion sizes and promotes mindful eating. Cooking methods such as steaming, boiling, and stir-frying are commonly used in macrobiotic cuisine. These methods are believed to preserve foods' natural flavors, textures, and nutritional integrity. Macrobiotics promote an awareness of the source and quality of food. Organic and locally sourced foods are often preferred, and sustainability and environmental considerations may be emphasized.

Practitioners of this lifestyle diet often emphasize the importance of mindful eating, including chewing food thoroughly to aid digestion and appreciate the flavors and textures. Becoming more aware and grounded in the moment while eating thoughtfully is ideal for rebuilding your relationship with food and home, and it can be nourishing rather than detrimental.

While a macrobiotic template can be used as a lifestyle diet to work in tune with the body, it can be confusing for beginners who don't understand the qualifiers that make a food Yin or Yang. Urban areas may be more likely to have macrobiotic restaurants, where one can try the cuisine and experience a different eating style. Alternatively, plenty of online resources and cookbooks are available for the macrobiotic lifestyle.

Similarly to this theory of yin and yang foods, all things have energy and can do specific things in the body. Yes, there is bioelectricity in your whole foods. Bioelectricity, the electrical activity in living organisms, plays a crucial role in health and nutrition. Foods contain bioelectrical properties that can influence bodily functions. The concept of electron transfer is central to understanding how antioxidants work. Electron donors, such as those found in plant-based foods, neutralize harmful free radicals by donating electrons, which helps protect cells from oxidative damage. Antioxidants, such as vitamins C and E, flavonoids, and carotenoids, are rich in these electron-donating properties and are predominantly found in fruits, vegetables, nuts, and seeds.

Electrons, the negatively charged subatomic particles, play a crucial role in chemical reactions, including those essential for nutrition and overall health. In the realm of nutrition, electron donors are substances capable of neutralizing free radicals by donating electrons. This donation helps prevent cellular damage, a process known as oxidation. Plant-based foods, which are rich in antioxidants, are excellent sources of electron donors. These antioxidants help maintain cellular health by balancing the electron transfer within the body, reducing oxidative stress.

Electron donors and takers are integral to understanding the role of antioxidants in nutrition. Free radicals, which are highly reactive molecules, cause cellular damage by stealing electrons from other molecules, leading to a chain reaction of cellular damage known as oxidative stress. Antioxidants, which are electron donors, neutralize these free radicals by donating electrons, thus stabilizing them and preventing further damage. Vitamins such as C and E, carotenoids, and flavonoids are well-known examples of antioxidants that act as electron donors, protecting cells from the harmful effects of oxidation.

Conversely, electron takers, or acceptors, are molecules that receive electrons and act as oxidizing agents. These agents play essential roles in various metabolic processes and cellular functions. For example, oxygen acts as an electron acceptor during cellular respiration, a process vital for energy production. While the presence of electron takers is necessary for certain metabolic functions, an imbalance, where oxidizing agents outnumber antioxidants, can lead to excessive oxidative stress and potential cellular damage.

Focusing on electron donors means incorporating foods with strong antioxidant properties in the context of nutrition. These foods help stabilize free radicals, thereby protecting cells from potential damage. For instance, berries like blueberries, strawberries, raspberries, and blackberries are rich in antioxidants like anthocyanins.

These compounds can donate electrons, effectively neutralizing free radicals and contributing to the maintenance of cellular health. Other plant-based foods, including leafy greens, nuts, seeds, and fruits, also offer antioxidant properties, promoting a balanced internal environment and overall well-being. Antioxidants act as electron donors to neutralize free radicals and are primarily found in plant-based foods, such as fruits, vegetables, whole grains, nuts, seeds, and herbs/spices.

These foods contribute to a diet that provides a balance of electron donors and takers, helping to maintain overall cellular health. While animal meat does not possess antioxidant properties, leafy greens, such as spinach, kale, Swiss chard, and other leafy greens, contain antioxidants like vitamins C, E, and beta-carotene that can act as electron donors. Oranges, lemons, grapefruits, and other citrus fruits are high in vitamin C, a potent antioxidant that can donate electrons to neutralize free radicals. Almonds, walnuts, chia seeds, flaxseeds, and sunflower seeds are rich in antioxidants like vitamin E and polyphenols, which can act as electron donors.

Green tea is known for its high content of polyphenols, including catechins, which have strong antioxidant properties and can act as electron donors. Dark chocolate, with a high cocoa content, is rich in flavonoids and antioxidants, which can donate electrons and provide health benefits. Turmeric, ginger, cinnamon, and cloves are examples of spices that contain antioxidants and can act as electron donors. Vibrantly colored vegetables like tomatoes, bell peppers, carrots, and sweet potatoes are rich in antioxidants like vitamin C and beta-carotene, which can donate electrons.

Finding a balance that works for you is vital. This means incorporating a variety of foods that meet your nutritional needs and bring you joy and satisfaction. A healthy diet is not about deprivation or strict rules; it's about enjoying a wide range of foods in moderation and finding pleasure in nourishing your body. As you explore new foods and recipes, keep an open mind and be willing to experiment. Try new vegetables, fruits, grains, and protein sources, and find ways to prepare them that appeal to your taste buds. Cooking at home can be a fun and creative way to discover new flavors and develop a deeper appreciation for the food you eat.

Over time, you'll discover that a diet rich in whole, nutritious foods can be both delicious and fulfilling, sustainably supporting your overall well-being. As you make gradual changes to your eating habits, you'll start to notice positive effects on your energy levels, mood, and overall health. You can develop a healthier, more intuitive relationship with food by prioritizing nutrient-dense foods and listening to your body's hunger and satiety signals. This holistic approach improves your physical health and enhances your emotional and mental well-being, leading to a more balanced and fulfilling life.

Consistently reaching for the best option available to you at any moment will yield better results than simply eating for convenience and familiarity. Giving your body an array of whole organic foods can reset its ability to process the availability of nutrients. Even if you do this briefly, you will feel lighter and more satisfied while not feeling overly full. Your body will immediately show results, from bathroom regularity to clearer-looking skin and less bloating. As your body shows signs of healing, it learns where to mine these nutritional gold nuggets. Your cravings will nudge you into a naturally tailored meal plan that caters to your needs as your body interprets a new palette of dietary options.

Your body instinctively selects foods with the highest returns. If you have delayed eating to the point where your body needs energy, it will crave high-calorie foods to sustain its functions. Alternatively, suppose you need more nutrition than you have been getting. You may crave a salad after a few days of consuming fast food because your body knows it can obtain antioxidants, amino acids, fiber, vitamins, and minerals from the greens. However, suppose your salad consists only of iceberg lettuce and cucumbers. In that case, you are not getting as many nutrients or calories as possible, leaving you hungry and likely to reach for salty or sugary snacks. Hence, when you are inclined to have a salad, it is an ideal opportunity to enrich your meal with various nutrients.

Try incorporating a mix of leafy greens and different toppings into your salads to do this. Adding superfoods such as pomegranate seeds, sunflower seeds, hemp seeds, and cooked quinoa to a salad of kale or other dark leafy greens, along with beets and avocado, chunks of sweet potato or roasted squash, and a hearty tahini or cashew-based dressing can elevate a lackluster salad into a nourishing meal that you will want to enjoy on repeat.

Adopting new foods that pack a higher nutritional punch is often crucial to breaking away from physical addictions to substances like dairy and sugar. This shift is necessary because these foods can trigger a reaction similar to withdrawal in the brain. Replacing common allergens with predominantly unprocessed foods can reprogram your metabolic system in just a few days.

The process is even more effective with daily probiotics from beverages like kombucha, top-quality probiotic supplements, or non-dairy yogurts. Additionally, research indicates that engaging with soil, particularly during childhood when the microbiome is still forming, can have a lasting positive impact on its healthful composition. This supports the idea that even modest home gardening provides fresh produce and benefits your overall health in a self-reinforcing loop.

Our lifestyle choices profoundly influence our mental and physical health and the overall functioning of our bodily systems. Many people struggle to attribute their challenges to the foods they eat because these foods have served them in the past. We develop emotional attachments to flavors, textures, and memories associated with certain foods. We associate these foods with our caregivers and honor them for the security, safety, and satiety they provide. People often favor information that reaffirms their preconceived beliefs and tends to ignore or dismiss information that contradicts them. This cognitive bias complicates the consideration of alternative dietary perspectives.

As civilization has evolved, diets have become complex, influenced by traditions and local foods. Yet, altering these patterns requires more than determination for individuals accustomed to unhealthy eating habits. Permanent change requires understanding the genuine benefits and potential harm of available foods. The adverse effects of certain foods are sometimes evident in weight gain, lethargy, mental cloudiness, excessive cravings, and digestive issues. Many people have trouble accepting that their current diet might be behind specific health issues, often because those foods did not seem to cause problems in younger years. The mindset of "I have been eating this my whole life; how can it suddenly be an issue?" is common, but the reality is that our bodies change over time, and what once worked may no longer be suitable.

People often use the fear of change as an excuse to avoid making dietary adjustments. However, our emotional attachment to specific foods can make it challenging to stop consuming them, even when they don't benefit our health. Food involves more than flavor and feel; it is tied to our memories and can sometimes satisfy us emotionally. Additionally, certain chemical additives in foods can lead to physical dependence. To break free from this, one must deliberately select healthier choices and persist in these habits until they become established. Remember, habits can change, and beliefs are merely thoughts we repeatedly think. Adventuring into new dietary territories should be an exciting way to explore self-care through what we eat, not a self-imposed contest about the ideal diet for optimal appearance.

Eating habits are intricately connected to emotional wellness, stress relief, and coping mechanisms. Changing our beliefs about food can disrupt these emotional ties, necessitating the discovery of new coping methods and the substitution of more healthful options. It is possible to shift how you perceive food from an emotional crutch into a means of self-nourishment. Discard emotional attachment to foods one by one by replacing them with a healthier version. You begin to look at food as a tool to nourish yourself from the inside out. Initially, this decision requires conscious effort.

With time and understanding of the truths behind your dietary choices, preferring more wholesome foods becomes second nature. Remember, diets are temporary, but a lifestyle is to be maintained for the long term.

Adopting new food beliefs can be an effort without a supportive environment or resources encouraging healthier options. The presence of aggressive advertising, pervasive food marketing, and ready access to unhealthy options can be significant barriers for some. Try following healthy eating accounts on social media and subscribing to wellness channels on YouTube. Changing your algorithm can increase exposure to positive media, reinforcing your daily goals.

The science behind the foods we eat can be complex and infinite, yet the most relevant ideals to empower you on your individual journey to wellness will naturally resound and reveal themselves. You will be transformed as you employ this new understanding of the power of what's on your plate.

5
THE HYPE ABOUT FASTING

The human body is a marvel of evolution, equipped with instincts and mechanisms honed over millennia to ensure survival. These primal instincts, which once guided our ancestors through the harsh realities of a world where food was scarce and life was unpredictable, still influence our behaviors today. Our cravings, responses to hunger, and environmental interactions are deeply rooted in these ancient survival mechanisms. Understanding and acknowledging these instincts can help us navigate the complexities of modern life, where abundance often leads to overindulgence, and convenience can mask the actual needs of our bodies.

In modern-day America, the pervasive presence of fast food establishments and the normalization of oversized meal portions have dulled our natural hunger signals and cravings. The ease of access to fast food drive-thrus and delivery services further complicates our ability to listen to our bodies' actual needs. However, skipping meals or delaying food intake can have its own consequences. When the brain senses a lack of nourishment, it craves the most accessible high-energy foods, typically those rich in fats, salts, and sugars. While these habits can be difficult to break, they are not permanent. One can recondition their physiological hunger responses by understanding how the body's energy needs fluctuate and responding with a well-timed snack or meal.

The Hype About Fasting

Humans have evolved mechanisms to cope with food shortages, a trait deeply embedded in our DNA. This evolutionary adaptation is still at play today, even though the modern world offers an abundance of food. The multi-billion-dollar diet industry often obscures these fundamental biological truths with its misleading claims and quick-fix solutions. To regain control, it's essential to understand and utilize these truths to our benefit without being swayed by the confusing and often contradictory messages found in media.

Our bodies require specific nutrients to synthesize, repair, and maintain cellular function. When faced with a calorie deficit, such as during fasting or skipping meals, the body initiates a series of adaptations to maintain energy balance and support vital functions. Metabolism adjusts by conserving energy, focusing on essential processes, and using stored fat for fuel. During fasting, insulin levels drop, prompting the body to rely on glycogen stores for energy before transitioning to fat metabolism. Additionally, growth hormone levels increase during this period, aiding in fat breakdown and muscle preservation.

By understanding these physiological responses, you can make more informed decisions about your eating habits. Rather than being controlled by external pressures or the convenience of modern food options, you can learn to work with your body's natural processes, ensuring that your energy needs are balanced and healthy. This approach helps maintain a healthy weight and supports overall well-being, as it aligns your eating habits with the body's innate rhythms and needs.

Intermittent fasting has gained significant traction in recent years and is touted as a miracle solution for weight loss, anti-aging, and overall wellness. However, many people approach it with misconceptions, believing that simply skipping a meal or two will yield transformative results. The reality is far more complex. The claims surrounding fasting often promise rapid weight loss and anti-aging effects. Still, these outcomes depend on a nuanced understanding of the body's physiological responses to prolonged periods without food. The alleged anti-aging benefits of fasting are primarily linked to the body's response to extreme depletion, where it is forced into a state of autophagy (cell repair and renewal) when it experiences a scarcity of nutrients.

To truly experience the full spectrum of fasting's benefits, including the production of growth hormones and the shedding of damaged cells, one must typically fast for 15 to 18 hours a day. This extended fasting period is necessary to trigger significant physiological changes in the body, particularly in cellular processes such as autophagy. However, this is a substantial portion of the day, making it difficult for most people to maintain a busy schedule while adhering to restrictive eating patterns. Moreover, when the eating window finally opens, consuming enough of the right foods to nourish and sustain the body effectively can be challenging. For many, this practice can be particularly detrimental, especially for individuals prone to eating disorders, those at risk for diabetes or hypoglycemia, and those who experience significant mood swings when hungry.

The negative effects of entering a starvation-like mode can manifest in various ways, including irritability, fatigue, cognitive challenges, and metabolic disruptions, all of which can significantly impact daily life. At the cellular level, fasting triggers a remarkable process known as autophagy. Autophagy is a natural mechanism by which cells remove damaged components, including misfolded proteins and dysfunctional organelles, and recycle them for energy and cellular repair. This process is akin to the body's internal recycling system, continuously working to maintain cellular health and vitality.

The term "autophagy" is derived from the Greek words for "self-eating," it is a finely tuned process that balances cellular growth and degradation. During times of stress or nutrient scarcity, such as fasting, cells increase autophagy to scavenge for resources, ensuring survival in challenging conditions.

Scientific research has shown that autophagy plays a crucial role in protecting against various diseases, including neurodegenerative disorders like Alzheimer's and Parkinson's. Studies have demonstrated that autophagy helps to clear away toxic proteins that accumulate in the brain, potentially reducing the risk of these debilitating conditions.

For example, a study published in the journal *Nature* found that enhancing autophagy in mice reduced the accumulation of amyloid-beta plaques, a hallmark of Alzheimer's disease, and improved cognitive function. Additionally, autophagy has been linked to improved metabolic health, as it enhances insulin sensitivity and reduces inflammation, both of which are critical factors in preventing metabolic diseases such as type 2 diabetes and obesity.

While fasting is a well-known trigger for autophagy, other lifestyle factors can also support this sought-after process. Regular exercise, for example, has been shown to stimulate autophagy by activating cellular stress responses that promote cellular cleanup and renewal. Exercise-induced autophagy is particularly important for maintaining muscle health and preventing the accumulation of damaged proteins that can lead to muscle atrophy.

A diet rich in nutrient-dense foods, packed with antioxidants and anti-inflammatory compounds, provides the essential building blocks for cellular repair and may enhance autophagy. Antioxidants such as resveratrol in grapes and berries and curcumin in turmeric have been shown to activate autophagy pathways, further supporting cellular health.

Intermittent fasting, a practice that involves cycling between periods of eating and fasting, has gained attention as a powerful tool for regulating autophagy and promoting cellular rejuvenation. Research has indicated that intermittent fasting can enhance the body's natural repair processes, reduce oxidative stress, and improve mitochondrial function, which is essential for energy production and overall cellular health. However, it is important to note that autophagy is not solely dependent on fasting or exercise. Quality sleep, effective stress management, and minimizing exposure to environmental toxins are critical in supporting cellular health and facilitating autophagy.

Quality sleep is crucial; during sleep, the body undergoes many of its repair processes, including autophagy. Disrupted sleep patterns have been linked to impaired autophagy and an increased risk of chronic diseases, including cardiovascular disease and diabetes. Studies have shown that sleep deprivation can lead to decreased autophagy activity, accumulating cellular damage over time. This underscores the importance of maintaining a consistent sleep schedule and ensuring the body receives the rest it needs to perform its essential repair functions.

Similarly, chronic stress can inhibit autophagy by increasing the production of cortisol, a stress hormone that can interfere with the body's natural repair mechanisms. Prolonged exposure to high levels of cortisol has been linked to a variety of health issues, including weight gain, impaired immune function, and increased inflammation. By managing stress through practices such as mindfulness meditation, yoga, and deep breathing exercises, individuals can support their body's ability to engage in autophagy and maintain cellular health. Research has shown that stress-reduction techniques can lower cortisol levels and enhance the body's resilience to stress, thereby promoting overall well-being.

People often turn to fasting as a weight loss tool after other methods have failed, viewing it as an extreme measure to achieve their goals. This demographic often starts with an unhealthy diet,

The Hype About Fasting

and the transition from consuming addictive, toxic food chemicals to a whole foods diet can provide more benefits than simply starving oneself. When forced into survival mode through prolonged fasting, the body can induce high cortisol levels, low blood sugar, drained adrenal function, dehydration, and metabolic dysfunction. These physiological responses are counterproductive to overall health and can exacerbate existing health conditions. For instance, elevated cortisol levels during fasting can lead to increased fat storage, particularly in the abdominal region, counteracting the desired weight loss effects.

The idea of "starvation diets," often repackaged as cleanses, weight loss strategies, or reset methodologies, is rooted in the belief that reducing food intake can catalyze weight reduction and detoxification. While some scientific evidence supports the benefits of intermittent fasting for metabolic health, it is important to understand that digestion and fiber fermentation are daily necessities for maintaining a healthy microbiome. The gut microbiome plays a crucial role in overall health, influencing everything from digestion and nutrient absorption to immune function and mental health. Studies have shown that prolonged fasting can disrupt the balance of beneficial bacteria in the gut, leading to dysbiosis and an increased risk of gastrointestinal disorders.

For example, a study published in *Cell Metabolism* found that intermittent fasting altered the gut microbiota composition in mice, leading to reduced diversity and an imbalance of beneficial bacterial species. These changes were associated with increased intestinal permeability, also known as "leaky gut," which can contribute to inflammation and a host of other health issues. This research highlights the importance of maintaining a balanced diet with sufficient fiber and prebiotics to support a healthy gut microbiome, even when practicing intermittent fasting.

Fasting has deep roots in ancient Buddhist philosophy, which is practiced as a spiritual discipline to diminish reliance on materiality and enhance spiritual connectedness. In these traditions, fasting is often seen as a way to purify the body and mind, allowing individuals to transcend physical desires and focus on spiritual growth. However, it is essential to recognize that the context in which fasting was originally practiced vastly differs from modern-day fasting trends. In the past, fasting was often accompanied by meditation, prayer, and other spiritual practices that provided a holistic approach to health and well-being.

While fasting can have beneficial outcomes in certain contexts, such as in cancer treatments when supervised by medical professionals, it is not a method to be undertaken lightly. Some research suggests that fasting may enhance the body's natural defenses against cancer by stimulating autophagy, promoting cellular repair, and potentially improving the effectiveness of conventional treatments like chemotherapy and radiation therapy. For example, a study published in *Science Translational Medicine* found that short-term fasting enhanced the sensitivity of cancer cells to chemotherapy in mice while protecting normal cells from the toxic effects of the treatment. These findings have led to increased interest in the potential role of fasting as an adjunct to cancer therapy. Still, more clinical trials are needed to evaluate these effects and establish guidelines for fasting in clinical practice.

Fasting should not be mistaken for a trendy diet or used as an excuse to avoid proper meal preparation. Like other diet trends, such as the Ketogenic diet, intermittent fasting, juice fasts, and soup diets, fasting often results in weight loss due to reduced calorie intake. However, this weight loss is usually temporary and often regained once the diet ends. The initial weight loss that occurs during fasting is more likely due to the reduction in calories rather than any unique metabolic advantage. Limiting eating to a short window naturally reduces calorie intake, but this is not a sustainable method for long-term weight management.

Moreover, the rapid weight loss associated with fasting can lead to a loss of muscle mass, which can negatively impact overall metabolic health.

Muscle tissue is metabolically active, meaning it burns more calories at rest compared to fat tissue. Losing muscle mass can slow the metabolism, making it more difficult to lose weight over time. Combining any weight loss strategy with resistance training and adequate protein intake is essential to preserve muscle mass and support metabolic health.

For those unfamiliar with their body's hunger signals, it can be challenging to distinguish true hunger from other sensations like thirst, stress, or boredom. Ignoring these signals can lead to negative consequences, such as disrupted energy levels, impaired cognitive function, and a slowed metabolism. This is particularly true when fasting is combined with intense exercise or high mental stress, both of which require a steady supply of glucose for optimal performance.

Claims have been made that fasting improves insulin sensitivity, regulates blood sugar levels, and reduces the risk of type 2 diabetes. But these benefits are frequently due to the cessation of processed sugar intake rather than fasting. Research has shown that reducing the consumption of refined sugars and processed foods can significantly improve metabolic health, independent of fasting. For instance, a study published in *The Lancet Diabetes & Endocrinology* found that individuals who replaced processed sugars with slow-digesting carbohydrates, such as whole grains and legumes, experienced significant improvements in insulin sensitivity and blood sugar control, even without changes in calorie intake.

While intermittent fasting has been linked with improved cardiovascular health, such as lower blood pressure and cholesterol levels, these effects are primarily due to eliminating unhealthy food groups rather than the absence of food. Studies have shown that diets rich in whole foods, including vegetables, fruits, whole grains, and healthy fats, are more effective at improving cardiovascular health than intermittent fasting alone. For example, the Mediterranean diet, which emphasizes the consumption of plant-based foods and healthy fats like olive oil, has been shown to reduce the risk of heart disease and stroke, independent of fasting.

The reduction in oxidative stress and inflammation seen in some fasting studies is often more about cutting out processed foods than the fasting itself. Chronic inflammation and oxidative stress are major factors behind conditions like heart disease, diabetes, and cancer. By steering clear of pro-inflammatory foods such as refined sugars, trans fats, and processed meats, people can significantly lower their levels of oxidative stress and inflammation, leading to better overall health. The shift toward whole, nutrient-rich foods plays a big role in supporting overall well-being by calming the body's inflammatory responses.

Intermittent fasting has also been linked to potential benefits for brain health, like improved cognitive function and protection against neurodegenerative diseases. However, these findings are still in the early stages, and more research is needed to fully understand how fasting affects the brain. It's also important to consider that the mental boost some people feel from fasting might be more about removing unhealthy foods from their diet rather than fasting itself.

Diets high in processed foods and refined sugars have been linked to memory issues and a higher risk of brain-related diseases. By cutting out these harmful foods, people might see an improvement in their mental clarity and overall cognitive function, independent of fasting. This shows that making healthier food choices can have a powerful impact on brain health and help protect against cognitive decline.

The Hype About Fasting

Intermittent fasting requires careful planning to avoid nutrient deficiencies. If the eating window is too narrow, there is a risk of not consuming enough essential nutrients, leading to potential health issues such as anemia, osteoporosis, and immune dysfunction. Nutrient deficiencies can have serious long-term consequences, including impaired cognitive function, weakened immune response, and increased risk of chronic diseases. Rather than cutting calories by eating less frequently, consider the benefits of eating small, balanced meals throughout the day. This approach allows you to meet your body's nutritional needs without feeling deprived or overly hungry.

Fasting can also take a mental toll, leading to an unhealthy fixation on food and a sense of deprivation. Eating should be an opportunity to nourish your body with a wide range of nutrients, not a way to conform to restrictive diets. For individuals with a history of eating disorders or those at risk of developing an unhealthy relationship with food, intermittent fasting can exacerbate these issues. It is crucial to approach fasting with the right mindset, prioritize overall health, and consult a healthcare professional if needed. The psychological impact of restrictive eating patterns should not be underestimated, as it can lead to disordered eating behaviors and a negative relationship with food.

Additionally, certain populations, such as pregnant or breastfeeding women, individuals with medical conditions, or those on specific medications, should avoid fasting or consult a doctor before attempting it. Pregnant women, for instance, require a steady intake of nutrients to support fetal development, and fasting could potentially lead to nutrient deficiencies that harm both the mother and the baby. Similarly, individuals with medical conditions such as diabetes, hypoglycemia, or adrenal insufficiency may experience adverse effects from fasting, including dangerously low blood sugar levels and impaired adrenal function.

EATING LESSONS

For others, fasting may trigger overeating or binge-eating behaviors during the eating window, negating the potential benefits. It's important to approach the eating period with mindfulness and make nutritious food choices that support overall health. Binge-eating during the eating window can lead to overconsumption of calories and weight gain, counteracting the intended effects of fasting. Additionally, consuming large quantities of food quickly can stress the digestive system, leading to discomfort, bloating, and impaired nutrient absorption.

When it comes to digestion or when you're not particularly hungry, consider alternatives like drinking Kombucha or fresh green juices made from fruits and vegetables. Carbohydrates, especially those from whole foods, are essential for maintaining your body's functions. Carbohydrates are the body's primary energy source, and depriving the body of carbs for extended periods can lead to fatigue, impaired cognitive function, and decreased physical performance.

In today's world, juice and smoothie bars have become popular, offering convenient and healthy options. Brands like Blueprint provide home-delivery juice kits, which are available at stores like Whole Foods. While commercial options like V8 are available, they often contain high sodium levels and are pasteurized, reducing their nutritional value. Freshly pressed juices are always a better option, as they retain more nutrients and enzymes that begin to degrade soon after juicing. There are many affordable options for those interested in juicing at home, and macerating juicers are particularly effective at extracting juice with minimal waste.

Learning to distinguish between eating out of boredom and eating in response to actual hunger is a crucial step toward developing a healthier relationship with food. Starting your day with a well-balanced meal, rather than relying on coffee to curb your appetite, sets a positive tone for the rest of the day. Being attuned to your body's hunger signals and eating before you're ravenous can help prevent the irritability, irrational thoughts, and emotional swings that often come with extreme hunger. Eating when you're truly hungry ensures that your body gets the necessary nutrients it needs to function at its best rather than being deprived of vital fuel.

Contrary to outdated beliefs, eating after 8 pm does not automatically lead to weight gain. The body continues to burn calories during sleep, using this time to carry out many of its repair and healing processes. Sleep is essential for tissue repair, memory consolidation, and hormone regulation, and consuming the right nutrients before bed can support these critical functions.

Research shows that late-night eating does not inherently cause weight gain unless it leads to an overall increase in calorie consumption. A balanced, pre-planned meal before bed is acceptable as long as it fits your daily caloric needs. However, it's important to be mindful of alcohol consumption in the evening, as it can quickly increase your calorie intake and negatively affect sleep quality. Alcohol can disrupt sleep by causing fragmented rest and reducing the time spent in deep, restorative sleep. Moreover, alcohol is high in empty calories, which can contribute to weight gain if consumed excessively.

For those interested in enhancing muscle growth and overall health, especially during the night, studies suggest that consuming branched-chain amino acids (BCAAs) before bed can promote muscle growth. BCAAs are essential amino acids that are crucial for muscle protein synthesis, and taking them before sleep can aid in muscle recovery and growth. Since the body undergoes repair during sleep, a nutritious evening meal that includes an extra 400 to 500 calories can support better recovery and overall health. It's important to ensure this evening meal is balanced, including protein, healthy fats, and slow-digesting carbohydrates, to provide sustained energy throughout the night.

EATING LESSONS

If you crave something sweet after dinner, consider healthier alternatives like coconut yogurt. Coconut yogurt is rich in probiotics, which support gut health and can be enhanced with fresh fruits, nuts, and seeds for added nutrients and flavor. Making coconut yogurt at home allows you to control the ingredients, avoiding the added sugars and preservatives often found in store-bought versions. For a more indulgent treat, you can make "nice cream" by blending frozen bananas with other fruits, nut butter, or coconut milk, creating a creamy, dairy-free dessert that satisfies your sweet tooth without traditional ice cream's added sugars and unhealthy fats.

Understanding the difference between eating for nourishment and eating out of habit or boredom is critical to maintaining a healthy relationship with food. Eating in response to hunger, rather than waiting until you're extremely hungry, helps prevent overeating and ensures a steady supply of nutrients throughout the day. Ignoring hunger signals can lead to poor food choices and a cycle of restrictive eating followed by binge eating, disrupting metabolism and negatively impacting overall health.

While intermittent fasting can offer health benefits in supervised medical settings, it is not a universal solution and may not be suitable for everyone. Achieving a healthy diet is more about balance, variety, and consistency than drastic measures or restrictive eating patterns. By focusing on whole, nutrient-dense foods, paying attention to your body's hunger cues, and incorporating regular physical activity and stress management practices, you can support your overall health and well-being without resorting to extreme dieting or fasting.

6
WHAT'S WITH FIBER, THO?

Exploring the mysteries of dietary fiber often seems like a task left for moments of digestive distress. Yet, fiber is more than a remedy for digestional discomfort and a fundamental component of a healthy diet. It acts as the unseen threads that hold food's moisture and flesh together, working silently in the background to unleash vital nutrients as you chew. Fiber can be thought of as nature's packaging, enveloping the essential elements of nourishment. While fruits and vegetables are abundant in fiber, meats such as beef, pork, and poultry are lacking in this crucial component. Fiber is essential for maintaining regular bowel movements and preventing constipation. A diet deficient in fiber slows digestion, depriving stools of bulk and making their passage through the digestive system difficult and uncomfortable.

High-protein diets, particularly those rich in meat, can lead to increased water loss through urine, resulting in dehydration. Dehydration can cause stools to become firm and difficult to pass, which may lead to constipation and toxicity in the bowel. Protein digestion, unlike the digestion of carbohydrates and fats, requires a significant amount of water. Proteins are broken down into their constituent amino acids through hydrolysis reactions, which depend on water and place a considerable burden on the liver.

Fiber is an often-overlooked component of a healthy diet, yet its role in our well-being is indispensable. Found primarily in plant-based foods such as vegetables, fruits, legumes, and whole grains, fiber offers a multitude of benefits that extend beyond simple digestion. It is the structural framework of plants, the part that gives them shape and resilience. When we consume fiber, we take in this structure, which acts as a broom, sweeping through our digestive tract to maintain cleanliness and order.

The digestive system relies on fiber to function smoothly. Soluble fiber, which dissolves in water, forms a gel-like substance in the stomach. This gel slows down digestion, allowing for a more gradual absorption of nutrients and helping regulate blood sugar levels. For example, oats, apples, and beans are rich in soluble fiber, which can bind to cholesterol and reduce its absorption into the bloodstream. This action can lower the levels of LDL cholesterol, often referred to as "bad" cholesterol, reducing the risk of heart disease. Studies have shown that diets high in soluble fiber can lead to a significant decrease in LDL cholesterol, helping to prevent cardiovascular issues.

Insoluble fiber, on the other hand, does not dissolve in water. It adds bulk to the stool and aids in moving waste through the intestines. This is crucial for preventing constipation and promoting regular bowel movements. Vegetables like broccoli, whole grains like wheat, and the skins of fruits like apples and pears are excellent sources of insoluble fiber. By providing bulk, insoluble fiber helps food pass more quickly through the stomach and intestines, preventing the kind of slow movement that can lead to constipation and other digestive issues.

Both types of fiber play a significant role in maintaining a healthy gut. They serve as prebiotics, which are food for the beneficial bacteria in our intestines. When these bacteria digest fiber, they produce short-chain fatty acids like butyrate, which nourish the cells lining the colon and help reduce inflammation. These fatty acids can also improve the barrier function of the gut, preventing toxic substances from entering the bloodstream and causing systemic inflammation.

What's With Fiber, Tho?

Research has shown that a healthy gut microbiome, supported by a high-fiber diet, can lower the risk of inflammatory diseases and improve immune function.

The fermentation of fiber by gut bacteria not only produces beneficial short-chain fatty acids but also lowers the pH of the colon. A lower pH creates an environment that discourages the growth of harmful bacteria, thus protecting against infections and promoting overall gut health. Studies indicate that individuals with a high intake of dietary fiber have a more diverse gut microbiota, which is associated with better health outcomes. A diverse microbiome is more resilient to disruptions and more capable of withstanding challenges, such as those posed by antibiotics or a poor diet.

Fiber also plays a crucial role in regulating appetite and weight management. High-fiber foods tend to be more filling than low-fiber foods, which can help control hunger and reduce overall calorie intake. This is partly due to the fact that fiber slows the rate of digestion, which means that food remains in the stomach longer, promoting a sense of fullness. The gel-like substance formed by soluble fiber can also delay the emptying of the stomach, which further enhances satiety. By making us feel full longer, fiber can help prevent overeating and assist in maintaining a healthy weight.

In addition to promoting fullness, fiber-rich foods are often lower in calories. Vegetables, fruits, and whole grains are nutrient-dense but not energy-dense, meaning they provide essential vitamins and minerals without a high-calorie count. This makes them an ideal choice for those looking to manage their weight without sacrificing nutrition. The bulk provided by fiber also means that these foods take up more space in the stomach, leading to a natural reduction in food intake and a lower overall caloric consumption.

A high-fiber diet is also associated with a reduced risk of type 2 diabetes. The ability of fiber to regulate blood sugar levels is a key factor in this protective effect. By slowing the absorption of sugar into the bloodstream, fiber helps prevent the sharp spikes in blood glucose levels that can lead to insulin resistance, a precursor to type 2 diabetes. Research has shown that individuals who consume a diet high in fiber have a significantly lower risk of developing type 2 diabetes compared to those with low fiber intake.

The benefits of fiber extend to colon health as well. A high intake of dietary fiber is linked to a lower risk of developing colorectal cancer. Fiber helps to increase stool bulk and speed up the movement of waste through the intestines, which reduces the time that harmful substances are in contact with the colon lining. Furthermore, the short-chain fatty acids produced by the fermentation of fiber have been shown to have protective effects against cancer. Butyrate, in particular, has been found to inhibit the growth of cancer cells and promote the normal function of colon cells.

Fiber is also crucial for detoxification. By binding to toxins, waste, and excess hormones like estrogen, fiber helps remove these substances from the body. This detoxifying effect is particularly important for liver health, as the liver relies on the gut to excrete toxins. When fiber intake is low, the liver must work harder to process and eliminate toxins, which can lead to liver strain and a buildup of harmful substances. A diet rich in fiber can support the liver's natural detoxification processes and promote overall health.

Including a variety of fiber-rich foods in the diet ensures that the body receives all the different types of fiber, each with its unique benefits. Leafy greens, such as spinach and kale, are high in insoluble fiber, which helps maintain regular bowel movements. Fruits like apples and pears provide both soluble and insoluble fiber, making them excellent for overall digestive health. Legumes, including beans, lentils, and chickpeas, are among the best sources of soluble fiber, which can help regulate blood sugar and cholesterol levels.

What's With Fiber, Tho?

Whole grains, such as oats, brown rice, and quinoa, offer a balanced mix of soluble and insoluble fiber. These grains are also rich in essential nutrients like magnesium, zinc, and B vitamins, which support overall health and well-being. Nuts and seeds, including almonds, chia seeds, and flaxseeds, provide fiber along with healthy fats, making them a satisfying and nutritious addition to any diet.

Incorporating fiber-rich foods into the diet can be simple and enjoyable. Start the day with a bowl of oatmeal topped with fresh berries and nuts for a hearty, fiber-packed breakfast. Include a variety of colorful vegetables in meals, such as a salad with leafy greens, carrots, and bell peppers. Snack on fruits like apples, pears, or oranges, which provide natural sweetness along with fiber. Add legumes like lentils or black beans to soups, stews, and salads for a protein and fiber boost. Choose whole grain options, such as whole wheat bread, brown rice, or quinoa, over refined grains to increase fiber intake.

Transitioning to a high-fiber diet should be done gradually to allow the digestive system to adjust. Sudden increases in fiber intake can lead to bloating, gas, and discomfort. Drinking plenty of water is also important, as fiber absorbs water and needs adequate hydration to function effectively. Start by adding one or two high-fiber foods to your daily diet and gradually increase your intake over time. This approach will help your digestive system adapt and maximize the benefits of fiber.

Fiber is not just a dietary component; it is a cornerstone of health. From regulating digestion and supporting a healthy gut to protecting against chronic diseases and aiding in weight management, fiber plays a multifaceted role in promoting well-being. Embracing a diet rich in fiber from plant-based foods is a powerful way to support long-term health. By understanding the importance of fiber and incorporating a variety of fiber-rich foods into our diets, we can take significant steps toward a healthier, more balanced life.

The liver, often regarded as the body's detox powerhouse, processes everything we consume, neutralizing harmful substances and managing nutrient conversion. The liver not only processes amino acids but also transforms them into various substances necessary for bodily functions. Despite the liver's versatility, this process can be demanding.

Picture the liver as a tireless worker, constantly filtering and converting nutrients. A diet high in protein inundates this worker with an influx of materials that need to be broken down for digestion and utilization. To process proteins, the liver must remove nitrogen from amino acids in a step called deamination, which is crucial because free nitrogen is toxic. This nitrogen is then converted into urea, which the kidneys excrete.

The deamination of protein is an energy-intensive process, increasing the liver's workload. Over time, this persistent activity can lead to liver fatigue, much like an overworked employee struggling to maintain efficiency. A liver under continuous strain may become less effective at processing nutrients and detoxifying the body. As the digestive system works to break down food, water is absorbed from the gastrointestinal tract to help with nutrient absorption and overall digestion.

The higher protein content in meat affects water absorption, leading to firmer stools and a greater need for water to soften them. Meat can also act as a diuretic, further increasing water loss through urine, which may lead to dehydration, especially if there is inadequate water intake or a lack of fiber-rich vegetables in the diet.

A diet heavy in meat but low in fiber can disrupt the balance of the gut microbiome. The absence of dietary fiber means that beneficial gut bacteria lack essential nutrients, which can lead to an imbalance in gut flora and negatively impact digestive health. One of fiber's most significant benefits is its ability to regulate the digestion

What's With Fiber, Tho?

and absorption of nutrients, including proteins. Consuming fiber-rich plant foods such as beans, lentils, quinoa, and leafy greens slows the digestive process. This gradual digestion allows for a more controlled release of amino acids into the bloodstream, ensuring the liver receives a steady and manageable flow of nutrients instead of a sudden surge.

This controlled release helps reduce the liver's workload by preventing spikes in amino acid levels. By doing so, fiber enables the liver to perform deamination more efficiently, converting nitrogen into urea without becoming overburdened. The amino acid profiles of plant-based proteins offer additional advantages. While individual plant proteins may not always contain all the essential amino acids, combining different sources throughout the day can provide a complete protein profile. More importantly, plant proteins typically contain lower levels of methionine and other amino acids that, in excess, can increase the liver's workload.

Plant-based diets are naturally lower in saturated fats and cholesterol compared to animal-based diets. This reduction in harmful fats significantly lowers the risk of developing fatty liver disease, a condition where fat accumulates in the liver and impairs its function. Instead, plant-based diets are rich in unsaturated fats, which support liver health and promote overall cardiovascular wellness.

Excessive protein intake can also lead to an accumulation of ammonia, a byproduct of protein metabolism. Although the liver usually converts ammonia into urea efficiently, excessive protein can overwhelm this process, leading to a toxic buildup. This doesn't mean that protein should be avoided altogether. Proteins are essential, and understanding the demands they place on the liver can help guide dietary choices that support liver health. Incorporating a variety of protein sources, ensuring adequate hydration to assist the kidneys in flushing out urea, and pairing proteins with liver-friendly foods such as leafy greens, fruits, and vegetables can help manage the waste that results from meat breakdown.

The stomach produces hydrochloric acid and other digestive juices to aid in breaking down proteins, and these fluids are water-based. The production of these digestive fluids contributes to the body's overall water requirement during digestion. Meat is generally more challenging to digest than plant-based foods, taking longer to break down in the digestive system and potentially slowing overall digestion and bowel movements. Fiber is vital for a few reasons. The world of plant-based proteins is vast and varied, offering everything from beans and lentils to tofu and quinoa. These plant powerhouses are celebrated for their health benefits, as they are rich in fiber, vitamins, and minerals. But does the type of protein matter for liver health? It certainly does.

Plant-based proteins often come with fiber, antioxidants, and phytonutrients. Fiber plays a significant role in alleviating the liver's burden by aiding digestion, promoting gut health, and regulating the release of nutrients into the bloodstream. This gradual release helps maintain a balanced and less taxing influx of amino acids for the liver to process. Plant-based proteins differ from animal proteins in their amino acid profiles. Although plant proteins may not always offer complete amino acid profiles on their own, they often contain lower levels of methionine, an amino acid that, in excess, can increase the liver's workload. Combining different plant proteins throughout the day can provide all essential amino acids without overwhelming any single type.

There are other concerns with animal proteins, including the presence of saturated fats and cholesterol. Animal-based diets are often higher in these substances, which can contribute to fatty liver disease over time. Plant-based diets, rich in unsaturated fats and free from cholesterol, tend to be more liver-friendly and reduce the risk of fat accumulation in the liver. Incorporating a range of high-protein plant foods, such as lentils, chickpeas, tofu, quinoa, and nuts, can ensure a diverse nutrient intake and support liver health.

Fiber comes in various forms within plant-based foods, with the most commonly discussed being soluble and insoluble fiber. Beyond these, there are other types of fiber that play essential roles in health. Cellulose is the most abundant type of fiber found in plant cell walls, providing structure to plants. It is commonly found in vegetables, whole grains, and fruits. Hemicellulose, another major component of plant cell walls, is present in varying amounts in different plant foods and contributes to the overall fiber content of foods like whole grains, legumes, and some vegetables.

Pectin is a type of fiber found in fruits, particularly in the skins, and is responsible for the gel-like texture seen in jams and jellies. Apples, citrus fruits, and berries are rich sources of pectin. Beta-glucans, another type of fiber, are predominantly found in oats and barley. These fibers have been shown to have cholesterol-lowering properties and can help regulate blood sugar levels. Inulin is a soluble fiber that acts as a prebiotic, providing nourishment for beneficial gut bacteria. It is found in foods such as chicory root, Jerusalem artichokes, and onions.

Resistant starches resist digestion in the small intestine and, therefore, have a slower and more limited impact on blood sugar levels. Unlike other starches, they do not rapidly break down into glucose. Instead, they pass through to the large intestine, where they are fermented by gut bacteria. This fermentation process produces short-chain fatty acids, which offer various health benefits. Resistant starches are present in foods like plantains but can also be created by cooling and reheating certain starches. This process reduces the number of absorbable carbohydrates by turning them into resistant starches, which beneficial gut bacteria can then use as food.

Resistant starch can be created in grains or potatoes through cooking and cooling processes. Especially at the start of a new eating regimen, it can be helpful to change cooking methods to create these resistant starches. This will immediately affect gut health and help stabilize blood sugar levels. The fermentation process of resistant starch produces short-chain fatty acids and other byproducts, which affect blood sugar levels in several ways. Resistant starches release glucose more slowly into the bloodstream, resulting in a lower glycemic response compared to quickly digested carbohydrates. This helps stabilize blood sugar levels and provides sustained energy.

Including resistant starches in a meal can lower the overall glycemic load of that meal. Glycemic load considers both the glycemic index and the portion size of a food. Including resistant starches with other carbohydrates can reduce the overall glycemic load and potentially prevent blood sugar spikes. Resistant starches may also positively impact insulin sensitivity, the body's ability to respond to insulin and regulate blood sugar. By promoting beneficial changes in the gut microbiota and producing short-chain fatty acids, resistant starches can enhance insulin sensitivity and improve glucose metabolism.

The impact on the glycemic index can vary depending on the type and amount of resistant starch consumed, as well as individual factors such as metabolic health and the overall composition of the meal. Including a variety of whole foods rich in resistant starches, such as cooked and cooled potatoes, legumes, and whole grains, as part of a balanced diet can contribute to a lower glycemic response and help with blood sugar control.

There are common methods for creating resistant starches. One method is the cooking and cooling method. For grains like rice or pasta, cook the grains as usual and let them cool down to room temperature. Once cooled, the starch structure changes, and some starch becomes resistant to digestion. The cooled grains can be consumed as

What's With Fiber, Tho?

they are or reheated before consumption. For potatoes, cook them by boiling, steaming, or baking until fully cooked, then allow them to cool completely, either at room temperature or in the refrigerator. Cooling the potatoes forms resistant starch. The cooled potatoes can be eaten as they are or reheated before eating.

Coconut oil does play a role in increasing the resistant starch content of rice, in conjunction with the cooling and reheating process. Research has shown that adding a small amount of coconut oil to rice during cooking can enhance the formation of resistant starch, making it more beneficial for health.

When rice is cooked with coconut oil, the oil interacts with the starch molecules. During the cooking process, the starch granules absorb water and swell, a phenomenon known as gelatinization. The addition of coconut oil during this stage alters how these starch molecules reorganize during cooling. The oil creates a barrier, which makes it harder for digestive enzymes to break down the starch into glucose. This interaction is crucial because it sets the stage for the formation of resistant starch.

Once the rice is cooked with coconut oil, allowing it to cool completely and then refrigerating it for at least 12 hours promotes the formation of resistant starch. During the cooling phase, the starch molecules realign and form a crystalline structure that resists digestion. This type of starch is known as retrograded starch, and it remains even after the rice is reheated. Resistant starch, thus formed, is not digested in the small intestine. Instead, it reaches the large intestine, where it acts as a prebiotic, providing nourishment for beneficial gut bacteria. When gut bacteria ferment resistant starch, they produce short-chain fatty acids such as butyrate, which are associated with improved gut health, reduced inflammation, and better insulin sensitivity.

Studies have found that adding about a teaspoon of coconut

oil per half-cup of uncooked rice can significantly increase the formation of resistant starch. Research conducted in Sri Lanka demonstrated that rice cooked with coconut oil and then cooled for 12 hours before being reheated had 10-15% less digestible starch compared to rice prepared in the traditional way. This reduction in digestible starch means there is a corresponding increase in resistant starch, which can help reduce glycemic response and support metabolic health.

To take advantage of this process, one can add a teaspoon of coconut oil to boiling water for every half-cup of uncooked rice. After cooking the rice, it should be allowed to cool at room temperature and then refrigerated for at least 12 hours. Before eating, the rice can be reheated with the resistant starch remaining intact.

Using coconut oil in this way, combined with cooling and reheating, offers a practical method to increase resistant starch intake. This simple adjustment in cooking can lead to significant health benefits, including improved blood sugar control and enhanced gut health. By integrating coconut oil and this cooking method into daily dietary practices, it becomes possible to optimize the nutritional benefits of rice and promote better digestive and metabolic health.

The cooling and reheating processes alter the starch structure, converting some digestible starch into resistant starch. This resistant starch behaves differently in the digestive system compared to regular starch. It resists enzymatic digestion in the small intestine, meaning it reaches the large intestine intact, where it serves as a substrate for beneficial gut bacteria, promoting their growth and producing beneficial compounds like short-chain fatty acids. The amount of resistant starch formed and the specific effects on digestion can vary based on factors such as the type of starch, cooking methods, cooling duration, and individual differences in gut microbiota.

The retrogradation method, which involves cooling and then

reheating certain starchy foods, has been shown to increase the amount of resistant starch in foods like rice and bread. To create resistant starch using this method with rice, one would cook the rice as usual, allow it to cool completely, and then refrigerate it for at least 12 hours. After this cooling period, reheating the rice will enhance its resistant starch content. The same principle applies to bread: after baking, the bread should be allowed to cool completely, refrigerated for a minimum of 12 hours, and then reheated before consumption.

The transformation of regular starch into resistant starch during this process is due to the changes in the starch molecules as they cool. When starchy foods are heated, their starch molecules gelatinize, absorbing water and becoming more digestible. Upon cooling, these gelatinized starches can undergo a process called retrogradeation, where the starch molecules realign into a crystalline structure that resists digestion. This resistant starch does not break down in the small intestine but instead reaches the large intestine, where it serves as a substrate for beneficial gut bacteria. These bacteria ferment the resistant starch, producing short-chain fatty acids such as butyrate, which have been associated with various health benefits, including improved gut health, enhanced insulin sensitivity, and reduced inflammation.

While the type of fat used in bread can influence the texture and flavor, it is not a critical factor in the formation of resistant starch through the retrogradation process. Studies have shown that the key factors influencing the formation of resistant starch are the type of starch present in the food, the cooking method, and the cooling duration. Coconut oil or other fats do not significantly impact the creation of resistant starch; it is primarily the cooling and reheating process that matters.

However, the fat content can affect the overall digestion of the food and the glycemic response. Fats can slow down the digestion and absorption of carbohydrates, potentially leading to a more gradual release of glucose into the bloodstream. This can complement the effects of resistant starch, further stabilizing blood sugar levels.

It is important to note that not all bread will automatically become a significant source of resistant starch just by cooling and reheating. The amount of resistant starch formed can vary depending on the type of flour used and the specific ingredients in the bread. Whole grain or whole wheat bread, which contains higher levels of fiber and complex carbohydrates, may develop more resistant starch compared to white bread.

Additionally, the overall structure and water content of the bread can influence the degree of starch retrogradation. Research indicates that the cooling and reheating process itself is sufficient to enhance the resistant starch content in starchy foods like rice and bread. The presence of fat, such as coconut oil, is not necessary for this transformation, although it can play a role in modifying the digestion and absorption of these foods. To maximize the benefits of resistant starch, focusing on the cooling and reheating process is key, regardless of the type of fat used in preparation.

Lignin is another complex, non-carbohydrate fiber found in plant cell walls, present in high amounts in foods like whole grains, seeds, and vegetables. Different plant-based foods contain varying combinations and amounts of fiber types, and consuming a variety of fiber-rich foods ensures a diverse intake of these fibers, each offering distinct health benefits. Fiber acts as a buffer between the absorption of sugars into the bloodstream, essentially keeping everyone in line when nutrients are being absorbed.

Fiber plays a crucial role in removing toxins from the colon and feeding the microbiome, and it also helps create a feeling of fullness. Without fiber, it becomes easier to overeat because calories can be consumed in greater amounts, and they are quickly absorbed into

What's With Fiber, Tho?

the bloodstream, leaving the stomach empty and potentially causing feelings of hunger. When presented with high-calorie foods, it is best to fill the plate with three-quarters fiber-rich options like salad and roughage to balance the other foods being consumed.

Soluble fiber dissolves in water, forming a gel-like substance in the digestive tract, and is easily broken down by beneficial gut bacteria. Common sources of soluble fiber include oats, legumes like beans, lentils, and chickpeas, fruits such as apples, oranges, and berries, vegetables like carrots, broccoli, and Brussels sprouts, as well as chia seeds and flaxseeds. Soluble fiber provides multiple health benefits. It helps lower blood cholesterol levels by reducing the absorption of cholesterol from food, regulates blood sugar levels by slowing the digestion and absorption of carbohydrates, which can benefit individuals with diabetes, and promotes a healthy gut by serving as fuel for beneficial gut bacteria.

Insoluble fiber does not dissolve in water and passes through the digestive system largely intact, adding bulk to the stool and aiding in regular bowel movements, preventing constipation. Common sources of insoluble fiber include whole grains such as wheat, barley, and brown rice, nuts and seeds, vegetables like celery, cucumbers, and green beans, fruit skins, and seed shells. Insoluble fiber supports digestive health by providing roughage and helping to prevent or alleviate constipation. It also contributes to a sense of fullness, aiding in weight management by reducing excessive food intake.

Both soluble and insoluble fibers are important components of a healthy diet, and many plant-based foods contain a mix of both. To gain the benefits of both types, it is essential to consume a variety of fiber-rich foods. The recommended daily intake of fiber for adults is around 25 to 38 grams, though individual needs may vary. Prebiotic fiber serves as food for beneficial gut bacteria, supporting a healthy gut microbiome. Including prebiotic-rich foods in the diet can help maintain a balanced gut microbiome and improve overall digestive health.

Chicory root is one of the richest sources of inulin, a type of prebiotic fiber, and can be consumed as a supplement or added to foods and beverages. Garlic is not only a flavorful culinary ingredient but also a source of prebiotic fiber, specifically fructooligosaccharides (FOS). Onions contain fructooligosaccharides (FOS) and inulin, making them excellent prebiotic foods, while leeks, related to onions and garlic, also contain these prebiotics. Asparagus is rich in inulin and can be enjoyed in various ways, such as grilled, roasted, or steamed. Jerusalem artichokes, also known as sunchokes, are particularly high in inulin, making them a potent prebiotic source.

Bananas, especially unripe (green) ones, contain resistant starch, which acts as a prebiotic, supporting beneficial gut bacteria. Apples, particularly the skin, contain pectin, a type of prebiotic fiber. Dandelion greens are nutrient-rich leafy greens that provide prebiotic benefits. Barley is a whole grain that contains beta-glucans, a type of prebiotic fiber, and oats are also a good source of beta-glucans with prebiotic properties. Flaxseeds contain soluble fiber, including mucilage, which acts as a prebiotic in the gut. Certain types of seaweed, such as kelp and dulse, contain prebiotic fibers beneficial for gut health. Legumes, including beans, lentils, and peas, are rich in various types of prebiotic fibers, such as galactooligosaccharides (GOS) and resistant starch.

These foods help create a healthy gut by supporting good bacteria, which are important for digestion, immune function, and overall well-being. Including a mix of fiber-rich and prebiotic foods in your diet can keep digestion running smoothly, improve how your body absorbs nutrients, and keep your gut bacteria balanced. By understanding how important fiber is and what it does in our bodies, we can make better food choices that promote long-term health and vitality.

7
THROWING SHADE AT CARBS

"Carbs" have become a buzzword in the world of weight loss, with the media often portraying them as the enemy of a slimmer figure. This portrayal has led many to believe that cutting out carbohydrates altogether is the key to shedding pounds. Yet, carbohydrates are crucial nutrients that provide our bodies with energy, fuel brain function, and support overall health. They are the body's primary fuel source, playing an essential role in both physical performance and cognitive function.

The truth is that not all carbohydrates are created equal, and labeling them all as "bad" fails to recognize the important distinctions among them. The problem lies in how they're categorized. Simple carbohydrates, often found in sugary snacks, sodas, and processed foods, can lead to rapid spikes in blood sugar levels, resulting in weight gain and energy crashes. These simple carbs are digested quickly, causing a surge of glucose into the bloodstream, which triggers a rapid insulin response. This can lead to a cycle of spikes and crashes that leave us feeling tired and hungry soon after eating.

On the other hand, complex carbohydrates from whole foods like oats, sweet potatoes, lentils, and leafy greens are entirely different. These complex carbs are rich in essential nutrients and dietary fiber, which help regulate blood sugar levels, support digestion, and provide sustained energy throughout the day. The fiber content in these foods slows down the digestion and absorption of carbohydrates, leading to a more gradual release of glucose into the bloodstream. This not only helps prevent blood sugar spikes but also promotes a feeling of fullness, reducing the likelihood of overeating.

Carbohydrates have become a controversial topic in the world of nutrition, especially in the context of weight loss. They are often seen as the enemy, with many people believing that cutting out carbohydrates altogether is the key to shedding pounds. This perception has been fueled by various diets and media portrayals that label carbs as the primary culprit behind weight gain. Yet, carbohydrates are essential nutrients that provide our bodies with energy, fuel brain function, and support overall health. They are the body's primary fuel source, crucial in both physical performance and cognitive function.

To truly understand carbohydrates, it is essential to distinguish between different types and how they impact the body. Not all carbohydrates should be labeled as "bad" or harmful, as this fails to recognize the important distinctions among them. The real issue lies in how they are categorized and consumed. Simple carbohydrates, often found in sugary snacks, sodas, and processed foods, can lead to rapid spikes in blood sugar levels and contribute to weight gain and energy crashes.

On the other hand, complex carbohydrates from whole foods, like oats, sweet potatoes, lentils, and leafy greens, are entirely different. These complex carbs are rich in essential nutrients and dietary fiber, which help regulate blood sugar levels, support digestion, and provide sustained energy throughout the day.

By shunning all carbohydrates due to misconceptions, individuals may miss out on these vital, nutrient-rich foods, which are essential for a balanced diet. Understanding the difference between refined and whole-food carbohydrates can help people make smarter dietary choices that support both weight management and overall health. Embracing healthy carbs allows us to maintain our energy levels, support our body's needs, and achieve long-term wellness.

The glycemic index sheds light on this complexity, acting as a scientific tool akin to the "Scoville scale" for assessing how different carbohydrates impact blood sugar levels. When we consume carbs, they break down into glucose, our primary energy source. This glucose enters the bloodstream, either fueling immediate energy needs or being stored as glycogen in the liver and muscles. But when glycogen stores are full, any excess glucose undergoes de novo lipogenesis (DNL), converting into fat. It isn't carbs themselves but how carbs from processed sources affect our metabolism.

Opting for whole, nutrient-rich carbohydrate sources allows us to meet our energy needs without promoting excessive fat storage. It's about understanding the nuances and making informed choices about the types of carbs we consume to support optimal health. Rather than fearing carbohydrates, the focus should be on choosing those that offer more than just empty calories—carbs that nourish, sustain, and keep us moving forward with energy and vitality.

Carbohydrates are found in a wide variety of foods, from fruits and vegetables to grains and legumes. They come in three main types: sugars, starches, and fiber. Simple carbohydrates, or sugars, are quickly absorbed by the body, leading to rapid spikes in blood sugar levels. These are often found in processed foods like candies, pastries, and sodas. Complex carbohydrates, which include starches and fiber, are digested more slowly, providing a steady release of energy. These are found in whole grains, vegetables, and legumes.

The Glycemic Index (GI) is a measure that ranks foods based on how quickly they raise blood sugar levels. Foods with a high GI cause rapid spikes in blood sugar, while those with a low GI result in a slower, more gradual increase. Whole foods tend to have a lower

GI compared to processed foods, which can have a beneficial impact on overall health, particularly for managing weight and blood sugar levels.

Bread is a staple in many diets around the world, but not all bread is created equal. The difference between whole grain and white bread is significant when it comes to nutritional content and health effects. Whole grain bread is made from whole wheat grains that include the bran, germ, and endosperm.

The bran is the outer layer, which contains fiber, B vitamins, and minerals. The germ is the nutrient-rich core, packed with essential fatty acids, vitamin E, and B vitamins. The endosperm, the starchy middle layer, provides carbohydrates and some protein. Whole grain bread is rich in dietary fiber, which aids in digestion, helps regulate blood sugar levels, and keeps you feeling full longer. The presence of fiber also means a lower glycemic index, which prevents rapid blood sugar spikes.

In contrast, white bread is made from refined flour, which has been stripped of the bran and germ. This processing removes most of the fiber, vitamins, and minerals, leaving primarily the starchy endosperm. As a result, white bread has a higher glycemic index, causing quicker spikes in blood sugar levels. The lack of fiber also means that white bread is less filling, which can lead to overeating and subsequent weight gain.

Numerous studies have shown that diets high in whole grains are associated with a lower risk of heart disease, diabetes, and certain cancers. By choosing whole-grain bread over white, you are opting for a more nutrient-dense food that provides sustained energy and supports overall health. Whole grain bread not only keeps you fuller for longer periods but also helps maintain steady blood sugar levels, reducing the likelihood of cravings and energy crashes. The fiber content in whole-grain bread aids in digestion and promotes a healthy gut microbiome, which is crucial for overall health.

Potatoes are another common carbohydrate source that has been demonized, particularly in the context of weight loss. However, the way potatoes are prepared and consumed can significantly impact their health effects. Whole potatoes are a natural source of carbohydrates, rich in vitamins, minerals, and fiber, especially when the skin is left on. They are high in vitamin C, potassium, and vitamin B6, which support immune function, heart health, and brain development. Potatoes also contain resistant starch, a type of carbohydrate that acts like fiber. Resistant starch is not fully digested in the small intestine, reaching the colon where it feeds beneficial gut bacteria. This can improve gut health, increase feelings of fullness, and reduce blood sugar spikes.

Much of their nutritional value is lost when potatoes are processed into products like French fries, potato chips, or instant mashed potatoes. These products are often high in unhealthy fats, salt, and added sugars, making them calorie-dense and nutrient-poor. The processing also breaks down the resistant starch, removing the gut health benefits.

Additionally, processed potato products have a higher glycemic index, leading to rapid blood sugar spikes and crashes, which can increase hunger and lead to overeating. Opting for whole potatoes, especially those that are baked or boiled with the skin on, provides a nutritious, satisfying, and versatile food that fits well into a balanced diet. Whole potatoes are filling and provide a steady source of energy, making them an excellent choice for those looking to maintain a healthy weight and support overall health.

Rice is a dietary staple for much of the world's population and comes in various types, with brown and white rice being the most common. The difference between these two types lies in their processing and nutritional content. Brown rice is a whole grain, meaning it contains all parts of the grain—the bran, germ, and endosperm. It is rich in fiber, vitamins, and minerals, including magnesium, phosphorus, and B vitamins. Brown rice has a lower glycemic index compared to white rice, meaning it has a slower, less pronounced effect on blood sugar levels. The fiber content in brown rice aids digestion, helps maintain a healthy weight, and supports heart health.

White rice, like white bread, is refined, meaning the bran and germ are removed, leaving just the starchy endosperm. This process removes much of the fiber and nutrients, resulting in food that is less filling and higher on the glycemic index. White rice can cause rapid spikes in blood sugar levels, which is not ideal for those managing diabetes or trying to maintain a healthy weight.

While white rice is often enriched with vitamins and minerals, these added nutrients do not provide the same health benefits as those naturally present in whole grains. By choosing brown rice over white, you can increase your intake of fiber and essential nutrients, supporting better blood sugar control and overall health. Brown rice provides a steady source of energy and helps keep you feeling full, reducing the likelihood of overeating and supporting weight management.

Fruits are a natural source of carbohydrates, containing a mix of simple sugars (fructose) and dietary fiber. The fiber content in fruits slows down the digestion and absorption of sugars, preventing rapid spikes in blood sugar levels and providing a steady source of energy. In addition to fiber, fruits are packed with vitamins, minerals, antioxidants, and phytochemicals that offer a range of health benefits.

Eating whole fruits provides all the benefits of fiber and nutrients. The natural sugars in fruit are balanced by the fiber, which helps regulate the release of sugar into the bloodstream. This makes whole fruits a much healthier choice compared to fruit juices or dried fruits, which often lack fiber and have higher concentrations of sugar. Whole fruits such as apples, berries, oranges, and bananas provide important nutrients like vitamin C, potassium, and folate, which support immune function, heart health, and cell growth.

Processed fruit products, such as fruit juices, fruit snacks, and canned fruits with added sugars, often lose much of their fiber and nutritional value. These products can be high in added sugars, which contribute to rapid spikes in blood sugar levels and can lead to weight gain, insulin resistance, and other health issues. Even "100% fruit juice" can contain a high amount of natural sugars without the beneficial fiber to moderate its effects. Opting for whole fruits instead of processed fruit products ensures you are getting the full spectrum of nutrients and health benefits that fruits have to offer. Whole fruits are not only satisfying and delicious but also provide a range of health benefits that support overall well-being.

The key difference between whole foods and processed grains lies in their nutritional content and how they affect the body. Whole foods retain their natural fiber, vitamins, minerals, and other nutrients, making them more filling, nutrient-dense, and beneficial for health. The fiber in whole foods slows down digestion and absorption, helping to regulate blood sugar levels and keep you feeling full longer. This can prevent overeating and support weight management.

Processed grains, on the other hand, often have the bran and germ removed, leaving mainly the starchy endosperm. This refining process strips away much of the fiber, vitamins, and minerals, resulting in a food that is less satisfying and more likely to cause rapid spikes in blood sugar levels. Processed grains are also often enriched with synthetic vitamins and minerals to replace some of the nutrients lost during processing. Still, these added nutrients do not offer the same health benefits as those naturally present in whole grains.

Whole foods also provide a range of phytochemicals, compounds found in plants that have been shown to have various health benefits. These include antioxidants, which protect the body from damage caused by free radicals, and anti-inflammatory compounds, which can help reduce the risk of chronic diseases such as heart disease, cancer, and diabetes. In contrast, processed grains often contain added sugars, unhealthy fats, and preservatives, contributing to weight gain, inflammation, and other health problems. The lack of fiber and other nutrients in processed grains can also lead to overeating, as these foods are less filling and satisfying than whole foods.

One of the key components that sets whole foods apart from processed grains is fiber. Fiber is a type of carbohydrate that the body cannot digest, meaning it passes through the digestive system largely intact. There are two main types of fiber: soluble and insoluble. Soluble fiber dissolves in water and forms a gel-like substance in the digestive tract, which can help lower blood cholesterol levels and regulate blood sugar levels. Insoluble fiber does not dissolve in water and adds bulk to the stool, helping to prevent constipation and promote regular bowel movements.

Fiber plays a crucial role in maintaining a healthy digestive system and supporting overall health. It helps to regulate blood sugar levels by slowing down the absorption of sugars into the bloodstream, preventing rapid spikes and crashes in blood sugar levels. This can help reduce the risk of developing insulin resistance and type 2 diabetes. Fiber also promotes feelings of fullness and satisfaction, which can help prevent overeating and support weight management.

By choosing whole foods rich in fiber, such as whole grains, fruits, vegetables, and legumes, you can improve your digestive health, regulate blood sugar levels, and support overall well-being. These foods provide a wide range of nutrients that are essential for maintaining good health, including vitamins, minerals, antioxidants, and phytochemicals. In addition to their nutritional benefits, whole foods are often more satisfying and flavorful than processed foods, making them a more enjoyable, sustainable choice for long-term health.

Throwing Shade at Carbs

Carbohydrates are a vital part of a healthy diet, providing the energy and nutrients our bodies need to function optimally. While processed carbohydrates, such as refined grains and sugary snacks, can contribute to weight gain and other health problems, whole-food sources of carbohydrates offer a wealth of benefits.

By understanding the differences between whole and processed carbohydrates, we can make informed dietary choices that support our health and well-being. Embracing whole foods, rich in fiber and nutrients, allows us to enjoy the benefits of carbohydrates while avoiding the pitfalls of processed foods. By focusing on the quality of the carbohydrates we consume, we can achieve a balanced and healthy diet that supports our body's needs and promotes long-term wellness.

As we navigate the complex world of carbohydrates, it is important to remember that not all carbs are created equal. Whole foods, such as whole-grain bread, potatoes, brown rice, and fruits, offer a range of health benefits that processed grains cannot match. These foods provide essential nutrients, support digestive health, and help regulate blood sugar levels, making them an important part of a balanced diet. By choosing whole foods over processed grains, we can enjoy the energy and nourishment that carbohydrates provide while supporting our overall health and well-being.

By focusing on the quality of carbohydrates, we can better harness their benefits for overall health and well-being. Shunning all carbohydrates due to misconceptions may lead individuals to miss out on these vital, nutrient-rich foods, which are essential for a balanced diet. Understanding the difference between refined and whole-food carbohydrates can help people make smarter dietary choices that support both weight management and overall health. Embracing healthy carbs allows us to maintain our energy levels, support our body's needs, and achieve long-term wellness.

EATING LESSONS

The glycemic index sheds light on this complexity, acting as a scientific tool akin to the "Scoville scale" for assessing how different carbohydrates impact blood sugar levels. When we consume carbs, they break down into glucose, our primary energy source. This glucose enters the bloodstream, either fueling immediate energy needs or being stored as glycogen in the liver and muscles. But when glycogen stores are full, any excess glucose undergoes de novo lipogenesis (DNL), converting into fat. This process highlights that it isn't carbs themselves that are problematic but how carbs from processed sources affect our metabolism.

Opting for whole, nutrient-rich carbohydrate sources allows us to meet our energy needs without promoting excessive fat storage. It's about understanding the nuances and making informed choices about the types of carbs we consume to support optimal health. Rather than fearing carbohydrates, the focus should be on choosing those that offer more than just empty calories—carbs that nourish, sustain, and keep us moving forward with energy and vitality.

Upon carbohydrate ingestion, they are broken down into glucose, the body's primary fuel source. This glucose enters the bloodstream, serving immediate energy needs or being stored as glycogen in the liver and muscles. When glycogen reserves are full, excess glucose undergoes de novo lipogenesis (DNL), converting to fat. The vilification of carbohydrates is not universal. Instead, it hinges on discerning how distinct carbohydrates modulate blood glucose levels and metabolic pathways. Opting for whole, nutrient-rich carbohydrate sources allows for meeting energy demands without promoting excessive fat deposition. It's a matter of balance and informed decision-making regarding carbohydrate selection to support physiological needs optimally.

The calories we ingest from whole foods are more difficult to overeat because they are divinely designed, created "whole," and

Throwing Shade at Carbs

complete. This form is easy for our body to process. When we take food process it, and then eat it, it becomes something structurally different, and our bodies absorb it subsequently differently. Over an extended period of time, this can create minor imbalances that greatly impact our lives and bodies, leading to weight fluctuations, mood swings, irritability, vitamin deficiencies, nutritional gaps, candida overgrowth, type 2 diabetes, and gout.

Processing foods that contain sugar essentially extracts the sugar from the cellular encasing, making it readily available for absorption. Your body does that through digestion once it breaks away the fibers of a whole fruit or potato or beet, for example. This digestion process takes time and slowly trickles the sugars into your bloodstream rather than opening the floodgates and bombarding it. When we eat sugar without fiber, our body has to counteract it by releasing insulin. Insulin production is regulated by the pancreas and is associated with thyroid function. Too many instances of this cycle can permanently impair your thyroid's ability to manage these self-inflicted attacks.

Simultaneously, your brain, which functions on glucose, can be thrown off balance. The initial surge of sugar stimulates dopamine and serotonin transmitters, signaling that an effective fuel source has been found. However, this extreme reaction also creates a dependency similar to that of a drug. It is an intense chemical transaction that falls outside of the ideal functions of your body. The disruption in normal hormone production, such as leptin and ghrelin, further complicates the issue. Leptin, which signals satiety, may be suppressed, while ghrelin, which stimulates hunger, may be increased, contributing to overeating and weight gain.

Processed sugar affects the body much like a drug. When we examine how chronic sugar consumption disrupts hormone production, it becomes clear why so many people are confused about sugar and carbs. These hormones directly affect our ability to control our weight. Outside of the immediate negative effects of consumption, processed sugar may disrupt the normal regulation of appetite hormones. The result can be a vicious cycle of cravings, overeating, and weight gain.

When people forego carbs entirely or eat them at a minimum, they often rely on proteins and fats as the majority of their caloric consumption. As the body and brain require glucose to function, when it is not obtained from the diet, the body will convert other molecules to glucose. This is where the process of gluconeogenesis comes into play. Gluconeogenesis is a process by which the body synthesizes new glucose molecules from non-carbohydrate sources, such as amino acids from proteins and glycerol from triglycerides (a component of fats). This occurs primarily in the liver when blood glucose levels are low, such as during fasting or insufficient carbohydrate intake.

During gluconeogenesis, amino acids are converted into glucose through several enzymatic steps. The body prefers to use carbohydrates as its primary source of energy. Gluconeogenesis is a backup mechanism to ensure a steady supply of glucose for vital functions, particularly for organs that rely heavily on glucose, such as the brain. Compensating for the body's efforts to adjust to inadequate eating habits is taxing on the system. Allowing the body to function smoothly without these interruptions is ideal for sustaining long-term well-being.

The effects of improper eating are not impossible to overcome. The negative effects of past meals can often be mitigated with a plant-based diet. Although there can be "permanent damage" like type 2 diabetes, there are studies and testimonials from many people with food-related conditions that were deemed "permanent" who have been able to reverse or eradicate symptoms simply by changing their diet. Working with your body rather than against it allows for well-

Throwing Shade at Carbs

being that may have seemed unachievable. Over time and with consistency, the body can self-correct and achieve a state of wellness and homeostasis. Finding balance becomes easier when any common denominator of foods that works against your system's natural ideal functions is removed.

Whole foods, such as fruits, contain fructose along with dietary fiber. Fiber slows down the digestion and absorption of fructose, resulting in a slower and more controlled release of glucose into the bloodstream. This not only helps regulate blood sugar levels but also promotes a feeling of fullness, reducing the likelihood of overeating. Whole foods often provide essential vitamins, minerals, and phytochemicals alongside fructose. These nutrients are important for overall health and may help mitigate any potential negative effects of fructose. While carbohydrates can be converted into fat through de novo lipogenesis, and proteins can be used for gluconeogenesis under certain circumstances, the body has distinct metabolic pathways for each macronutrient. They are not all directly converted and stored as glucose or fat interchangeably.

The body has complex mechanisms to regulate energy storage and utilization based on dietary intake, energy needs, and metabolic priorities. When screening packaged food, it is important to look for sugar of any type, meaning any word that ends in "-ose," like sucralose or dextrose. Added sugars are not necessary in your diet, and this awareness can help prevent unnecessary consumption. Commercial foods are notorious for using cheap ingredients like sugars and oils as fillers and preservatives. They can sit on the shelf longer and, in turn, in your body longer. They can contribute to yeast overgrowths and, most of the time, come with low fiber content when added to foods.

When you eat an apple, it's a whole unit. It digests slowly as the fiber walls are broken down, and the sugars are absorbed slowly. When you eat food with low fiber, the sugar is absorbed quickly, and what cannot be stored in the liver or muscles as glucose is stored as fat. In addition to spiking your blood sugar and taxing your system to produce insulin, over time, a tired endocrine system can increase your risk of developing certain types of diabetes.

Strong signals for cravings should be used as a warning.

If your body is craving something intensely, it might actually be signaling a need for the opposite. This concept is rooted in macrobiotic eating, where eating the "opposite" of what you're craving can help bring balance. For example, some studies suggest that consuming vinegar before a high-carbohydrate meal can help lower post-meal blood sugar levels and improve insulin sensitivity. Alternatively, if you're following a high-fat, high-protein diet, and experience cravings, it might indicate that your brain and muscles are in need of glucose, suggesting it's time to incorporate more carbohydrates into your diet.

Apple cider vinegar "with the mother" is considered a living food. Similar to kombucha, it contains strains of probiotics. These probiotics consume sugar, which means that if you are eating sugar with probiotics, a small portion might be digested by the probiotics before it reaches your bloodstream. However, this isn't a solution to overeating sugar, as the amount processed by probiotics is minimal, and the digestion time in the stomach is not sufficient to significantly reduce sugar absorption.

Apple cider vinegar is theorized to help curb cravings for sweets by reducing blood sugar spikes and promoting better blood sugar control. The sour taste of vinegar might also psychologically satisfy the craving for sweets, providing a mental reset. While apple cider vinegar is not a cure-all for sugar cravings, it is a beneficial addition to the diet for other reasons. As a living food, it may offer potential health benefits, including supporting gut health and improving digestion.

Research on apple cider vinegar and its effects on sugar cravings is still in the early stages, and more studies are needed to confirm its efficacy. Natural foods can offer many benefits, but the most effective way to lose and maintain a healthy body weight is by creating a lifestyle that supports your body's needs. There is no miracle cure for weight gain found in a single supplement; effective weight management requires comprehensive changes to diet and lifestyle. Although adding apple cider vinegar, cayenne, and ginger can help stimulate metabolism and support better digestion, these should be used as part of a broader approach to healthy eating and living.

Non-nutritive sweeteners, such as stevia, monk fruit, erythritol, Splenda, and aspartame, are intensely sweet compounds. They activate the sweet taste receptors on your tongue, providing a sweet sensation without the added calories or carbohydrates of sugar. The intensity of the sweetness may differ from person to person, and some individuals may find that non-nutritive sweeteners have a different taste profile compared to sugar. Non-nutritive sweeteners are exceptionally low in calories or calorie-free, so they are often used as sugar substitutes. Since they are not metabolized in the same way as sugar, they generally do not contribute to energy intake or impact blood sugar levels. As a result, they may not provide the same feeling of satiety that can come from consuming calorie-containing foods.

Looking at the grams of sugar on a label is one thing, but how do you know what to do when it comes to eating out or regarding foods that don't have a label? There are apps that can scan food labels to help identify sugar content, as well as other nutritional information. These apps can be useful when you're shopping for groceries or even when eating out.

Downloading an app can be extremely helpful to someone ready to take control of understanding the breakdown of their eating, but it's not a catch-all. Meal tracking apps are especially useful in the beginning stages when someone is transitioning to a more purposeful diet. Before making any changes, it can be advantageous to understand the basics of what you are eating. Logging three days to a week of meals can provide a starting point for improvement based on what and when you have eaten.

This practice can reveal how you are naturally spreading out your meals and what the macro breakdown is. From there, you can fine-tune your meal plan to add or reduce caloric intake, fiber, macros, and meal timing. There will always be a variance between what your body absorbs nutritionally from the food you eat and what the food equates to compositionally when measured for calculating macros.

The act of eating and consuming food is not solely driven by taste or sweetness. Other factors, such as texture, aroma, and the overall sensory experience, contribute to the feeling of satisfaction and fullness after a meal. Non-nutritive sweeteners, being purely sweet, may not provide the same sensory experience as consuming foods that contain natural sugars or other nutrients. This may lead to a perception of feeling unsatisfied or craving additional food.

Glucose is a simple sugar that serves as the standard reference for the glycemic index (GI), with a GI of 100. It is the primary sugar found in the bloodstream and is commonly derived from corn starch through a refining process. Glucose is rapidly absorbed into the bloodstream, leading to a quick spike in blood sugar levels. This rapid absorption makes it a quick source of energy but can also contribute to blood sugar imbalances if consumed in excess.

Understanding the glycemic index of different sugars and sweeteners is essential for making informed dietary choices, as the GI measures how quickly a food raises blood sugar levels. Sucrose, commonly known as table sugar, has a GI of around 65-70. It is a disaccharide composed of one molecule of glucose and one molecule of fructose, typically derived from sugar cane or sugar beets. While it provides quick energy, sucrose lacks essential nutrients and is considered "empty calories."

Throwing Shade at Carbs

Honey, a natural sweetener produced by bees, primarily consists of fructose and glucose, giving it a variable GI that generally falls in the moderate range of 50 to 75. Honey also contains trace amounts of vitamins and minerals, such as vitamin C, calcium, and iron. Its antioxidant properties make it a slightly more nutritious option than refined sugars, but it should still be consumed in moderation due to its sugar content.

Agave nectar, derived from the sap of the agave plant, has a low to moderate GI, ranging from 15 to 30. Its low GI is due to its high fructose content, which can be beneficial for avoiding blood sugar spikes. However, the high fructose content may have other health implications if consumed excessively, such as contributing to insulin resistance and increased triglyceride levels. This makes it a controversial choice among sweeteners.

Cane sugar, another refined sugar from sugar cane, has a moderate GI similar to that of table sugar, around 65-70. Like sucrose, it provides quick energy but lacks significant nutrients, making it an "empty calorie" food.

Coconut sugar, derived from the sap of coconut palm trees, has a lower GI of about 35-55, which is lower than many other common sweeteners. This lower GI is attributed to the presence of inulin, a type of dietary fiber that slows glucose absorption. Coconut sugar contains small amounts of vitamins and minerals, such as iron, zinc, calcium, and potassium, making it a slightly more nutritious option. Despite its benefits, it is mostly sucrose and should be consumed in moderation.

Demerara sugar, a less refined form of cane sugar, has a GI similar to regular cane sugar, around 65-70. It retains some molasses, which gives it a slightly caramel-like flavor and a small amount of minerals, including calcium, iron, and potassium. While these minerals offer some nutritional benefits, the differences aren't significant enough to justify their consumption in large quantities.

Maple syrup, made from the sap of maple trees, has a lower GI than cane sugar, typically ranging from 54 to 68, depending on the grade. Maple syrup contains small amounts of minerals, including manganese, zinc, and calcium. These nutrients can provide health benefits, such as supporting bone health and immune function.

Molasses, a byproduct of the sugar refining process, has a GI of 55-65. It is richer in minerals compared to many other sweeteners, containing significant amounts of iron, calcium, magnesium, and potassium. These nutrients make molasses a more nutritious option among sweeteners, providing health benefits such as improved bone health and aiding in iron deficiency.

Corn syrup, derived from corn starch, has a high GI of around 100, similar to glucose in its effects on blood sugar. Corn syrup is primarily glucose and lacks significant nutritional value. Due to its high sugar content and lack of nutrients, it is not recommended as a primary sweetener, especially for those looking to manage their blood sugar levels.

Non-nutritive sweeteners such as stevia, monk fruit, and erythritol provide sweetness without calories and have a GI of 0. These sweeteners are suitable for those watching their blood sugar levels or seeking to reduce their calorie intake. Stevia, derived from the leaves of the Stevia Rebaudiana plant, has been shown to have potential health benefits, including blood sugar regulation and potential antioxidant properties. Monk fruit, derived from the fruit of the Siraitia Grosvenorii plant, contains compounds called Mogrosides, which provide sweetness without impacting blood sugar levels. Erythritol, a sugar alcohol, is absorbed into the bloodstream and excreted unchanged in the urine, making it a non-caloric option that does not affect blood sugar or insulin levels.

Lucuma, a fruit native to South America, has a low GI of 25-35, making it a low-glycemic sweetener option. Lucuma is known for its sweet flavor and provides various nutrients, including beta-carotene, iron, zinc, and vitamin C. These nutrients contribute to its antioxidant properties, supporting immune health and reducing inflammation.

Chicory root fiber, also known as inulin, has a very low GI and is often used as a low-glycemic sweetener or prebiotic fiber source. Inulin supports beneficial gut bacteria and adds dietary fiber without significantly raising blood sugar levels. It is low in calories and does not significantly impact blood sugar, making it a good choice for those looking to manage their blood sugar levels and improve gut health. Additionally, inulin provides a source of dietary fiber without adding a significant amount of digestible carbohydrates to the diet, making it a beneficial addition to a balanced diet.

Each of these sweeteners offers unique properties that can influence health results. Making informed choices about which sweeteners to use can help to manage blood sugar levels, provide essential nutrients, and contribute to overall well-being. By understanding the glycemic index and nutrient content of various sweeteners, people can make choices that align with their dietary and health goals.

Starch and sugar are both carbohydrates, but they have distinct structures and functions in the body. Starch, a complex carbohydrate found in grains, tubers, and legumes, serves as a plant's energy storage molecule. It comprises long chains of glucose molecules with two main components: amylose and amylopectin. Sugar refers to simpler carbohydrates like sucrose, fructose, and glucose, which are sweet-tasting and readily absorbed for energy.

When starch-containing foods are cooked or exposed to temperature changes, a process called gelatinization occurs.

Starch granules absorb water and swell during gelatinization, leading to the thickening or gel formation observed in cooked starchy foods. This process also breaks down starch chains into simpler sugar molecules, making them more accessible for digestion.

Starch is broken down into sugars through digestion in the body. Enzymes like amylase are present in saliva, and the digestive system breaks down starch into maltose and then glucose. This glucose can be absorbed into the bloodstream and used for energy.

Consuming starch that converts to sugar can contribute to weight gain if consumed excessively or in a calorie surplus. When we consume carbohydrates, including starches, our body breaks them into glucose for energy. Any excess glucose beyond what the body needs for immediate energy is stored as glycogen in the liver and muscles. Once glycogen stores are full, surplus glucose is converted into fat and stored in adipose tissue, leading to weight gain over time.

Weight gain is influenced by various factors, including overall calorie intake, the balance of macronutrients (carbohydrates, fats, and proteins), physical activity level, and individual metabolic factors. It's not solely the conversion of starch to sugar that causes weight gain but rather the overall energy balance.

A process called "resistant starch" can be utilized to make starch more resistant to digestion and lower its impact on blood sugar levels. Resistant starch is a type of starch that resists digestion in the small intestine and behaves more like dietary fiber. Instead of being broken down into simple sugars, resistant starch passes through the small intestine. It undergoes fermentation in the large intestine, which can have beneficial effects on gut health.

There are several ways to make starch resistant: Cooking and cooling starchy foods like potatoes, rice, or pasta causes the starch structure to change, making some of it resistant to digestion. This is known as retrogradation. Certain food processing techniques, such as extrusion or heat-moisture treatment, can alter the structure of starch and increase its resistance to digestion. Some foods, such as green bananas, raw oats, and legumes, naturally contain resistant starch. These foods can be integrated into the diet to increase resistant starch intake.

Multiple clinical studies have investigated the effects of resistant starch on body weight and fat storage. Most researchers found that incorporating resistant starch into the diet resulted in increased fat oxidation (burning of fat for energy) and reduced fat storage, improving body composition and weight loss.

Instead of using the carbs for instant energy, your body will likely burn fat stores because the glucose chains have become inaccessible. For those struggling with transitioning their macro-balance, increasing the number of resistant starches can shift to fat-burning for energy conversion, where carbohydrates are less available, incorporating resistant starch into your diet as an additional food source for your microbiome. Ketosis is a metabolic state in which the body primarily relies on ketones for fuel instead of glucose. Following a very low-carbohydrate, high-fat ketogenic diet typically achieves this metabolic state. Since resistant starch is a type of carbohydrate, it may not be compatible with achieving and maintaining a state of ketosis.

Although resistant starch is resistant to digestion in the small intestine, the gut bacteria can still break down resistant starch into glucose during fermentation in the large intestine. This glucose can be absorbed into the bloodstream and potentially disrupt the ketosis process by providing a source of glucose that the body can use for energy instead of relying on ketones.

In a traditional ketogenic diet, the primary energy source comes from fats, with a limited intake of carbohydrates to promote ketosis. Carbohydrate sources in a ketogenic diet are typically low in digestible carbohydrates, such as leafy greens, non-starchy vegetables, and lesser amounts of low-glycemic fruits. These sources are chosen to minimize the impact on blood glucose and insulin levels, thus promoting ketosis.

If the goal is to achieve and maintain a state of ketosis, it is generally recommended to limit carbohydrate intake, including resistant starch, as it may interfere with the process. Suppose the intention is not specifically to enter ketosis but to incorporate resistant starch for potential health benefits such as improved digestion and gut health. In that case, it can be included in a balanced diet.

When cooked potatoes are refrigerated, the cooling process causes the starches in the potatoes to undergo retrogradation, making them more resistant to digestion. Similarly, when cooked rice is cooled in the refrigerator, it can develop resistant starch through retrogradation.

Reheating the chilled rice may reduce the amount of resistant starch formed. Legumes like beans, lentils, and chickpeas can also contain resistant starch when cooked and then cooled, making them suitable for salads or cold side dishes. Refrigerating cooked pasta can also lead to the formation of resistant starch. The formation of resistant starch after refrigeration is influenced by various factors, including how the food was cooked, how long it's been stored, and individual differences in starch content. Reheating these cooled foods might decrease the amount of resistant starch they contain.

Including cooled, cooked foods in your meals can still offer some benefits of resistant starch, which can benefit your microbiome. The amount of resistant starch may vary, but incorporating these foods into your diet can still contribute to overall gut health.

These techniques and food choices can influence health. Making informed choices about which carbohydrates and sweeteners to use and understanding the impact of processing and preparation methods can help manage blood sugar levels, provide essential nutrients, and contribute to overall well-being. By recognizing the complexity of carbohydrates and sweeteners and their varying effects on metabolism and health, you can make dietary choices that support your sweetest, highest-vibrational lifestyle.

8
THE LIES THEY TOLD YOU ABOUT PROTEIN

Amino acids are the essential building blocks of our cells. One of the biggest misconceptions is that we need protein when, in reality, we need nine specific amino acids. These amino acids are fundamental to life, and every living thing with cells contains them. A protein is simply a structure made of amino acids bonded together. This explains why genuine cases of protein deficiency are rare, even among those following a vegan or vegetarian diet. The common belief that you need entire protein blocks to build muscle is misleading; what you truly need are the individual amino acids.

If you consume a diverse array of nuts, grains, fruits, vegetables, and legumes, your body receives the necessary components to rebuild and repair muscle tissue. Whole plant foods offer easily absorbable nutrients with fewer personal and environmental drawbacks. By diversifying your diet to include a variety of plant-based foods, you ensure a balanced intake of essential amino acids. The human body is adept at mixing and matching these amino acids to meet its needs, even when they are not consumed in a single meal. This adaptability is why it's entirely possible to get all the essential amino acids required for health from a plant-based diet.

Historically, economic constraints have driven the working class to rely on grains, potatoes, and limited animal products, elevating the perceived value of meat, cheese, and other costly foods. Mainstream diets' emphasis on protein has further fueled this perception.

However, many people are unaware of how much protein they actually need and are confused about the quality of protein, from its sources to the hidden dangers associated with certain foods.

A food's classification as a protein source is not solely based on its presence of amino acids but also on the composition and concentration of essential amino acids it provides. Proteins are made up of various combinations of amino acids, and essential amino acids are those that the body cannot produce on its own and must obtain from the diet.

To be recognized as a complete protein, a food must deliver all nine essential amino acids in adequate amounts and proportions. These crucial amino acids are histidine, isoleucine, leucine, lysine, methionine, phenylalanine, threonine, tryptophan, and valine. When a food contains these necessary amino acids in sufficient quantities, it is deemed a complete protein. The exact balance of amino acids required to be classified as a complete protein varies depending on the specific amino acid needs of the human body. The essential amino acids, which cannot be synthesized by the body and must be obtained from the diet, have dietary reference intake (DRI) values established by various health organizations.

Consuming animal meat not only puts strain on your liver and kidneys but also introduces heme iron into your system. Some theories suggest a link between heme iron and cancer. During digestion, heme iron can interact with compounds like nitrites and nitrates found in meat to form N-nitroso compounds, some of which are known carcinogens and may increase the risk of cancer, especially colorectal cancer.

Heme iron can also facilitate the creation of free radicals and boost oxidative stress, which can harm cells and DNA. Chronic inflammation, which can be triggered by heme iron, is another factor linked to cancer development. High consumption of red and processed meats, which are rich in heme iron, may negatively affect the gut microbiota composition. Changes in the gut microbiota have been linked to various health conditions, including colorectal cancer.

Especially when cooked at high temperatures, meat can produce pro-carcinogenic compounds, such as heterocyclic amines (HCAs) and polycyclic aromatic hydrocarbons (PAHs). These compounds are formed during cooking and may contribute to cancer risk.

While there is no universally agreed-upon standard for the exact proportion of each essential amino acid required in a complete protein, one commonly used reference is the amino acid profile of human milk or egg protein. These profiles are considered to represent optimal amino acid ratios for human nutrition.

Because the conglomerations that subsidize the meat, dairy, and poultry industries have built their food pyramid around these animal foods, there has been a lot of confusion about what protein is, how it is measured, and how much we need. The comparisons of "adequate levels" of amino acids in foods to be classified as a "complete protein source" are somewhat blurred by an ideal. The companies that oversee calculating these daily intakes and allowances must have a comparison to which they measure a complete protein.

This is calculated based on two things. One being a chicken's egg and a human mother's breast milk. Neither of these are everyday foods for adults, but one is the unborn embryo of a chicken, and the other is a substance for a newborn infant. Because these are unrealistic to base what a protein is, some plant-based food sources look as though they are lacking, but the reality is that you have been persuaded to believe things that aren't truths.

Let's compare a chicken embryo to a serving of raw oats. By the rules governing food classification, the egg is considered a complete protein, while oats are not.

But when we place them side by side, it becomes evident that oats are by no means inferior. Your body doesn't require every amino acid in large quantities with each meal as long as you consume a variety of foods. Interestingly, oats provide more amino acids per serving, have greater bioavailability, and lack the harmful cholesterol and hormones found in eggs. Additionally, oats are rich in antioxidants, healthy fats, and fibers that nourish.

Here is a comparison of the amino acid content in one cup of raw oats and one cooked egg:

- Oats (1 cup raw) Egg (1 large, cooked)
- Histidine 0.483 g 0.159 g
- Isoleucine 0.593g 0.613 g
- Leucine 1.015g 0.906 g
- Lysine 0.760g 0.757 g
- Methionine 0.322 g 0.393 g
- Phenylalanine 0.870g 0.608 g
- Threonine 0.500g 0.503 g
- Tryptophan 0.209g 0.093 g
- Valine 0.721g 0.806 g

As you can see, the oats have similar, if not more, amino acids, and they are available without the seal of a protein bond. Typically, a food is considered a complete protein source if it provides adequate amounts of all nine essential amino acids in proportions that meet or exceed the dietary reference intake (DRI) values or are similar to those found in the reference protein. On the other hand, if a food is deficient in one or more essential amino acids, it is classified as an incomplete protein.

Incomplete protein sources can still contribute to the overall protein intake and provide essential amino acids when combined with other complementary protein sources. The concept of combining complementary proteins refers to consuming different foods that, when combined, provide a balance of essential amino acids. For example, legumes (such as beans or lentils) are typically low in the amino acid methionine but are rich in lysine. Grains, on the other hand, are lower in lysine but higher in methionine. By combining legumes and grains in a meal, you can obtain a more complete amino acid profile. Our bodies synthesize eleven of the amino acids; the other nine we source from the foods we eat.

These nine are listed with the amount you need. Histidine is found in quinoa, chickpeas, soybeans, and lentils. To calculate the recommended daily intake for a 150 lb. (approximately 68 kg) adult with 20 percent body fat, you would follow these steps: Calculate the lean body mass (LBM) by subtracting the body fat from the total body weight: LBM = Body weight - (Body weight *Body fat percentage) LBM = 150 lb. - (150 lb 0.20) = 120 lb (approximately 54.4 kg)* Multiply the LBM by the recommended histidine intake per kilogram of body weight: Histidine intake = LBM *14 mg/kg Histidine intake = 54.4 kg* 14 mg/kg = 761.6 mg (approximately 0.76 g). Therefore, for a 150 lb adult with 20 percent body fat, the recommended daily intake of histidine would be approximately 0.76 grams.

Leucine can be found in vegan food sources, including soybeans, lentils, peanuts, chickpeas, quinoa, brown rice, and pumpkin seeds. Leucine intake is usually expressed as a ratio to the total protein intake. The general recommendation for leucine is about 2-3 grams per meal or a total daily intake of around 10-14 grams for adults.

Lysine is found in vegan food sources, including legumes such as lentils, chickpeas, black beans, quinoa, tempeh, tofu, seitan, and hemp seeds. The recommended daily intake of lysine for adults is approximately 12 mg per kilogram of body weight. For a 150 lb adult (approximately 68 kg), this would amount to around 816 mg adult (approximately 68 kg), this would amount to around 816 mg (0.82 g).

Methionine is found in vegan food sources, including legumes such as soybeans, lentils, and chickpeas, seeds such as sesame seeds, chia seeds, pumpkin seeds, and whole grains such as quinoa and brown rice. There is no specific daily recommendation for methionine alone. However, the recommended daily intake of methionine plus cysteine, another sulfur-containing amino acid, is approximately 19 mg per kilogram of body weight. For a 150 lb adult (approximately 68 kg), this would be around 1.292 g (1292 mg).

Phenylalanine is found in vegan food sources, including legumes, nuts such as almonds, peanuts, and walnuts, seeds such as pumpkin seeds, chia seeds, flaxseeds, quinoa, and tofu. There is no specific daily recommendation for phenylalanine alone. The daily recommended intake for phenylalanine plus tyrosine, an amino acid produced from phenylalanine, is approximately 25 mg per kilogram of body weight. For a 150 lb adult (approximately 68 kg), this would be around 1.7 g (1700 mg).

Threonine can be found in vegan food sources, including legumes, nuts, seeds, whole grains, and quinoa. The recommended daily intake of threonine for adults is approximately 15 mg per kilogram of body weight. For a 150 lb adult (approximately 68 kg), this would be around 1020 mg (1.02 g).

Tryptophan can be found in vegan food sources, including legumes and seeds such as pumpkin seeds and chia seeds, oats, quinoa, tofu, and spirulina. The recommended daily intake of tryptophan for adults is approximately 4 mg per kilogram of body weight. For a 150 lb adult (approximately 68 kg), this would be around 272 mg (0.27 g).

Valine can be found in food sources such as legumes, whole grains, seeds, nuts, and soy products. The recommended daily intake

The Lies They Told You About Protein

of valine for adults is approximately 26 mg per kilogram of body weight. For a 150 lb adult (approximately 68 kg), this would be around 1.768 g (1768 mg).

The determination of what constitutes an "adequate proportion" of amino acids in a food to be considered a complete protein source is based on amino acid composition and their relative amounts in comparison to the human body's needs.

Comparison of quinoa and chicken:

1 cup cooked quinoa:
- Histidine: Approximately 0.70 grams
- Isoleucine: Approximately 1.03 grams
- Leucine: Approximately 1.76 grams
- Lysine: Approximately 1.64 grams
- Methionine: Approximately 0.63 grams
- Phenylalanine: Approximately 1.28 grams
- Threonine: Approximately 0.94 grams
- Tryptophan: Approximately 0.19 grams
- Valine: Approximately 1.18 grams

VS.

5-ounce (100-gram) serving of cooked chicken breast:
- Histidine: Approximately 0.56 grams
- Isoleucine: Approximately 1.08 grams
- Leucine: Approximately 1.77 grams
- Lysine: Approximately 2.16 grams
- Methionine: Approximately 0.69 grams
- Phenylalanine: Approximately 1.21 grams
- Threonine: Approximately 1.07 grams

- Tryptophan: Approximately 0.29 grams
- Valine: Approximately 1.08 grams

These are very comparable sources of amino acids. But when we compare them side by side on a macronutrient level, you will see that the chicken shows a much higher content for protein. This is because chicken breast is a structural composition made of amino acids. The way a house can be a structure made of brick. Just because the label says there are however many grams of protein doesn't mean your body will absorb those direct "protein for protein" the way people have been convinced. In fact, your body can break down about 10-25 grams of protein per 1-2 hours, and the rest will be converted to fat. Yes, fat.

The idea of a "complete protein" is that it contains all nine essential amino acids in one. But our bodies are complex machines, and as long as you eat a somewhat diversified array of plants, you will likely ingest all nine of those amino acids easily.

Proteins are broken down into amino acids during digestion. These amino acids are primarily used for building and repairing tissues, enzymes, and hormones. In certain circumstances, when the body needs energy and doesn't have sufficient carbohydrates or fats available, amino acids can be converted into glucose through a process called gluconeogenesis.

When you are eating a protein, it has to have all of the amino acids to create the muscle structure, for example, a chicken breast. Yes, you are getting quantities of the nine essentials, but you are also bombarding your body with all of the excess amino acids that you don't need; therefore, it is taxing on the liver. It makes more sense to eat a variety of vegetables to reach that goal without excess.

Meat also has free-floating hormones, which are of the animal variety, so we can absorb them. This doesn't only apply to poultry, though; hormones in poultry farming have been banned in the US, and naturally occurring hormones still exist. And beef is a different story. The U.S. does permit the use of hormones such as estradiol, progesterone, testosterone, and zeranol, which are approved for use in beef cattle to promote growth and improve feed efficiency. In short, eating grams of straight protein is one way to get amino acids, in the same way that you can catch tuna with a net, but you're also going to catch a lot of stuff you don't need in that net. Eating more natural plant options increases the availability to your system of a variety of nutrients, enzymes, vitamins, and minerals; these are called phytonutrients.

Let's do another amino profile comparison:

1 cup of hemp seeds to 1 cup of steak
Hemp seeds are considered a reliable source of essential amino acids, providing a well-balanced profile of amino acids. Here is an approximate breakdown of the essential amino acid content per 3 tablespoons (30 grams) of hemp seeds:
- Histidine: Approximately 0.76 grams
- Isoleucine: Approximately 0.95 grams
- Leucine: Approximately 1.69 grams
- Lysine: Approximately 0.92 grams
- Methionine: Approximately 0.70 grams
- Phenylalanine: Approximately 1.07 grams
- Threonine: Approximately 0.72 grams
- Tryptophan: Approximately 0.26 grams
- Valine: Approximately 1.13 grams

Hemp seeds are also rich in other non-essential amino acids and provide a good balance of omega-3 and omega-6 fatty acids. Additionally, hemp seeds are a source of minerals such as magnesium, phosphorus, and zinc.

VS.

30 grams of cooked beef steak:
- Histidine: Approximately 0.46 grams
- Isoleucine: Approximately 0.80 grams
- Leucine: Approximately 1.48 grams
- Lysine: Approximately 1.56 grams
- Methionine: Approximately 0.54 grams
- Phenylalanine: Approximately 1.08 grams
- Threonine: Approximately 0.76 grams
- Tryptophan: Approximately 0.14 grams
- Valine: Approximately 1.08 grams

As you can see, the profiles are similar. But eating steak has some drawbacks. A lot, actually. High saturated fat content: Beef, especially fatty cuts, can be high in saturated fat. Consuming excessive amounts of saturated fat has been linked to an increased risk of cardiovascular diseases.

Beef is a source of dietary cholesterol. High intake of dietary cholesterol, especially when combined with saturated fat, may contribute to elevated blood cholesterol levels in some individuals. Cattle production has a significant environmental impact, including deforestation, greenhouse gas emissions, and water usage. Large-scale beef production is associated with deforestation of land for cattle grazing and the emission of methane, a potent greenhouse gas.

The use of antibiotics in livestock farming, including beef production, can contribute to the development of antibiotic-resistant bacteria, posing a public health concern. Red meat includes beef, pork, lamb, and goat. The International Agency for Research on Cancer (IARC) classifies red meat as a Group 2A carcinogen, indicating that it is "probably carcinogenic to humans."

There is evidence suggesting an association between red meat consumption and colorectal cancer. Possible explanations for this association include the presence of certain compounds in red meat, such as heme iron and heterocyclic amines formed during cooking at high temperatures. The intestine lining is absorbent, and the longer these decaying foods sit in our system, the more harmful they become.

Most people sear, broil, and grill their meat, and this in and of itself escalates the carcinogenic properties. High-temperature cooking methods, such as grilling, broiling, or frying, can lead to the formation of harmful compounds. For example, heterocyclic amines (HCAs) and polycyclic aromatic hydrocarbons (PAHs) can form when meat is exposed to high temperatures. In animal studies, these compounds have been shown to have mutagenic and carcinogenic properties. Heterocyclic amines are created in a chemical reaction when meat is cooked; the proteins and creatines in the meat have a reaction that makes this. While baking, stewing, and slow cooking lessen this particular reaction, it does not mitigate the other harmful potential side effects.

Heme iron, found predominantly in animal-based foods like red meat, poultry, and fish, is known for its high bioavailability and is absorbed more efficiently by the body than non-heme iron. The absorption rate of heme iron typically ranges from 15-35%, whereas non-heme iron, found in plant-based sources such as beans, lentils, spinach, raisins, and spirulina, is absorbed at a lower rate, usually between 2-20%. This difference in absorption efficiency is often cited as a reason to consume heme iron to maintain adequate iron levels.

However, faster absorption does not necessarily equate to being healthier. Despite its efficient absorption, heme iron poses potential health risks that should not be overlooked. During digestion, heme iron can react with compounds like nitrites and nitrates, which are commonly found in processed meats, to form N-nitroso compounds. These compounds are recognized carcinogens that can damage the lining of the colon, promoting the development of cancerous cells. Studies have shown a clear association between high heme iron intake and an increased risk of colorectal cancer. This risk is particularly concerning given the typical Western diet, which is high in red and processed meats.

Heme iron also contributes to the formation of free radicals, unstable molecules that can cause oxidative stress and damage to cells, proteins, and DNA. This oxidative stress is a key factor in the development of various chronic diseases, including cancer and cardiovascular disease. The pro-oxidant nature of heme iron suggests that while it is a vital nutrient, its high intake can initiate and exacerbate processes leading to disease.

High consumption of heme iron has been linked to increased levels of inflammation in the body. Chronic inflammation is a known driver of cancer development and progression. It can lead to DNA damage, promote the growth and survival of cancer cells, and create an environment conducive to cancer development. The inflammatory response triggered by heme iron adds to its potential carcinogenic effects, further complicating its role in human health.

The consumption of high amounts of heme iron, particularly from red and processed meats, has been shown to disrupt the balance of the gut microbiota. A healthy gut microbiome is essential for maintaining overall health, including digestion, immune function, and even mental health. Disruptions to this delicate balance can lead to inflammation and other changes that may increase the risk of cancer, especially in the colon.

On the other hand, non-heme iron from plant-based sources offers a safer and healthier alternative. Although it is absorbed at a slower rate, this type of iron does not have the same associations with cancer risk as heme iron. The slower absorption rate of non-heme iron can actually be beneficial, as it provides a more steady and controlled release of iron into the body, reducing the likelihood of iron overload and the associated oxidative stress. Foods rich in non-heme iron, such as beans, lentils, spinach, quinoa, raisins, nuts, seeds, and spirulina, are also packed with other beneficial nutrients like fiber, vitamins, minerals, and antioxidants that support overall health.

The presence of these additional nutrients in plant-based iron sources helps enhance their absorption and utilization in the body. For instance, vitamin C, found in many fruits and vegetables, can significantly enhance the absorption of non-heme iron. Consuming a varied diet rich in these plant-based foods not only ensures adequate iron intake but also provides a host of other nutrients that contribute to overall health and well-being.

Incorporating a variety of iron-rich plant foods into the diet can help maintain healthy iron levels without the risks associated with heme iron. While it might take a bit more planning to ensure sufficient iron intake from plant sources, the benefits far outweigh the potential health risks associated with heme iron. By focusing on a diet that includes a diverse array of whole, plant-based foods, individuals can support their health and reduce the risk of chronic diseases, all while meeting their body's iron needs in a safe and sustainable way.

It's important to note that the classifications by the IARC do not imply that consuming these meats guarantees the development of cancer. The risk is associated with long-term, frequent consumption of processed or red meats, and other factors such as overall dietary patterns, lifestyle, and genetic predisposition also play a role. While meat has little insoluble fiber to help move it through the body, as it sits in your intestines, it can continue to decay inside of you, which can create toxins and difficult bowel movements. When red meat is cooked or metabolized in the body, it can lead to the formation of certain compounds, including N-nitroso compounds and heterocyclic amines, which have been linked to carcinogenesis. The heme iron itself may also promote oxidative stress and inflammation, which can contribute to cellular damage and the development of cancer. Low-fiber foods paired with fiber-rich foods can be helpful to balance this. Eating a whole food in its complete package, i.e., unprocessed, is the best way to eat it because you are digesting the whole package as it was designed by nature to be eaten.

Your body is under enough daily stressors that I can't advise adding to them a controversial protein source. While there is nothing wrong with calculating protein grams in your macros, it isn't so dire if you don't mind hitting your macro goals. Creating a lifestyle means replacing your habits with healthier ones, one at a time, so that you can gradually create a lifestyle where you can focus on enjoying your life and your health instead of constantly struggling with food, weight, and illness.

Metabolic processes associated with high-protein diets can have indirect effects on the body's pH regulation. For example, the breakdown of proteins results in the production of nitrogenous waste products, such as urea, which is excreted by the kidneys. This excretion process can potentially influence the overall acid-base balance in the body.

Furthermore, some animal-based foods, such as certain types of processed meats, can contain additives or preservatives that may have an impact on health. Excessive consumption of these processed meats, along with an imbalanced diet overall, can potentially lead to health issues, including disturbances in pH balance. While the body has systems in place to rectify imbalances within, the constant taxation of negative-impact foods makes it difficult for all other systems to carry out their ideal regeneration if the body is constantly out of whack. The longer time spent out of balance with your body creates more time for illness and disease to accrue.

Diets rich in high-fat and animal protein content bear a significant load of cholesterol and sodium and fall short of providing the dietary fiber vital for a balanced intestinal microbiome, placing undue strain on the body's hepatic and renal systems. While such diets, including the ketogenic and Atkins diets, may lead to short-term weight loss, the detrimental effects of adhering to these dietary patterns far exceed the benefits of any weight loss achieved in the interim. The consumption of saturated animal fats in excessive quantities is associated with a wide array of health risks, including heart disease, high cholesterol, and other cardiovascular issues. These fats can contribute to the buildup of plaque in arteries, leading to atherosclerosis and an increased risk of heart attacks and strokes.

Saturated fats, commonly found in red meat, butter, cheese, and other animal products, are known to raise low-density lipoprotein (LDL) cholesterol levels in the blood. Elevated LDL cholesterol is a significant risk factor for cardiovascular disease because it promotes the formation of fatty deposits in the arteries. Over time, these deposits can harden and narrow the arteries, a condition known as atherosclerosis, which can restrict blood flow to the heart and brain. This narrowing increases the risk of heart attacks, strokes, and peripheral artery disease. Research has consistently shown a link between high intake of saturated fats and increased levels of LDL cholesterol, underscoring the importance of limiting these fats in the diet to maintain cardiovascular health.

In addition to the cardiovascular risks, excessive intake of saturated fats has been linked to obesity and type 2 diabetes, further compounding the risk of chronic illnesses. High-fat diets can contribute to weight gain because fats are calorie-dense, providing more than double the calories per gram compared to carbohydrates and proteins. Obesity is a major risk factor for type 2 diabetes, a condition characterized by insulin resistance and high blood sugar levels. Studies have shown that diets high in saturated fats can impair insulin sensitivity, making it more difficult for the body to regulate blood sugar levels. This can lead to the development of type 2 diabetes, a condition that is associated with numerous complications, including heart disease, kidney failure, and nerve damage.

Moreover, high-fat, low-fiber diets can negatively impact the gut microbiome, the community of trillions of microorganisms that reside in the digestive tract. A healthy gut microbiome is essential for digestion, immune function, and overall health. Dietary fiber, found in fruits, vegetables, whole grains, and legumes, serves as a prebiotic, providing food for beneficial gut bacteria. These bacteria ferment the fiber, producing short-chain fatty acids (SCFAs) that have anti-inflammatory effects and support gut health. Diets low in fiber, such as those high in animal fats and proteins, can disrupt the balance of the gut microbiome, leading to a decrease in beneficial bacteria and an increase in harmful bacteria. This imbalance has been linked to a range of health issues, including inflammation, impaired immune function, and an increased risk of gastrointestinal disorders such as irritable bowel syndrome (IBS) and inflammatory bowel disease (IBD).

The impact of high-fat diets on the liver and kidneys also raises concerns. Diets high in saturated fats can lead to the accumulation of fat in the liver, a condition known as non-alcoholic fatty liver disease (NAFLD). NAFLD can progress to more severe liver damage, including inflammation, fibrosis, and cirrhosis. The liver plays a critical role in metabolizing fats, and an excessive intake of saturated fats can overwhelm the liver's capacity to process them, leading to the buildup of fat within liver cells. This can impair liver function and increase the risk of liver disease.

Similarly, high-protein diets can strain the kidneys, especially in individuals with pre-existing kidney conditions. The kidneys are responsible for filtering waste products from the blood, and high protein intake increases the production of urea, a waste product of protein metabolism. This places additional stress on the kidneys, which must work harder to eliminate the excess urea. Over time, this increased workload can lead to kidney damage, particularly in those with reduced kidney function. Research has shown that long-term high-protein diets can accelerate the progression of chronic kidney disease (CKD) and increase the risk of kidney stones due to the higher excretion of calcium and other minerals in the urine.

The high sodium content often found in animal-based diets can contribute to hypertension (high blood pressure), a major risk factor for heart disease and stroke. Sodium, commonly found in processed meats and salty snacks, can cause the body to retain water, increasing blood volume and, consequently, blood pressure. High blood pressure puts added strain on the heart and blood vessels, increasing the risk of heart attacks, strokes, and kidney damage. Reducing sodium intake, along with limiting saturated fats, is essential for maintaining cardiovascular health and preventing chronic diseases.

While high-fat, high-protein diets may offer short-term weight loss benefits, they pose significant risks to long-term health. The excessive intake of saturated fats, cholesterol, and sodium, combined with a lack of dietary fiber, can lead to a range of health issues, including cardiovascular disease, obesity, type 2 diabetes, liver and kidney damage, and gut dysbiosis. A balanced diet that includes a variety of nutrient-dense foods, such as fruits, vegetables, whole grains, lean proteins, and healthy fats, is essential for promoting overall health and reducing the risk of chronic diseases. By focusing on the quality and diversity of the foods we eat, we can support our bodies' natural ability to maintain health and well-being, ensuring a longer, healthier life.

9
OMEGA WARS

Oils and fats, whether hidden or obvious, play a significant role in our diets, contributing nine calories per gram compared to the four calories per gram found in carbohydrates and proteins. This high caloric density is why many calorie-restrictive diets advise caution with fat intake. However, it's not just the oils we add to our salads or use in cooking that contribute to our fat consumption; hidden oils in processed and convenience foods can also sneak in unwanted calories and unhealthy fats. As modern humans, we face an abundance of these hidden oils, from cooking to pre-packaged meals, making it challenging to moderate our fat intake.

Interestingly, our brains are wired to appreciate the energy density that fats provide. When we consume foods rich in fats, the molecules signal to our brain that we're getting a substantial energy source. This is a primal instinct, a leftover survival mechanism from times when high-calorie foods were scarce. The brain essentially celebrates the finding of a calorie-dense food source, which would keep our metabolism humming and stave off potential starvation. This is why eating fats, even in small amounts, can lead to feelings of satiety and satisfaction that are harder to achieve with just carbohydrates or proteins.

The difference between fats found in whole, minimally processed foods like olives, coconuts, avocados, nuts, and seeds and the extracted oils that flood many of our modern dishes is crucial. Eating closer to the source, opting for whole foods instead of processed ones, is a timeless principle that can guide us toward healthier dietary choices. Whole foods contain not only fats but also fiber, vitamins, minerals, and antioxidants, which are often lost during the processing and extraction of oils. Consuming energy-dense foods, including those with added oils, can lead to a feeling of fullness and satisfaction. Our brains, built for survival, celebrate a win when they detect a food source capable of keeping our metabolism out of starvation mode.

The original form of dietary fat was in fatty foods like whole olives, coconut meat, avocados, nuts, and seeds. Today, however, we have extracted these oils and allowed them to permeate nearly every processed food product. This shift from whole food fats to extracted oils has led to what could be considered dietary pollution, contributing to a range of health issues from obesity to heart disease. Eating closest to the source is always the best rule of thumb, not only for the nutritional benefits but also for the flavor and enjoyment of food. Fats, including oils, contribute significantly to the flavor and mouthfeel of foods. They enhance dishes' taste, texture, and aroma, making eating more enjoyable. The presence of oil in foods can activate taste receptors, which may enhance the overall sensory experience and increase the perceived satisfaction from the meal.

Moreover, fats have been found to affect satiety and hunger-regulating hormones. When we consume fats, they trigger the release of certain hormones, such as peptide YY (PYY) and cholecystokinin (CCK), associated with feelings of fullness and decreased appetite. These hormonal responses can enhance satisfaction and reduce hunger after consuming oil-containing foods. Fat-rich foods, including those with added oils, tend to slow down gastric emptying, which is the process of food moving from the stomach to the small intestine. This delayed gastric emptying can prolong the feeling of fullness and contribute to a sense of satisfaction after a meal.

The shift in dietary fats since the 1950s, when lard was a common cooking ingredient, reflects our evolving understanding of nutrition. Lard was once used extensively in baking, frying, and cooking. As the detrimental effects of this rendered animal fat became known, many people began replacing it with other cooking oils, sprays, and butter. With the exception of bacon fat taking its place, Americans have made a confused effort to find the best fats for the kitchen.

However, this shift raises the question: are these fats hurting more than they are helping? What does fat do to our body, for good, for evil, and for the sake of understanding?

Although the media was influential in spreading the information that lard is not ideal for ingesting, people haven't fully embraced the concept that the lard they avoid is ever-present in the animal foods they eat.

Lard is rendered animal fat, and when you eat a burger or pork, it is layered with this fat. When ingested, lard or other animal fats are metabolized similarly to different types of dietary fats. The body breaks down fats into fatty acids, which are then absorbed and utilized for energy or stored as body fat. Excess consumption of lard, combined with an overall high-calorie diet, can lead to weight gain and potential health consequences associated with an unhealthy diet.

Some research suggests that not all saturated fats are equal, and that specific food sources and the overall dietary context play a role. For instance, sources of saturated fat from processed meats and high-fat dairy products have been associated with a higher risk of disease. Lard is a type of animal fat that is high in saturated fat. Diets high in saturated fat have been linked to an increased risk of cardiovascular disease. Saturated fats can raise levels of LDL cholesterol (often referred to as "bad" cholesterol) in the blood, which can contribute to the development of atherosclerosis and heart disease.

Animal fats, including lard, contain cholesterol. Seafood, particularly salmon and shrimp, is exceedingly high in saturated fat. High dietary cholesterol intake has been associated with increased blood cholesterol levels in some individuals. Elevated levels of LDL cholesterol are a risk factor for cardiovascular disease. Consuming excessive amounts of animal fat, including lard, as part of a high-calorie diet can contribute to weight gain and obesity. Obesity is a risk factor for various health conditions, including heart disease, type 2 diabetes, and certain cancers. Animal fats, including saturated fats found in lard, can raise LDL (low-density lipoprotein) cholesterol levels in the blood.

Saturated fats are typically solid at room temperature and more oxidation-resistant than unsaturated fats. When consumed in excess, saturated fats can increase LDL cholesterol levels in the blood. Cholesterol, including LDL cholesterol, is transported in the blood by lipoproteins. LDL cholesterol is often referred to as "bad" cholesterol because elevated levels of LDL can contribute to the development of atherosclerosis, which is the build-up of plaque in the arteries. Cells throughout the body have LDL receptors on their surface. These receptors bind to LDL particles and take cholesterol from the bloodstream into the cells. However, when there is an excess of LDL cholesterol in the blood, it can lead to an overload of cholesterol in cells, particularly in the walls of the arteries.

In atherosclerosis, the excess LDL cholesterol that accumulates in the arterial walls can trigger an inflammatory response. Over time, this can lead to the formation of fatty deposits, known as plaques, in the arteries. These plaques can narrow the arteries and impede blood flow, increasing the risk of cardiovascular diseases such as heart attacks and strokes.

In the United States, the market for cooking oils is flooded with numerous options, and not all of them are what they claim to be. Fake oil blends—often marketed as pure or extra-virgin olive oil—are a growing concern among consumers and regulators alike. These oils are frequently diluted with cheaper, lower-quality oils such as soybean, canola, or sunflower oil, yet are sold at a premium price. In some cases, these blends are mixed with partially refined olive oils or even colorants and flavorings to mimic the taste and appearance of genuine olive oil. The result is a product that not only lacks the authentic flavor and health benefits of true extra-virgin olive oil but may also pose health risks due to the presence of oxidized or contaminated oils.

Regulatory oversight and testing have revealed that a significant percentage of olive oils on supermarket shelves in the U.S. do not meet the purity standards set by the International Olive Council. Consumers who believe they are purchasing high-quality, health-promoting olive oil may instead be buying a mixture of low-grade oils. This deception undermines consumer trust and can have economic consequences for honest producers of genuine olive oil. To safeguard against fake oil blends, consumers are advised to buy from reputable brands, look for certification seals from recognized quality standards organizations, and be wary of prices that seem too good to be true. Educating oneself on the sensory characteristics of real olive oil, such as its flavor, aroma, and texture, can also help in identifying authentic products.

These seals indicate that the oil has been tested and verified to meet specific quality and purity standards. For example, the USDA Organic Seal guarantees that the oil is made from organically grown ingredients without synthetic pesticides or fertilizers. The Non-GMO Project Verified label ensures that the product does not contain genetically modified organisms, which can be a concern for some consumers. Additionally, the International Olive Council (IOC) certification is specifically important for olive oil, indicating that the product meets strict international standards for quality and authenticity.

Another important label to look for is the Protected Designation of Origin (PDO) or Protected Geographical Indication (PGI), which signifies that the oil comes from a specific region known for its high-quality production methods, like certain types of olive oil from Italy, Spain, or Greece. Consumers should also check for the California Olive Oil Council (COOC) seal when buying extra virgin olive oil from California, as it guarantees the oil meets rigorous testing standards. To further protect themselves, consumers should read ingredient lists carefully, avoiding products labeled simply as "vegetable oil" or those that list multiple types of oils, which could indicate blending.

Choosing oils that come in dark glass bottles can also help maintain the oil's integrity by protecting it from light, which can degrade quality. By being mindful of these labels and taking steps to verify the authenticity of the cooking oils they purchase, consumers can better ensure they are getting a high-quality product that is pure and unadulterated.

The term "seed oil" can be confusing, as it encompasses a variety of vegetable-based, often refined oils. These include canola, soybean, corn, cottonseed, grapeseed, safflower, sunflower, rice bran, and peanut oils. These oils are packaged separately from their source, unlike the nut and seed oils found naturally separated at the top of your tahini or peanut butter. Commercial seed oils are manufactured through synthetic chemical extraction, which sometimes includes additional processing like bleaching and deodorizing. These oils are then used in food products. If tampered with, these oils can cause inflammation in the body and an imbalance of Omega 6.

The oils naturally found in seeds, when they come out naturally upon crushing, are in direct proportion with fiber and minerals and have beneficial effects on the body. But when these oils are extracted, further processed, and then added unnecessarily into common foods that people consume throughout the day, the sheer number of Omegas goes up exponentially, as does inflammation within the body. Avoiding foods that have seed oils on the label is wise.

Embrace the naturally occurring seed oils from whole nuts and seeds. The difference in the effects of processed seed oils and whole seeds on inflammation in the body is primarily due to their fatty acid composition and how they are processed and consumed. Processed seed oils, such as soybean oil, corn oil, and sunflower oil, are high in omega-6 fatty acids. While omega-6 fatty acids are essential for the body and have some health benefits, excessive consumption of these fatty acids relative to omega-3 fatty acids can lead to an imbalance in the omega-6 to omega-3 ratio.

Making your own cooking oil at home can be a rewarding way to ensure purity, quality, and control over the ingredients you use. The process of making homemade cooking oil generally involves extracting oil from seeds, nuts, or fruits such as olives, coconuts, or sunflowers. One of the simplest methods to make oil at home is through cold pressing, which involves crushing the chosen material using a mechanical press.

For example, to make olive oil, fresh olives are washed and crushed into a paste, which is then pressed to extract the oil. Similarly, for nut oils like almond or walnut oil, the nuts are crushed, and the resulting paste is pressed to release the oil. A more straightforward method involves using a high-speed blender or food processor, where you can blend seeds or nuts until they release their oils. The mixture is then strained through a fine mesh or cheesecloth to separate the oil from the solids.

Another method for making oil at home is infusion, where a base oil like olive or sunflower oil is infused with flavors from herbs, spices, or other flavorings. This process doesn't actually extract oil but instead flavors it, providing a simple way to create unique, flavored cooking oils. Regardless of the method, it's essential to use fresh, high-quality ingredients and to store the oil properly in a cool, dark place to prevent it from going rancid. Making your own cooking oil can be an enjoyable and satisfying process, allowing you to create custom oils tailored to your culinary needs and preferences, free from additives and unwanted blends.

A diet high in omega-6 fatty acids and low in omega-3 fatty acids has been associated with increased inflammation in the body. The body metabolizes omega-6 fatty acids into pro-inflammatory compounds, such as arachidonic acid, which can contribute to inflammation when not balanced with anti-inflammatory compounds from omega-3 fatty acids. Processed seed oils are more susceptible to oxidation when exposed to heat, light, and air during processing and cooking. Oxidized fats can generate harmful free radicals and inflammatory compounds in the body.

Some processed seed oils can undergo partial hydrogenation to increase their shelf life, resulting in the formation of harmful trans fats, which are known to promote inflammation and contribute to chronic diseases. Whole seeds, such as chia seeds, flaxseeds, and hemp seeds, contain a balanced ratio of omega-6 to omega-3 fatty acids. They are rich in alpha-linolenic acid (ALA), a plant-based omega-3 fatty acid with anti-inflammatory properties. Whole seeds also contain natural antioxidants, such as vitamin E and polyphenols, which can help protect against oxidative stress and inflammation in the body. They also are a reliable source of dietary fiber, vitamins, minerals, and other beneficial nutrients.

Fiber has been shown to have anti-inflammatory effects and can support digestive health. Minimally processed when consumed in their whole form, whole seeds preserve their natural nutrients and health-promoting compounds. Opt for raw nuts and seeds, as heat treatment can destroy nutrients. This isn't easy to do in the US as all California almonds are required to be heat treated, thus destroying their ability to sprout. Spanish-imported Almonds may be sourced as an alternative. Monounsaturated fats are considered the most beneficial for human health. They have been associated with several health benefits, including improved heart health and reduced risk of chronic diseases.

Food sources of monounsaturated fats include olive oil, avocado, nuts (such as almonds, cashews, and peanuts), and seeds (such as flaxseeds and chia seeds). It's no coincidence that the most beneficial fats for humans are those that the body can process and utilize in many avenues of the body; they are found in nuts, seeds, plants, and fruits such as avocados. The understanding that animals are living beings that are not intended to be consumed by humans helps explain why animal fats have so many adverse health effects.

The modern food landscape, influenced by government policies, agricultural practices, commercial farming incentives, and market forces, often prioritizes profit over health. This has led to a proliferation of highly processed foods designed more as money-making novelties than as nutrition sources. These foods prey on the naivety of the human condition, making it essential for individuals to take responsibility for their dietary choices and understand the impact of what they consume.

Your "eating" mindset is a personal thing that becomes a set of ideals in adulthood. Depending on how you were fed, what you ate, and what comforted you, these formative memories around food and the care you were given will shape your adult mindset. Everyone knows someone who hates peas because they were forced to eat them as a child. Everyone knows someone who reaches for the ice cream when "things" are "bad". And everyone knows someone who's "annoying" to go out with because they have to ask a lot of questions or modify menu items to eat somewhere.

There are social and personal reasons why people make the food choices they make. Still, like anything else, from finances to mortgages and interest rates, the landscape has changed. The added information is in, and it's up to the individual to reevaluate their ideas about what is going into one's body. This goes beyond choosing a salad over a burger for the sake of calorie counting. This transformation begins with an understanding of food's effects on you. It would be an injustice to yourself if you find you are not at the level of health you want to be at if you don't know the truth, and you bear the consequences.

Polyunsaturated fats are also considered healthy and are divided into two main types: omega-3 fatty acids and omega-6 fatty acids. Both types are essential for the body and play important roles in various bodily functions. Omega-3 fatty acids are mainly known for their anti-inflammatory properties and cardiovascular benefits. Flaxseeds, chia seeds, walnuts, and certain vegetable oils (such as soybean oil and sunflower oil) are good sources of omega-3s.

Saturated fats have been the subject of much debate in the past. While they were once widely regarded as detrimental to health, the understanding of their impact has evolved. Saturated fats are generally considered neutral in terms of their effect on health when consumed in moderation. Sources of saturated fats include animal fats (such as fatty cuts of meat, poultry with skin, and full-fat dairy products) and some plant-based sources (such as coconut oil and palm oil).

Trans fats are considered the least beneficial and should be avoided as much as possible. These fats are artificially created through a process called hydrogenation, which converts liquid vegetable oils into solid fats. Trans fats have been shown to raise LDL cholesterol levels, increase the risk of heart disease, and have detrimental effects on overall health. Trans fats are primarily found in processed foods, commercially baked goods, fried foods, and some margarine.

When it comes to cooking with fats and oils, it's important to consider their smoke points, stability, and nutritional profiles. Extra virgin olive oil is widely considered one of the healthiest oils. It is rich in monounsaturated fats, which have been associated with heart health. It has a relatively low smoke point, making it suitable for low to medium-heat cooking or as a finishing oil in salad dressings and dips.

One of the least processed types of cooking oil that is commonly available and non-GMO is extra virgin olive oil. Extra virgin olive oil is made from the pressing of olives and does not undergo significant refining processes. It retains the natural flavors, aroma, and nutritional benefits of olives. It is vital to choose a reputable brand to ensure the oil is truly extra virgin and not blended with lower-quality oils.

Another option is cold-pressed or expeller-pressed oils, such as cold-pressed avocado oil or cold-pressed coconut oil. These oils are mechanically extracted without the use of excessive heat or chemical solvents, preserving more of their natural properties. Flaxseed oil, for example, is not ideal for high-heat cooking due to its low smoke point and delicate nature. Its smoke point is relatively low, typically around 225°F (107°C), which means it can easily break down and produce smoke at high temperatures. When flaxseed oil reaches its smoke point, it can develop an unpleasant taste and potentially release harmful compounds.

Instead of using flaxseed oil for cooking, it is best to consume it in its raw or unheated form to maximize its nutritional benefits. Flaxseed oil is a rich source of alpha-linolenic acid (ALA), an omega-3 fatty acid, and has potential health benefits, such as reducing inflammation and supporting heart health. You can drizzle flaxseed oil over salads, add it to smoothies, or use it as a finishing oil for dishes. For cooking purposes, it is advisable to choose oils with higher smoke points, such as avocado oil, coconut oil, or refined olive oil. These oils can withstand higher temperatures without breaking down or producing harmful byproducts.

It's worth noting that the term "non-GMO" refers to the genetic modification of the source crop rather than the processing method of the oil itself. So, when selecting a non-GMO oil, it's important to look for oils derived from non-GMO plant sources, such as non-GMO soybean oil or non-GMO sunflower oil. Keep in mind that even minimally processed oils, including non-GMO options, can still undergo some processing steps to extract and refine the oil. If you're looking for the least processed option overall, you may consider oils that are minimally refined, such as unrefined or virgin oils, which undergo fewer processing steps and retain more of their natural characteristics.

Always check the product labels and look for oils that are labeled as "cold-pressed," "extra virgin," "unrefined," or "virgin" to ensure a less processed and non-GMO option. Avocado oil is another healthy choice for cooking. It has a high smoke point and is rich in monounsaturated fats, vitamins, and minerals. Avocado oil is versatile and can be used for high-heat cooking, such as sautéing or roasting. Coconut oil, a highly saturated fat, has gained popularity in recent years. It has a relatively high smoke point and is suitable for medium to high-heat cooking. However, due to its high saturated fat content, it is advised to be used in moderation.

Canola oil is low in saturated fat and high in monounsaturated fats. It has a moderately high smoke point and is a versatile option for various cooking methods, including sautéing, baking, and grilling. Canola oil is derived from the seeds of the canola plant, a variety of rapeseed that has been bred to have lower levels of erucic acid and glucosinolates. The name "canola" is a contraction of "Canada" and "ola," which means oil. Canola oil was developed in Canada in the 1970s through selective breeding to create a rapeseed oil with improved nutritional characteristics.

The main difference between traditional rapeseed oil and canola oil lies in their chemical composition. Conventional rapeseed oil contains higher levels of erucic acid, a type of monounsaturated omega-9 fatty acid, and glucosinolates, which are sulfur-containing compounds responsible for the characteristic pungent taste and odor of cruciferous vegetables. Canola oil, on the other hand, has been selectively bred to have significantly reduced levels of erucic acid and glucosinolates, making it milder in flavor and odor. Canola oil's lower levels of erucic acid make it more suitable for human consumption, as a high intake of erucic acid has been associated with potential health concerns. Canola oil has a favorable fatty acid profile, with a relatively high content of monounsaturated fats, including oleic acid, and a balanced ratio of omega-6 to omega-3 fatty acids.

Canola oil is derived from the rapeseed plant but is specifically bred to have lower levels of erucic acid and glucosinolates, making it a healthier and more versatile cooking oil than traditional rapeseed oil. Canola/rapeseed (Brassica napus, Brassica rapa, and Brassica juncea of canola quality) is the world's second-largest oilseed crop. The primary product of canola/rapeseed is vegetable oil (40% by seed weight), and the protein-rich meal (38% protein by meal weight) is a coproduct. Nutritionally, canola/rapeseed proteins are comparable with soybeans and contain more sulfur amino acids than many other oilseed meals. Current knowledge of canola/rapeseed protein is extensive. However, the main emphasis of research in the past has been the use of meal protein in animal feed rather than food-grade protein products.

Grapeseed oil has a high smoke point and is relatively neutral in flavor. It is rich in polyunsaturated fats, particularly omega-6 fatty acids. It can be used for high-heat cooking and in salad dressings. Peanut oil has a high smoke point and a neutral flavor, making it suitable for high-heat cooking methods like deep frying. It contains monounsaturated fats and is commonly used in Asian cuisine. Butter and ghee (clarified butter) are derived from milk and are primarily composed of saturated fats. While they add flavor to dishes, they have relatively low smoke points and are better suited for low to medium-heat cooking or as toppings.

It's important to note that heating oils at high temperatures can cause chemical changes in their molecular structure, potentially leading to the formation of harmful compounds. This process is known as oxidation. Oils with low smoke points, such as extra virgin olive oil, are more prone to oxidation at high temperatures. When cooking at high temperatures, it's recommended to choose oils with higher smoke points, such as avocado oil, peanut oil, or canola oil. Additionally, it's essential to avoid reusing oils for frying as it further increases the production of harmful compounds.

Grapeseed oil is made by pressing the oil from the seeds of grapes. It predominantly comprises polyunsaturated fats, particularly omega-6 fatty acids. It contains a good balance of linoleic acid (an essential omega-6 fatty acid) and alpha-linolenic acid (an essential omega-3 fatty acid). However, it is vital to maintain a balanced ratio of omega-6 to omega-3 fatty acids in the diet, as excessive omega-6 intake relative to omega-3s may promote inflammation in some individuals. Grapeseed oil contains antioxidants, such as vitamin E and various phenolic compounds, associated with potential health benefits, including reducing inflammation and protecting against oxidative stress. Grapeseed oil has a high smoke point, which makes it suitable for high-heat cooking methods such as stir-frying, sautéing, and baking. Its high smoke point means it can withstand temperatures before breaking down and producing smoke. Grapeseed oil has a mild and neutral flavor, which makes it versatile for use in various culinary applications, including salad dressings, marinades, and cooking oil.

Grapeseed oil is relatively high in omega-6 fatty acids compared to other oils, and excessive consumption of omega-6 fatty acids relative to omega-3s may have adverse health implications for some individuals. It's recommended to consume a variety of fats and oils in moderation as part of a balanced diet. The balance between omega-6 and omega-3 fatty acids is important for maintaining overall health. While omega-6 and omega-3 fatty acids are necessary for the body, an imbalance can lead to certain health concerns.

Omega-6 fatty acids, when metabolized in the body, can give rise to pro-inflammatory molecules called eicosanoids. In contrast, omega-3 fatty acids are involved in producing anti-inflammatory eicosanoids. An excessive intake of omega-6 fatty acids relative to omega-3s can tip the balance towards a pro-inflammatory state, potentially promoting chronic inflammation. Chronic inflammation is associated with various health conditions, including cardiovascular disease, arthritis, and certain cancers.

In modern Western diets, the typical ratio of omega-6 to omega-3 fatty acids is much higher than optimal for health. While estimates vary, it is generally recommended to maintain a balance of omega-6 to omega-3 fatty acids between 4:1 and 1:1. However, the typical Western diet may have a ratio as high as 16:1 or even higher. This imbalance may contribute to inflammation and increase the risk of chronic diseases.

Omega-6 and omega-3 fatty acids compete for the same enzymes in the body for metabolism. When omega-6 fatty acids dominate the diet, they may possibly outcompete omega-3s, reducing the incorporation and utilization of omega-3 fatty acids in the body. This further exacerbates the imbalance between the two fatty acid types. These fatty acids are not inherently evil or unhealthy. They play crucial roles in the body's physiological processes. The key is maintaining a balanced intake of omega-6 and omega-3 fatty acids to promote overall health and minimize the risk of chronic inflammation. It's recommended to consume a variety of healthy fats and oils, including sources of omega-6 fatty acids (such as grapeseed oil) and omega-3 fatty acids (such as walnuts, chia seeds, and flaxseeds).

By opting to eat raw foods, salads, and foods cooked in other ways, you can still reap the benefits of oils with a lower heat point by drizzling them over the foods as a dressing. Certain types of fish, specifically larger predatory fish, may be more likely to contain higher levels of heavy metals like mercury due to bioaccumulation in their tissues. However, most fish oil supplements are typically derived from smaller fish species known to have lower levels of heavy metal contamination.

The problem is that marketing has made it seem like fish oil is the only way to get omegas. There are superior, less processed forms available. While eating whole foods for these beneficial oils is ideal, those who are advised by their doctor to add fish oil supplements are probably not using a food coach or a dietician to monitor their macros. There are healthier, more bio-available options for these lipids. EPA (eicosapentaenoic acid) and DHA (docosahexaenoic acid) are primarily found in marine sources such as fish and algae.

However, vegan sources are available that can provide EPA and DHA. These sources include algal oil, which is derived from algae and is a direct source of EPA and DHA. Algae are the source of omega fatty acids in the marine food chain, and certain algae species are cultivated specifically for their high EPA and DHA content. Algal oil supplements are available in the form of capsules or liquid and can provide an alternative source of these essential fatty acids for vegans.

Some species of seaweed and microalgae naturally contain small amounts of EPA and DHA. While the levels of EPA and DHA in these plant-based sources are generally lower compared to fish or algal oil supplements, regularly incorporating them into your diet can contribute to your overall omega-3 intake. Alternatively, two tablespoons of chia seeds in your smoothie, salad, etc., is a much less expensive and natural option with the additional gut benefits that a processed fish oil capsule of unknown origin can provide. This is all about making the best decision for your health. And the whole food option is always going to be the best for bio validity because it is a food in its purest form.

Palm oil is extracted from the fruit of the oil palm tree (Elaeis guineensis). The oil palm tree produces large clusters of fruit, and the flesh of the fruit is used to extract palm oil. The palm fruit contains both the pulp and the palm kernel, and palm oil is obtained from the pulp. Coconut oil, on the other hand, is extracted from the meat (also known as the kernel or copra) of mature coconuts, which come from the coconut palm tree (Cocos nucifera). The meat is typically dried and then pressed to extract the oil.

Although palm oil and coconut oil are derived from palm and coconut trees, they have different compositions and properties. Palm oil is predominantly saturated fat, while coconut oil is high in saturated fat but contains a significant number of medium-chain triglycerides (MCTs), specifically lauric acid. These oils' different fatty acid profiles contribute to variations in their culinary applications and potential health effects.

The controversy surrounding seed oils stems from the fact that they are often refined oils created through synthetic chemical extraction methods that sometimes include additional processing like bleaching and deodorizing. These include canola, soybean, corn, cottonseed, grapeseed, safflower, sunflower, rice bran, and peanut oils. Seed oils are typically high in polyunsaturated fatty acids (PUFAs), specifically omega-6 fatty acids. While omega-6 fatty acids are essential for the body, excessive consumption of omega-6 fatty acids, relative to omega-3 fatty acids, may contribute to an imbalance in the body's fatty acid profile. This imbalance has been associated with increased inflammation and potentially adverse health effects.

The processing methods used to extract and refine seed oils can affect their nutritional profile and stability. High-temperature processing methods and the use of chemical solvents in extraction may lead to the formation of trans fats or the degradation of beneficial compounds. Opting for cold-pressed or minimally processed seed oils may be preferable. The impact of seed oils on health can vary among individuals depending on factors such as overall diet, lifestyle, genetic factors, and existing health conditions. Some individuals may tolerate and benefit from moderate consumption of certain seed oils, while others may choose to limit or avoid them.

Not all seed oils are the same, and their nutritional profiles can vary. Some seed oils, such as flaxseed oil or chia seed oil, are higher in omega-3 fatty acids and may offer certain health benefits. Avoid heavily processed seed oils like soybean oil, which is commonly used and heavily processed, often extracted using high-temperature mechanical methods, followed by refining, bleaching, and deodorizing processes. Corn oil is another widely used seed oil that typically undergoes significant processing, including extraction using solvents and refining processes. Canola oil is derived from the seeds of the canola plant, which is a variety of rapeseed. It often undergoes extensive processing, including solvent extraction, refining, and deodorizing.

Less processed or minimally processed seed oils include extra virgin olive oil, which is minimally processed and extracted solely through mechanical means. It is obtained from the fruit of the olive tree and is known for its health benefits. Flaxseed oil, derived from the seeds of the flax plant, is typically cold-pressed or undergoes minimal processing to preserve its nutrient content, including omega-3 fatty acids. Hempseed oil is obtained from the seeds of the hemp plant and is often cold pressed, which helps retain the natural qualities of the oil. Chia seed oil is extracted from chia seeds using a cold-pressing method, which helps maintain its nutritional properties.

Sesame oil is often considered a healthy option due to its rich content of monounsaturated and polyunsaturated fats, including omega-6 fatty acids. These fats can help promote heart health by reducing bad cholesterol (LDL cholesterol) levels and improving the balance between LDL and good cholesterol (HDL cholesterol). Sesame oil contains natural antioxidants, including sesamol and sesaminol, which have been shown to have protective effects against oxidative stress and inflammation in the body. These antioxidants may contribute to various health benefits. Sesame oil is also a good source of several essential nutrients, including vitamin E, which is an antioxidant that helps protect cells from damage. It also contains minerals such as calcium, iron, and magnesium.

Some studies suggest that certain components of sesame oil, such as sesamin, may have anti-inflammatory effects. This could potentially benefit individuals with conditions related to inflammation, although further research is needed to understand these effects fully. Sesame oil adds a distinctive flavor to dishes and is commonly used in Asian cuisine. It can be used for stir-frying, sautéing, and as a flavorful dressing or marinade for salads and other dishes.

Black sesame seeds and white sesame seeds have different pigmentation due to variations in their seed coats. Black sesame seeds are darker in color due to the presence of pigments like melanin and anthocyanins. Black sesame seed oil is often considered to have higher antioxidant content compared to white sesame seed oil. The dark color of black sesame seeds indicates the presence of antioxidants, including anthocyanins, which have potential health benefits. Black sesame seed oil may have a slightly stronger, nuttier flavor compared to white sesame seed oil. The flavor difference is subtle and may not significantly impact the nutritional composition.

Both black and white sesame seed oil contain similar amounts of healthy fats, including monounsaturated and polyunsaturated fats. They are also good sources of vitamin E, which is an antioxidant that helps protect cells from damage. Black sesame seeds are often associated with various health benefits in traditional medicine systems, including promoting hair health and preventing premature greying. These claims are mainly anecdotal and have not been extensively studied or supported by scientific evidence.

While black sesame seeds and black sesame oil contain minerals such as iron, calcium, magnesium, and zinc, which are essential for overall health. There is a big difference in the process of extruding soybean oil and sesame oil. If you can make it at home, it is likely a more wholesome choice when it comes to food. You can start with the base of sesame seeds at home, and pulverize them in a food mill, coffee grinder, or high-speed blender. This opens the cell wall up, making butter. This then will separate, the oil rising to the top and then can be poured off and used in dressings, for cooking, marinades, etc.

Nuts and seed oils should be kept in a cool dark place as they are perishable. The best way to determine what is best for you is to detox all of the garbage foods and reintroduce whole options one at a time until your body has an opportunity to recover from the assault and addiction of these negative impact food and readjust to foods that will increase your wellness. Cacao butter, also known as cocoa butter, is a type of vegetable fat extracted from cacao beans.

Cacao butter has a relatively high smoke point, which is the temperature at which the fat starts to break down and produce smoke. The smoke point of cacao butter is typically around 375°F to

392°F (190°C to 200°C), depending on the specific product and quality. This makes it suitable for various cooking methods, including sautéing, baking, and frying at moderate to high temperatures. Cacao butter has a distinct chocolate aroma and flavor, which can impart a unique taste to the dishes it is used in. This can be desirable in certain recipes, particularly those that benefit from a hint of chocolate flavor.

Solid at room temperature, cacao butter melts at slightly above body temperature. This characteristic can provide a smooth and creamy texture to recipes when it is used as a fat ingredient. It is free from cholesterol and contains trace amounts of vitamins and minerals. However, it is important to note that cacao butter is a calorie-dense fat, so it should be consumed in moderation as part of a balanced diet. While cacao butter can be used for cooking at higher temperatures, it is worth considering the overall flavor and aroma it imparts to the dish. It is often used in desserts, confections, and chocolate-based recipes to take advantage of its unique properties.

Additionally, oils like shea, coconut, and cocoa can be used topically. Once you know this, the number of unnecessary ingredients on your moisturizer's label could help you understand why your skin never really feels dewy, glowing, and fully quenched. Simply blending a solid at room temperature "butter" with one part oil liquid at room temperature will give you a perfect all-purpose moisturizer that should whip up in your mixing bowl like whipped cream does, as you can whip anything with a fat content. Adding a bit of Arrowroot powder can take out some of the greasy feeling.

If you are concerned about getting this on your clothes, use it sparingly, or use it before bed. Your skin is your body's largest organ, and it will absorb all the chemicals in your creams and lotions, so give yourself a chance to thrive and remove as many chemicals from your daily interactions as you can.

Fats and oils shouldn't be feared, they play a significant role in our diets, influencing not only our health but also the enjoyment of food. Understanding the difference between various types of fats, their sources, and how they are processed can help us make better dietary choices. By focusing on whole, minimally processed foods and balancing our intake of different types of fats, we can support our health, reduce the risk of chronic diseases, and enjoy the flavors and textures that fats bring to our meals

10
EAT BEFORE YOU'RE HUNGRY, DRINK BEFORE YOU'RE THIRSTY

A sophisticated network within us orchestrates a symphony of hormones and signals, constantly communicating with the gut to gauge satiety or hunger. This intricate system is crucial for maintaining the delicate balance necessary to keep our body's complex processes finely tuned for synthesis, repair, and overall function at the cellular level. Despite their complexity, these signals are often overlooked in the fast-paced, convenience-driven world we live in today, leading to poor dietary choices and imbalanced eating habits. Understanding these signals and responding to them appropriately is key to maintaining not just our weight but our overall health.

When the body experiences hunger, it sends out signals in the form of hormones, like ghrelin, often referred to as the "hunger hormone." Ghrelin is secreted by the stomach and stimulates appetite by signaling the brain's hypothalamus, which regulates hunger and energy balance. Its levels rise before meals and decrease after eating. However, when we ignore these signals or wait too long between meals, the body can enter a state of energy conservation, often resulting in muscle breakdown and fat storage. This process is known as metabolic adaptation, an evolutionary mechanism designed to help humans survive periods of food scarcity.

The body's primary goal during periods of prolonged fasting or significant caloric deficits is to preserve energy for essential functions, such as maintaining brain and organ function. This survival mechanism can be traced back to our ancestors, who faced frequent famines and relied on stored body fat and muscle tissue for energy during these times. Unfortunately, in today's world, where food is abundant but often nutritionally poor, this response can have unintended consequences, including loss of muscle mass and increased fat storage.

Waiting too long to eat triggers the brain's survival instincts, making us crave high-calorie foods that are rich in fat, sugar, and salt—nutrients that provide quick energy and are easily stored as fat. This is why, after hours of not eating, people often find themselves reaching for candy, chips, or fast food. These cravings are not merely a lack of willpower but are driven by biological signals meant to ensure our survival.

However, this cycle can be reversed by understanding and responding to these hunger signals in a timely and balanced manner. By eating small, balanced meals every few hours, you send a clear message of abundance to your brain. This abundance signals your body that it no longer needs to conserve energy, which can lead to increased energy levels, improved skin, nails, and hair, reduced fat stores, and increased muscle growth when paired with appropriate exercise. Developing these habits requires consistent effort. It is estimated that it takes about 30 repetitions of a new behavior to form a habit, making the practice of eating regularly an investment in long-term health.

Research supports the idea that eating every few hours can help stabilize blood sugar levels, prevent metabolic slowdown, and promote fat loss while preserving muscle mass. When you consume food, blood glucose levels rise, providing energy. The pancreas releases insulin, which helps transport glucose into cells, where it is used for energy. If you go too long without eating, blood glucose levels drop, leading to hypoglycemia, which triggers hunger and cravings for quick-energy foods, often high in sugar and fat.

Maintaining stable blood sugar levels by eating frequently can reduce the risk of insulin resistance, a condition where cells become less responsive to insulin, leading to higher blood sugar levels and an increased risk of type 2 diabetes. Moreover, regular eating helps keep the metabolism active. When the body receives food consistently, it doesn't feel the need to store fat for future energy use, thus supporting weight management efforts.

Understanding hunger signals is akin to listening to a car's engine. If you ignore the fuel warning light, the car will eventually run out of gas and stop. Similarly, when the body sends out hunger signals that are ignored, it will continue to function for a while, but eventually, it will start to conserve energy, leading to a metabolic slowdown. By responding to these signals promptly with balanced, nutrient-rich meals, you prevent the need for drastic measures to recover from a state of depletion.

Ignoring hunger signals and allowing yourself to become overly hungry increases the likelihood of overeating or choosing high-calorie, low-nutrient foods. This is a natural response driven by the body's attempt to prevent starvation by clinging to calories. Although this survival mechanism served our ancestors well, it is largely misunderstood and often counterproductive in modern society, where food is readily available.

The modern food environment is flooded with advertisements for diet products, supplements, and weight-loss procedures, contributing to a multi-billion-dollar industry that often obscures the fundamental truths of how our bodies function. Understanding these truths is the first step toward leveraging our innate evolutionary mechanisms for our benefit. By learning to recognize and respond to hunger signals appropriately, you can achieve a healthier, more balanced approach to eating that supports both immediate and long-term health.

At first, trusting your body's signals may seem counterintuitive, especially if past experiences with cravings have led to weight gain or other health issues. However, by learning to listen to and interpret these signals correctly, you can harness the power of your body's natural hunger cues. Your eyes, brain, and stomach are key players in selecting the nourishment that will enable your body to thrive at its optimal weight.

Rigid meal plans aren't necessary for a lifetime of health. While they can serve as a useful jumpstart for those new to balanced eating, a more flexible approach is often more sustainable. The goal is to understand and respond to your body's needs rather than adhering strictly to a prescribed set of rules. This flexible approach allows for the occasional indulgence without guilt or fear of derailing progress.

Eating to fuel strength, rather than just to lose weight, is a critical shift in mindset. Traditional diet and exercise regimens often emphasize cardio workouts and diets high in protein, low in carbohydrates, and sparse in fats. Intermittent fasting has also gained popularity. Despite the myriad of approaches to weight loss, a comprehensive understanding remains elusive for many. It is true that consuming fewer calories than one expends will lead to weight loss, but the quality of those calories and the balance of macronutrients are what is important to achieve genuine satiation.

Each calorie consumed should be viewed as an opportunity to infuse nutrition into your bloodstream and introduce diverse fibers into your microbiome. Think of yourself as a prudent shopper with a fixed budget, striving to get the most nutritional value for your money. The goal is to maximize the nutritional content of every calorie, ensuring that each meal is a balanced combination of fats, proteins, and carbohydrates that fuels strength and health rather than simply aiming for thinness.

For instance, a banana is a healthy snack choice, but pairing it with nut butter provides a balance of fats, carbohydrates, and proteins, creating a more satisfying and nutrient-dense snack. Including all macronutrient groups, fats, carbohydrates, insoluble fibers, and proteins, at each meal allows your brain to check all its nutritional boxes, reducing the prospect of cravings and overeating.

Eating plain celery or carrot sticks will not leave you feeling satisfied, no matter how many you eat. However, adding a dip like hummus, rich in protein and healthy fats, not only makes these snacks more enjoyable but also helps stabilize blood sugar levels over a longer period, thanks to the fiber's effect on slowing carbohydrate absorption. The practice of food combining and pairing foods that digest at different rates results in prolonged fullness, significantly reducing the impulse to make poor food choices due to hunger.

When you eat foods high in protein and fiber, which digest slowly, your stomach releases a hormone called Peptide YY, which signals the brain to reduce hunger and increase feelings of satiety. Fats, while less time-intensive to digest, provide a higher calorie density and stimulate the release of another hormone, Cholecystokinin, which also promotes feelings of fullness. By understanding and aligning with your body's natural messaging system, you can create a rhythm of eating that prevents hunger from becoming overwhelming and reduces the risk of overeating.

Carbohydrates are often misunderstood, especially processed carbohydrates that, when consumed in isolation or in large amounts without the balancing effects of fiber or protein, can cause blood sugar spikes and crashes. These fluctuations can lead to increased calorie intake and persistent hunger. In contrast, whole foods like fruits, vegetables, and whole grains contain insoluble fiber, which slows carbohydrate absorption and provides a steady, sustainable energy source.

Including a balance of fats, carbohydrates, and fiber with every meal or snack can prevent constant thoughts about food after eating. These thoughts often arise when we eat based on mood rather than true hunger and fail to meet our body's nutritional needs. The aim should be to nourish the body, not just to satisfy fleeting cravings. Creating a routine that prioritizes wellness is a fundamental form of self-care. The food you choose to eat is at the heart of your self-care practice, influencing your health, energy levels, and overall well-being.

Your eating habits as an adult are often shaped by dietary patterns established during childhood. This makes it important to re-assess the habits you've developed over the years and determine which ones genuinely serve your well-being. Rather than sticking to outdated habits that may not benefit you, consider adopting new practices that align with your current health goals.

Many people develop poor eating habits due to convenience or societal pressures, leading to the consumption of processed foods high in additives and low in nutrients. These foods are designed to be addictive, making it easy to fall into a cycle of sugar cravings and energy crashes. Such patterns often begin in childhood and continue into adulthood, leading to a state of unwellness that can become normalized over time.

Setting personalized daily calorie targets is a crucial step in managing your diet and ensuring that you meet your nutritional needs without overeating. By planning meals and visualizing your daily intake, you gain control over your diet, making it easier to avoid impulsive food choices driven by hunger or convenience. Instead of running around all day, skipping meals, and then reaching for pizza and ice cream in a state of ravenous hunger, a more structured approach to eating can help you maintain steady energy levels throughout the day.

An ideal meal plan template for someone looking to restructure their eating patterns might involve consuming 20 to 30 grams of protein every two to three hours. Depending on your lifestyle and preferences, this could take the form of three meals and three snacks, six small meals, or four meals and two snacks. Regular protein intake helps stabilize blood sugar levels, supports muscle repair and growth, and promotes satiety, reducing the likelihood of overeating at any given meal.

Twenty grams of protein from plant-based sources can come from a variety of foods, each contributing different amino acid profiles. For example, one cup of cooked lentils provides about 18 grams of protein and contains a good mix of essential amino acids, particularly lysine, which is often lacking in cereal grains. While lentils are low in methionine, they pair well with grains like rice, which is lower in lysine but higher in methionine, creating a complementary protein profile.

Another source, quinoa, contains all nine essential amino acids and provides around 8 grams of protein per cooked cup. Thus, two and a half cups of quinoa would give you approximately 20 grams of protein with a balanced amino acid profile. Quinoa is a particularly valuable food for those on a plant-based diet because it is a complete protein, which means it has an adequate proportion of all essential amino acids.

Tofu, made from soybeans, is another excellent plant-based protein source. A half-cup serving of tofu can provide around 10 grams of protein. Two half-cup servings, therefore, offer 20 grams of protein and a well-rounded amino acid profile. Soy protein is one of the few plant-based proteins that are considered complete, making tofu, edamame, and other soy products ideal for meeting amino acid needs.

Chickpeas are also a valuable protein source. One cup of cooked chickpeas offers around 15 grams of protein, and consuming about one and a half cups would yield roughly 20 grams of protein. Chickpeas are rich in lysine but, like lentils, are lower in methionine. Pairing chickpeas with grains such as quinoa or whole wheat can balance out the amino acid profile, ensuring that all essential amino acids are consumed.

Nutritional guidelines are often based on a 2,000-calorie-per-day diet, which is intended for the average active person. However, individual needs vary, and this standard may not be appropriate for everyone. A sedentary person consuming 2,000 calories a day, especially from highly processed foods, may find themselves in a state of sluggish metabolism and poor digestion.

Processed foods often lack the essential nutrients and fiber needed to support optimal health, leading to a cascade of negative effects on well-being. Including a variety of colorful fruits and vegetables in each meal or snack is another important strategy for maintaining a balanced diet. Different colors in fruits and vegetables often indicate different nutrients, such as vitamins, minerals, and antioxidants, which are essential for a well-balanced body chemistry. For example, orange foods like carrots and sweet potatoes are rich in beta-carotene, which the body converts into vitamin A, essential for vision and immune function. Green vegetables like spinach and broccoli are packed with folate, which supports cell function and tissue growth. By diversifying your intake of these foods, you ensure that your body receives a broad spectrum of nutrients, supporting overall health and vitality.

Salads that include a variety of vegetables, seeds, nuts, and a protein source like grilled tofu or tempeh can serve as a filling, nutrient-packed meal that supports metabolic health. Simple snacks like crudité platters with hummus or homemade plant-based mozzarella offer fiber, protein, and healthy fats, helping to stabilize blood sugar levels and prevent energy crashes. Indulging in treats like tahini brownies, made with nutrient-dense ingredients like sesame seeds, provides not only satisfaction for a sweet tooth but also a dose of calcium and healthy fats.

Smoothie bowls, thick and creamy, topped with nut butter and seeds, can be a delightful way to incorporate fruits, protein, and healthy fats into your diet, providing sustained energy and nutrients. Spaghetti squash with fresh pesto and marinara is a low-carb, fiber-rich alternative to pasta that still satisfies the craving for Italian flavors. Garlic asparagus and zucchini offer a flavorful, nutrient-dense side dish that supports digestion and immune health.

Simple snacks like air-popped popcorn, when sprinkled with nutritional yeast and Harissa spices or drizzled with maple syrup and paired with grapes, can satisfy both savory and sweet cravings without the need for processed snacks. For heartier meals, BBQ-baked tofu with roasted sweet potatoes and massaged kale offers a balanced, protein-rich, and flavorful dish that supports muscle health, digestion, and overall vitality.

By integrating these practices into your daily routine, you not only satisfy your hunger but also nourish your body with the nutrients it needs to thrive. This approach to eating aligns with your body's natural rhythms and supports long-term health, helping to prevent the metabolic slowdown that can occur with poor dietary habits. Emphasizing whole, nutrient-dense foods and regular, balanced meals ensures that your energy levels remain stable, your metabolism functions efficiently, and your body is equipped to perform at its best, day in and day out.

Changing your eating patterns requires a shift in mindset. Many individuals ignore their actual cravings for whole foods, replacing them with chemically-laden processed items that leave the body feeling tired, sluggish, and still hungry. To break this cycle, it's essential to start listening to your body's signals. Instead of reaching for the nearest convenient snack, take a moment to ask yourself why you want a particular food, what specific flavor you're craving, and how you can satisfy that craving with whole, nourishing food. For example, if you find yourself craving something sweet, consider whether your body might be asking for natural sugars found in fruits rather than processed snacks. By tuning into these signals, you honor your body and begin to shift your eating habits toward true nourishment rather than empty calories.

To make your body the best tool it can be to ward off disease and maintain overall health, it's crucial to remove every obstacle. This involves not only changing what you eat but also how you think about food and self-care. Sometimes, negative habits develop when we don't fully value ourselves, leading us to make choices that don't serve our well-being. The time has come to learn how to properly nourish yourself, recognizing that every choice you make has an impact on your health.

Creating a grocery list focused on whole foods is a smart step to take before shopping. This approach helps prevent impulse buys, which often lead to overspending or failing to purchase the necessary items for a complete meal. Shopping or dining out on an empty stomach usually results in poor choices, driven by the body's urgent need for calories.

When you approach even a minimal level of starvation, your body cries out for energy. Without a plan in mind, you might end up buying a variety of foods that you later regret yet feel obligated to consume because they're already in your pantry. This lack of planning not only affects your diet but can also lead to a cycle of unhealthy eating.

Hunger can significantly impact your mood, often leading to irritability or impatience. The common 4 o'clock slump is a familiar experience for those who skip meals. Ignoring hunger can result in fatigue, weakness, and difficulty concentrating. In these situations, many people reach for a second coffee or an energy drink. While this may temporarily dampen hunger signals, it increases cortisol levels and disrupts your metabolism, guaranteeing that once the caffeine wears off, you'll face insatiable hunger.

Consuming food before the onset of hunger is an exercise in mindfulness and self-awareness. This practice allows you to distinguish true hunger from emotional cravings and make informed choices about nourishing your body. It's like filling your car's fuel tank with the right type of gasoline before it runs low, ensuring that your body remains in optimal condition rather than waiting until it's running on empty.

Start caring for your body with the same diligence, if not more, that you apply to other aspects of your life. Breaking free from patterns of mindless eating, whether it's grabbing whatever is convenient, succumbing to the allure of prepackaged snacks, or delaying meals until hunger becomes overwhelming, requires mindfulness and intention. Consider a scenario where you're pressed for time, and hunger strikes. It's easy to reach for a caffeinated drink to keep your energy up, temporarily dulling the hunger. Instead, try choosing food in its purest form, opting for single ingredients that are naturally delicious even on their own.

Take traditional pizza, for example. Imagine eating uncooked flour with a spoon. It's hardly appetizing, right? A crust made from cauliflower, however, is a far superior choice, as cauliflower is inherently flavorful and enjoyable even without added ingredients. The market and online platforms are filled with alternatives for traditional pizza, offering responsible ways to satisfy your cravings. By indulging in a more wholesome version, you can enjoy your favorite foods whenever the urge strikes, with the awareness that it's not the indulgence itself but the manner of its preparation that truly matters.

This approach allows you to satisfy your desires while prioritizing your health. By choosing nourishing, natural ingredients over processed options, you align your eating habits with the care and respect you naturally extend to other aspects of your life. In doing so, you create a sustainable path to well-being where you can enjoy your favorite foods without compromising your health.

Knowing how not to eat is half the equation; knowing how much, how often, and what to eat to achieve and maintain your ideal weight is the other half. With a better understanding of which foods you need to replace and what your calorie needs are to live, look, and feel your best, you can create a new norm and a new series of habits that become a lifestyle where you find your ideal weight. The only way to lose weight is by creating a calorie deficit, either by decreasing your daily overall calorie intake or increasing your metabolic rate through exercise. This is why the nutrition in the foods you choose to eat is so important. Both burning calories and increasing muscle mass are integral to burning more overall calories, even while at rest.

Understanding your macronutrient requirements is crucial to achieving your fitness goals, whether you aim to shed pounds or bulk up. Limiting fat intake to 30% of daily calories, with saturated fats making up no more than 10%, is a good starting point for calculating your needs.

Next, determine your protein intake. A simple method is to use your target weight—provided it's not more than 20 to 30 pounds away from your current weight. For example, if you're aiming for a target weight of 150 pounds, you should aim for 150 grams of protein per day. Since protein provides 4 calories per gram, you can multiply your target protein intake by this number to get your daily calorie target from protein. To evaluate the protein content in food, check nutrition labels. For an item with 20 grams of protein, expect about 80 calories from protein. However, some foods contain more than just protein. For instance, peanut butter is high in protein but also rich in fat. Remember to account for the calories from fat towards your daily fat allowance, even though the food also provides protein.

For carbohydrates, understanding the difference between refined and complex carbohydrates is key. Traditional wheat pasta is mainly a carbohydrate source, but alternatives like chickpea pasta offer higher protein content. When choosing carbohydrates, opt for those that provide fiber, such as whole grains, fruits, and vegetables, to help stabilize blood sugar levels and support digestion.

A less stringent way of tracking your meals while transitioning to healthier eating is to take photos of everything you eat. If you plan on recording it in an app or a journal for macro-based meal tracking, keeping a photo file can help you remember what you ate when you have time to log it.

This creates accountability toward your future self when you look back on it, even if you aren't using a tracking app. You are more likely to succeed if you create accountability, even if you reflect on your days or weeks' meals just by the vibe of the photos.

Accountability to others, such as a trainer, spouse, or workout buddy, is a great tool for creating a support system. However, the most powerful form of accountability is to develop it within yourself. Taking pictures of what you eat in a day and reviewing them at the end will help you make better choices more often because you have to acknowledge your choices.

It is vital to take the time to reflect on your journey. Progress happens incrementally, and it's easy to miss how far you've come if you don't stop to take stock. Acknowledging your small victories can be the fuel you need to keep going. Use your meal photos, journal entries, or tracking apps not just as tools for accountability but as a way to celebrate how much you've accomplished. These milestones, no matter how small, are stepping stones toward the larger goals you're aiming for.

Forgiving yourself for past mistakes is another essential part of the process. The road to healthier habits is rarely a straight line, and there will be setbacks. Instead of letting these moments derail your progress, use them as learning opportunities. Ask yourself what triggered the lapse, what you can do differently next time, and how you can move forward with renewed commitment. By treating yourself with kindness and understanding, you foster resilience, which is key to long-term success.

As you continue to develop these habits, you'll find that they start to become second nature. What once required conscious effort will gradually become automatic. This is the beauty of consistency; it rewires your brain and body to align with your new lifestyle. Over time, the healthier choices you make today will shape the person you become tomorrow.

Remember, you are not alone in this journey. Connecting with others, whether through social media communities, support groups, or friends and family who share your goals, can provide the encouragement and motivation you need to stay on track. Share your successes, seek advice during challenges, and offer support to others in return. Together, you can create a network of positive reinforcement that makes it easier to stick to your goals and enjoy the process.

In conclusion, anticipating hunger and planning meals and

snacks is not just about controlling what you eat; it's about empowering yourself to make choices that support your health and well-being. By understanding your body's signals, setting realistic goals, and creating a supportive environment, you can break the cycle of poor eating habits and establish a sustainable, balanced approach to nutrition. This process requires time, patience, and commitment, but the rewards—a healthier, stronger, and more vibrant you—are well worth the effort. Embrace the journey, celebrate your progress, and keep moving forward with confidence and determination. By doing so, you honor yourself and your body, laying the foundation for a lifetime of health and wellness.

11
KNOW YOUR CRAVINGS

Mapping the intricate landscape of our cravings is like navigating a vast terrain where the mind and body communicate through the gut-brain axis, a complex superhighway of signals that dictates the foods we reach for to satiate our deepest desires. When the mind's longing for a particular taste melds with real or perceived hunger, signals are sent to the gut, urging you to fulfill that craving. This intricate dialogue is not one-sided; our gut's microbiome can send its own powerful messages back to the brain, influencing our cravings based on the type of gut bacteria we are hosting.

Our physical form communicates its needs through cravings, which are shaped by the sustenance we regularly consume. If one's diet is dominated by processed meats, cheeses, sugary beverages, and alcohol, especially in evening meals, this shapes the body's expectations. The body starts to believe these are the only options available, and as a result, individuals adhering to such dietary patterns seldom yearn for items like steamed broccoli or fresh salads because these aren't recognized as typical offerings. This indicates a disordered gut microbiome, necessitating a dual rehabilitation approach that involves reintroducing foods rich in nutrients and fiber to revitalize your cells and microbiome.

When we consume food or drink, the molecules interact with these receptors, initiating a sequence of taste transduction, a transformation of chemical stimuli into electrical signals. These signals travel through our taste nerves to the brain's gustatory cortex for processing, alongside contributions from the olfactory cortex for smell and the somatosensory cortex for texture and temperature. While this may sound intricate, it all happens without us even realizing it, creating an electrical interpretation of our foods, from the initial taste to the mouthfeel and aroma.

This multisensorial dance informs your brain's perception of flavor, rounding out taste with smell, texture, temperature, and visual cues. Moreover, altering just one element, such as the color of a familiar food under a different light, can significantly impact our ability to perceive its flavor, demonstrating the significance of presentation. Your brain is wired to detect and avoid potential spoilage in food, often flagged by changes in color. This protective response is designed to keep you from consuming anything that might be harmful.

There is a misconception that consuming animal products automatically provides all the necessary nutrients. In reality, the nutrients present in animal muscles do not always translate efficiently into our bodies. Animal products lack phytonutrients and living enzymes that are found in plant-based foods. While meat might appear to be a complete nutritional source, it is misleading to assume that it alone supports optimal health.

Incorporating some vegetables or salads into a meat-heavy diet might offer a modest improvement by adding fiber and some essential nutrients. However, transitioning from meat to a more diverse range of whole foods is more effective for a truly balanced diet. Emphasizing whole, minimally processed foods ensures a more comprehensive intake of nutrients, supporting overall health and well-being.

The body can express a craving or desire for a specific micronutrient through various signals. These signals can be both physical and psychological. For example, you may crave citrus fruits when you need vitamin C or leafy greens when you lack iron.

Sometimes, specific nutrient deficiencies can affect hunger

Know Your Cravings

and appetite. For instance, a deficiency in certain minerals or vitamins may lead to increased appetite or persistent feelings of hunger, which can be the body's way of signaling a need for those nutrients.

Changes in mood or energy levels can also be linked to nutrient deficiencies. For example, low levels of iron may lead to fatigue and cravings for iron-rich foods.

Sometimes, the body may develop cravings for certain foods rich in the desired micronutrient. These cravings can vary from person to person and may reflect the body's attempt to obtain the missing nutrient. It's important to note that while cravings can sometimes signal a specific nutrient deficiency, they can also be influenced by various other factors, including emotional and environmental cues.

The element of the unknown, the willingness to try new things, is often lost as we age. Until we introduce or revisit a food, it remains an enigma. Our bodies are unaware of what nutrients it possesses until it hits the tongue and, subsequently, the intestines. Some vitamins are absorbed through the mouth via sublingual absorption, while others are absorbed in the small intestine. Adding colorful organic vegetables is the best way to get nutrients that your body can absorb into your bloodstream.

Additionally, these foods provide the necessary fiber for their complex role in our wellness. Incorporating these foods regularly allows your body to file a memory of what this food offers and how it can request it in the form of a craving.

Cravings intertwine psychological and physiological strands in the human mind and body. These impulses, often sparked by our emotional landscape, habitual patterns, or the body's plea for particular nutrients, require understanding if we are to master them. Delving into the physiological aspects of cravings reveals the role of nutrient deficiencies and hormonal fluctuations in triggering these urges. Recognizing the connection between certain cravings and the body's need for specific nutrients can empower individuals to make informed dietary choices that address these underlying needs.

Stress is a significant factor that influences cravings. When we are stressed, the body releases cortisol, a hormone that increases appetite and can lead to cravings for high-calorie foods. This response is deeply rooted in our evolution, where stress often meant physical danger, and the body needed extra energy to cope. However, in today's world, where stress is more likely due to emotional or psychological pressures, this same response can lead to unhealthy eating patterns.

Understanding the role of stress in cravings can be crucial for managing these physiological triggers. A study conducted at the University of California, San Francisco, found that women who were stressed were more likely to crave and consume high-calorie, sweet foods than those who were not stressed. This study highlights the importance of managing stress to control cravings and maintain a healthy diet.

Many of us find ourselves at the mercy of these siren calls for comfort foods during moments punctuated by stress, boredom, or strong emotions. Understanding the true meaning or cause behind these cravings and mapping the unique constellation of personal triggers provides the knowledge to disarm these temptations.

Food journaling can be an effective tool in this journey. By writing down the foods consumed and the emotions felt at the time, one can bring accountability to the process and discern patterns that link emotional states to cravings. This practice can lead to greater self-awareness, enabling individuals to make better choices and reduce the instinct to self-medicate with food. When true hunger arises, we can redirect these cravings to serve us, taking command in the dance of desire and satiation, turning a potential foe into an ally in the pursuit of well-being.

Know Your Cravings

When we eat, we do not simply feed our stomachs or satisfy our brain's reward system; we also nourish the microscopic inhabitants of our gut. Cravings and emotional eating can become intertwined when the microbiome is not properly nourished, influencing mood and behavior. Research has shown that gut bacteria can impact your emotions, with some strains linked to anxiety and depression. Sometimes, the brain seeks dopamine, which can be synthesized by consuming sugary treats, perpetuating a vicious cycle of sugar addiction. This creates an insulin dependency issue and a dopamine reward cycle and feeds harmful bacteria while healthy bacteria starve on a different diet.

Many beneficial bacteria in the gut, such as Bifidobacteria and Lactobacilli, ferment dietary fiber and resistant starches. These components, known as prebiotics, serve as food for the beneficial bacteria in the gut. A study published in the journal Gastroenterology found that individuals with a diet high in prebiotics had lower levels of cortisol and reported feeling less stressed compared to those with a diet low in prebiotics. This suggests that nourishing the gut microbiome can play a role in reducing stress-related cravings.

Consistently eating too much white sugar can disrupt the delicate balance of the microbiome, potentially leading to various health issues. Maintaining a balanced diet of fiber, fruits, vegetables, and probiotic foods is essential to support a healthy gut microbiome. However, the prior cravings diminish as you start replacing these cravings with whole foods. The sugary cake no longer tastes the same. Your desires begin to steer toward healthier desserts such as avocado chocolate mousse and dense date brownies, neither of which are harmful when sweetened with dates, applesauce, maple syrup, or coconut sugar.

Erratic eating habits and suboptimal dietary choices condition your body to crave foods higher in calories, largely because it does not recognize the wealth of existing food options. You're not yet proactive in staving off hunger by offering nutritious snacks readily. When ravenous hunger strikes, the inclination is to reach for calorie-dense options, a body's desperate measure born out of ignorance of the next meal's timing. This often leads to dietary decisions that birth regret.

Some diet coaches advocate for moderation, suggesting that if you want a piece of cake or pizza, have a small piece. However, this approach may not work in the long term. It does not train your mind to seek healthier, nutrient-dense foods. You are still giving your body foods because they have an addiction to calorie density or because they are craving a nutrient that you haven't given yourself an opportunity to source from a healthier place.

Instead of resorting to temporary fixes like Lactaid before ingesting cheese, consider a holistic perspective on wellness, which advises eliminating foods that impede your body's functionality. If you acknowledge symptoms for what they are signals. Choose not to mask them, and you orient your body toward maintaining homeostasis.

Understanding healthier options for your cravings begins by trying alternatives. For chocolate cravings, address magnesium deficiencies with green leafy veggies, seeds, nuts, beans, and fruits. Choose high-quality carob or cacao instead of lower-quality chocolates, as these are nutrient-rich. Combat cravings for fatty or oily foods by increasing your intake of calcium-rich foods like spinach, collard greens, and broccoli. This may include creating a balanced diet plan, introducing healthy snacks, building resilience to emotional triggers, and fostering a supportive network for accountability and encouragement. Integrating mindfulness practices, physical activity, and stress-reducing techniques can significantly contribute to a holistic approach to managing cravings.

For example, bread cravings might indicate a nitrogen deficiency, which can be addressed by incorporating oatmeal, greens, and legumes into your diet. Cravings for salty snacks could point to a chloride deficiency, which can be managed by adding sea salt, celery, and tomatoes to your meals. Cravings for sweets often signal an underlying blood sugar imbalance or a need for chromium, which can be met by consuming cinnamon, grapes, and sweet potatoes.

Cravings for alcohol, on the other hand, might indicate a protein deficiency, which can be addressed by focusing on protein-rich plant foods like legumes, beans, lentils, and leafy greens. These foods provide the amino acids necessary for maintaining muscle mass, repairing tissues, and supporting overall health. Additionally, cravings for alcohol may be linked to deficiencies in certain vitamins and minerals, such as B vitamins, magnesium, and zinc, which can be replenished by consuming a diverse diet rich in whole, unprocessed foods.

Potassium, another essential nutrient that helps regulate fluid balance, muscle contractions, and nerve signals, can be sourced from a variety of plant foods, including seaweed, bananas, sweet potatoes, and citrus fruits. Meanwhile, if you find yourself reaching for sugary snacks or caffeine, you may be experiencing a glutamine deficiency. Glutamine is an amino acid that plays a vital role in immune function and intestinal health. To address this, consider incorporating root vegetable broths, such as those made from carrots, parsnips, and beets, as well as fresh-pressed vegetable juices, which can provide a quick and natural source of glutamine.

By understanding the underlying nutritional needs driving cravings and opting for healthier alternatives, you can satisfy your body's requirements without relying on potentially addictive substances or unhealthy food choices. This approach not only helps in breaking unhealthy habits but also supports overall well-being by ensuring a balanced intake of essential nutrients.

A craving or desire to chew on ice is a classic sign of iron deficiency, which can be addressed by legumes, dried fruits, and greens.

Yearnings for pasta or other baked goods might be satiated with a focus on chromium-rich foods like cinnamon, grapes, and onions. Opt for whole ingredients; if an item on the ingredients list is not something you would consume alone, seek better alternatives.

When you contemplate cravings objectively, you understand the complex interplay between the nutrients your body seeks and the foods that deliver them. If you crave a banana cream pie, perhaps it is potassium the body is after; add avocado, spinach, watermelon, coconut water, sweet potato, or butternut squash to satisfy both the craving and the body's nutritional requirements.

The tongue is a pivotal sensor in flavor interpretation, but taste perception is a complex process that intertwines with other senses and neural activities. When your eyes perceive food, your brain kicks into gear, assessing and recognizing its nutritional value. Taste transduction is the biochemical process where taste receptors convert chemical signals from foods into electrical signals that travel to the brain, crafting an intricate flavor perception.

Much like how a subwoofer enhances the depth of bass in music, your sense of smell amplifies taste. The olfactory system plays a crucial role, as smell and taste are intertwined in the overall perception of flavor. Each taste bud is equipped with specialized cells known as taste receptors, capable of recognizing the primary flavors: sweet, sour, salty, bitter, and umami.

The element of the unknown, the willingness to try new things, is often lost as we age. Until we introduce or revisit a food, it remains an enigma. Our bodies are unaware of what nutrients it possesses until it hits the tongue and, subsequently, the intestines. Some vitamins are absorbed through the mouth via sublingual absorption, while others are absorbed in the small intestine. Adding colorful organic vegetables is the best way to get nutrients that your body can absorb into your bloodstream.

Whole Foods provides the necessary fiber for its complex role in our wellness. Incorporating these foods regularly allows your body to file a memory of what this food offers and how it can request it in the form of a craving.

Cravings intertwine psychological and physiological strands in the human mind and body. These impulses, often sparked by our emotional landscape, habitual patterns, or the body's plea for particular nutrients, require understanding if we are to master them. Delving into the physiological aspects of cravings reveals the role of nutrient deficiencies and hormonal fluctuations in triggering these urges. Recognizing the connection between certain cravings and the body's need for specific nutrients can empower individuals to make informed dietary choices that address these underlying needs.

Stress is a significant factor that influences cravings. When we are stressed, the body releases cortisol, a hormone that increases appetite and can lead to cravings for high-calorie foods. This response is deeply rooted in our evolution, where stress often meant physical danger, and the body needed extra energy to cope. However, in today's world, where stress is more likely due to emotional or psychological pressures, this same response can lead to unhealthy eating patterns.

Understanding the role of stress in cravings can be crucial for managing these physiological triggers. A study conducted at the University of California, San Francisco, found that women who were stressed were more likely to crave and consume high-calorie, sweet foods than those who were not stressed. This study highlights the importance of managing stress to control cravings and maintain a healthy diet.

Many of us find ourselves at the mercy of these siren calls for comfort foods during moments punctuated by stress, boredom, or strong emotions. Understanding the true meaning or cause behind these cravings and mapping the unique constellation of personal triggers provides the knowledge to disarm these temptations.

Food journaling can be an effective tool in this journey. By writing down the foods consumed and the emotions felt at the time, one can bring accountability to the process and discern patterns that link emotional states to cravings. This practice can lead to greater self-awareness, enabling individuals to make better choices and reduce the instinct to self-medicate with food. When true hunger arises, we can redirect these cravings to serve us, taking command in the dance of desire and satiation, turning a potential foe into an ally in the pursuit of well-being.

When we eat, we do not simply feed our stomachs or satisfy our brain's reward system; we also nourish the microscopic inhabitants of our gut. Cravings and emotional eating can become intertwined when the microbiome is not properly nourished, influencing mood and behavior. Research has shown that gut bacteria can impact your emotions, with some strains linked to anxiety and depression. Sometimes, the brain seeks dopamine, which can be synthesized by consuming sugary treats, perpetuating a vicious cycle of sugar addiction. This creates an insulin dependency issue and a dopamine reward cycle and feeds harmful bacteria while healthy bacteria starve on a different diet.

Many beneficial bacteria in the gut, such as Bifidobacteria and Lactobacilli, ferment dietary fiber and resistant starches. These components, known as prebiotics, serve as food for the beneficial bacteria in the gut. A study published in the journal Gastroenterology found that individuals with a diet high in prebiotics had lower levels of cortisol and reported feeling less stressed compared to those with a diet low in prebiotics. This suggests that nourishing the gut microbiome can play a role in reducing stress-related cravings.

Consistently eating too much white sugar can disrupt the

delicate balance of the microbiome, potentially leading to various health issues. Maintaining a balanced diet of fiber, fruits, vegetables, and probiotic foods is essential to support a healthy gut microbiome. However, the prior cravings diminish as you start replacing these cravings with whole foods. The sugary cake no longer tastes the same. Your desires begin to steer toward healthier desserts such as avocado chocolate mousse and dense date brownies, neither of which are harmful when sweetened with dates, applesauce, maple syrup, or coconut sugar.

    Erratic eating habits and suboptimal dietary choices condition your body to crave foods higher in calories, largely because it does not recognize the wealth of existing food options. You're not yet proactive in staving off hunger by readily offering nutritious snacks. When ravenous hunger strikes, the inclination is to reach for calorie-dense options, a body's desperate measure born out of ignorance of the next meal's timing. This often leads to dietary decisions that birth regret.

    Some diet coaches advocate for moderation, suggesting that if you want a piece of cake or pizza, have a small piece. However, this approach may not work in the long term. It does not train your mind to seek healthier, nutrient-dense foods. You are still giving your body foods because they have an addiction to calorie density or because they are craving a nutrient that you haven't given yourself an opportunity to source from a healthier place.

    Instead of resorting to temporary fixes like Lactaid before ingesting cheese, consider a holistic perspective on wellness, which advises eliminating foods that impede your body's functionality. If you acknowledge symptoms for what they are—signals—and choose not to mask them, you orient your body toward maintaining homeostasis.

    Understanding healthier options for your cravings begins by trying alternatives. For chocolate cravings, address magnesium deficiencies with green leafy veggies, seeds, nuts, beans, and fruits.

Choose high-quality carob or cacao instead of lower-quality chocolates, as these are nutrient-rich. Combat cravings for fatty or oily foods by increasing your intake of calcium-rich foods like spinach, collard greens, and broccoli. This may include creating a balanced diet plan, introducing healthy snacks, building resilience to emotional triggers, and fostering a supportive network for accountability and encouragement. Integrating mindfulness practices, physical activity, and stress-reducing techniques can significantly contribute to a holistic approach to managing cravings.

For example, bread cravings might indicate a nitrogen deficiency, which can be addressed by incorporating oatmeal, greens, and legumes into your diet. Cravings for salty snacks could point to a chloride deficiency, which can be managed by adding sea salt, celery, and tomatoes to your meals. Cravings for sweets often signal an underlying blood sugar imbalance or a need for chromium, which can be met by consuming cinnamon, grapes, and sweet potatoes.

When you crave cheese, it might be an essential fatty acid deficiency urging you to consume flax oil or chia seeds. Calcium deficiency can be supplemented with the intake of legumes and greens, and for alcohol cravings, consider that a protein deficiency may require a focus on legumes and greens. Potassium can be sourced from seaweed and citrus fruits, whereas glutamine deficiencies might propel you toward root veggie broths and fresh-pressed vegetable juices.

A craving or desire to chew on ice is a classic sign of iron deficiency, which can be addressed by legumes, dried fruits, and greens. Yearnings for pasta or other baked goods might be satiated with a focus on chromium-rich foods like cinnamon, grapes, and onions. Opt for whole ingredients; if an item on the ingredients list is not something you would consume alone, seek better alternatives.

When you contemplate cravings objectively, you understand

the complex interplay between the nutrients your body seeks and the foods that deliver them. If you crave a banana cream pie, perhaps it is potassium the body is after; add avocado, spinach, watermelon, coconut water, sweet potato, or butternut squash to satisfy both the craving and the body's nutritional requirements.

The tongue is a pivotal sensor in flavor interpretation, but taste perception is a complex process that intertwines with other senses and neural activities. When your eyes perceive food, your brain kicks into gear, assessing and recognizing its nutritional value. Taste transduction is the biochemical process where taste receptors convert chemical signals from foods into electrical signals that travel to the brain, crafting an intricate flavor perception.

Flavor is an amalgamation of taste, smell, texture, temperature, and visual cues. Disorientation in one aspect, such as sight, can alter the perceived flavor. The art of cooking and food development involves creating a harmonious blend of tastes, contrasting elements, and layering techniques to enhance the overall gastronomic experience. Fresh ingredients and proper consideration of texture and temperature play significant roles in flavor appreciation.

A fascinating study conducted by the Crossmodal Research Laboratory at the University of Oxford found that changing the color of a food item can significantly alter its perceived taste. Participants who consumed a strawberry-flavored mousse under red, green, and white lighting reported different taste intensities despite the flavors being identical. This study underscores the importance of sensory cues in how we experience cravings and satisfaction from food.

Understanding this intricate ballet of sensations and brain processes highlights the importance of choosing wisely when indulging in flavors and texture in foods, aiming for nutritionally dense, well-balanced meals that satisfy both the palate and the body's demands. Your brain is wired to detect and avoid potential spoilage in food, often flagged by changes in color. This protective response is designed to keep you from consuming anything that might be harmful. Creating appealing flavors involves various techniques, whether in culinary pursuits or food development. Upon consumption of high-fat, sugar, carbohydrates, and alcohol, the brain's reward circuits are activated, creating a habitual pattern only you possess the power to alter.

You may not immediately observe the internal shifts, but your microbiome can regenerate into a healthier version by eliminating processed and unhealthy foods and replacing them with fiber-laden fruits, vegetables, and legumes. Once you consistently offer nourishment to your body, a natural balance ensues, and past cravings can be modified with more wholesome alternatives. Envision replacing the craving for an afternoon pizza with sundried tomatoes, basil, and garlic pesto spread over a rice cake paired with a slice of tofu, a simple and work desk-friendly preparation.

You can absolutely savor the foods you love with a healthy lifestyle. For instance, chocolate can be a healthy part of each meal. Cravings, like those for chocolate, are really your body signaling its needs. In this case, it may be indicating a need for magnesium. This is the true purpose of cravings. They are a hint from your body regarding its requirements at the micronutrient level.

Practical exercises such as mindfulness techniques, creating a supportive environment, and incorporating balanced meals with essential nutrients can significantly curb cravings. You might yearn for chocolate, which can be a constructive craving. Chocolate contains magnesium, which your body might need, illustrating how cravings should ideally function as a signal from your body, drawing a parallel between nutrient deficiencies and food associations. Magnesium is involved in regulating various hormones, including those that control the menstrual cycle. It helps balance estrogen and progesterone, two key hormones in menstruation. Imbalances in these hormones can contribute to irregular menstrual cycles, PMS (premenstrual syndrome), and other menstrual symptoms.

Both pregnancy and menopause can be stressful times for many women due to the physical and emotional changes associated with these life stages. Magnesium has a calming effect on the nervous system and helps to regulate stress hormones like cortisol. Adequate magnesium levels may help to reduce stress and anxiety levels during menopause, promoting a sense of calm and well-being. Never feel bad about craving something that clearly has a high concentration of one or two vitamins or minerals, as that is your biggest clue to what your body needs.

Cravings and emotional eating are interconnected challenges. An improperly nourished microbiome can harm your emotional well-being because the bacteria in your gut influence your mood. It is not wrong to have a bad day and seek comfort in a slice of cake, but it is essential to understand that your brain is craving dopamine, and sugar triggers its release, fostering a sugar addiction. This perpetuates an unhealthy cycle requiring you to adopt a different strategy to conquer cravings.

A personal technique I use to decipher my cravings stems from a lesson I learned at fifteen while working at the local health food store, "Sprouts." A conversation between a customer and my boss focused on the health implications of adding milk and sugar to coffee. My boss challenged the customer to drink her usual three cups of coffee without the additives and place milk and sugar in a separate cup. As my boss predicted, the customer preferred the sweetened milk over plain coffee when she returned the next day. This exemplifies how cravings are not always apparent. They often arise from the body's plea for fuel. While not everyone wants to eat breakfast, note that if you crave sugary drinks in the morning, you most likely didn't eat enough carbohydrates to refuel your muscle and liver glycogen. You may interpret that craving for food incorrectly as a desire for sugar.

If the customer had started her day with a nourishing breakfast, she might not have craved the caloric components of her coffee. Her body was signaling a need for energy, and her reliance on the coffee's calories, specifically the creamer and sugar, suddenly made perfect sense. Identifying signals and comprehending food cravings is vital for improving decision-making abilities.

If you find yourself craving banana cream pie, it could be a sign that your body wants more potassium. A creamy banana shake made with coconut and soymilk can satisfy your nutritional needs, offering fiber, protein, and fats—the same building blocks of the treat you desire. Give your body a chance to soak in these nutrients and let your microbiome find equilibrium. Soon, you may prefer the banana smoothie over the pie. Breaking out of the cycle of "just a little bit" keeps you away from high-calorie, low-nutrient traps and aligns your hunger with nutritious satisfaction.

To truly nourish yourself, it's important to develop a mindset that prioritizes self-care and values the act of eating as an opportunity to fuel your body and support your health. This mindset shift involves seeing food not as a reward or a punishment but as a source of nourishment and energy. When you approach eating with this perspective, you're more likely to make choices that align with your long-term health goals rather than giving in to short-term cravings or emotional impulses.

Cultivating a positive relationship with food also involves letting go of the guilt and shame associated with eating. Many people struggle with feelings of guilt after eating certain foods, particularly those that are perceived as "bad" or "unhealthy." This negative self-talk can lead to a cycle of restrictive dieting followed by binge eating, which is not only unhealthy but also damaging to your self-esteem.

Instead of labeling foods as "good" or "bad," try to adopt a more balanced perspective. All foods can fit into a healthy diet in moderation, and it's important to listen to your body's cues and enjoy your food without guilt.

Incorporating more variety into your diet is another way to enhance your relationship with food. Eating a wide range of foods ensures that you're getting a diverse array of nutrients, which supports overall health. It also keeps your meals interesting and enjoyable, making it easier to stick to a healthy eating plan. Experimenting with new recipes, trying different fruits and vegetables, and exploring cuisines from different cultures can make eating more exciting and satisfying.

One practical way to ensure variety in your diet is to eat a rainbow of fruits and vegetables. Different colors in produce often correspond to different nutrients, so by including a range of colors on your plate, you can be sure you're getting a broad spectrum of vitamins, minerals, and antioxidants. For example, red foods like tomatoes and strawberries are rich in lycopene, an antioxidant that supports heart health. Orange foods like carrots and sweet potatoes are high in beta-carotene, which is vital for eye health. Green foods like spinach and broccoli provide folate, which is essential for cell function and tissue growth. Purple foods like blueberries and eggplant contain anthocyanins, which have anti-inflammatory properties. By eating a variety of colors, you're nourishing your body and making your meals more visually appealing and enjoyable.

Addressing cravings is another crucial aspect of managing hunger and maintaining a healthy diet. Cravings are a natural part of the human experience and don't necessarily have to be wrong. However, it's important to distinguish between cravings that arise from true hunger and those that are driven by emotional or psychological factors. When you experience a craving, take a moment to check in with yourself. Are you truly hungry or seeking comfort, distraction, or stress relief? If it's the latter, consider whether there might be a healthier way to address those needs, such as going for a walk, talking to a friend, or engaging in a hobby you enjoy.

A common challenge arises when cravings for vitamins and minerals from natural sources, like fresh berries or citrus, are misinterpreted as cravings for similar-tasting but less nutritious options, such as sour or fruity gummy candies. This misreading can occur because our brains have learned to associate sweet and fruity flavors with a quick release of dopamine, a neurotransmitter involved in pleasure and reward. However, while candies may mimic authentic fruit flavors, they lack the fiber, vitamins, and other beneficial compounds that whole fruits offer. To align your cravings with your nutritional needs, giving yourself the most wholesome version of the flavors you are craving is essential.

When you choose fresh fruit over gummy candy, you satisfy your taste buds and provide your body with the essential nutrients it craves. The fiber in fruit slows down the absorption of sugar, preventing the rapid spike and crash in blood sugar levels that candy can cause. This steadier release of energy helps maintain satiety and reduces the likelihood of overeating. Moreover, consuming whole foods like fruit can lead to a more fulfilling eating experience because they offer a complex array of tastes, textures, and nutrients that candies simply cannot replicate.

If you find yourself craving something sweet after dinner, consider healthier alternatives like coconut yogurt. Coconut yogurt is rich in probiotics, which support gut health, and can be topped with fresh fruits, nuts, and seeds for added nutrients and flavor. Making your coconut yogurt at home allows you to control the ingredients and avoid added sugars and preservatives in store-bought versions. For a more indulgent treat, you can create "nice cream" by blending frozen bananas with other fruits, nut butter, or coconut milk for a creamy, dairy-free dessert that satisfies your sweet tooth without the added sugars and unhealthy fats in traditional ice cream.

If the craving persists and you decide to indulge, try to do so mindfully. Rather than eating mindlessly, savor the experience. Pay attention to the food's flavors, textures, and sensations, and enjoy it without guilt. You may find that by eating mindfully, you can satisfy your craving with a smaller portion than if you were eating out of habit or distraction. Additionally, consider healthier alternatives to your cravings. For example, if you're craving something sweet, try a piece of dark chocolate or a fruit-based dessert instead of a sugary snack. If you're craving something salty, opt for roasted nuts or air-popped popcorn with a sprinkle of nutritional yeast instead of chips. By finding healthier ways to satisfy your cravings, you can enjoy the foods you love while still supporting your health goals.

Finally, it's important to recognize that building and maintaining healthy eating habits is a journey, not a destination. It's normal to have setbacks and slip-ups along the way, but what matters most is your overall progress and commitment to your health. Be patient with yourself, and remember that every small step you take toward healthier eating is a victory. Over time, these small changes add up, leading to lasting improvements in your health and well-being. Improving dietary consistency and making healthier food choices are crucial steps because inconsistent eating habits can train your body to crave high-calorie foods. When your diet lacks variety and nutritious options, your body becomes less familiar with these foods, leading to increased cravings for calorie-dense, less beneficial options. This cycle is further reinforced when high-fat, sugar-rich, carb-heavy, and alcoholic foods stimulate the brain's reward center, creating a pattern of cravings that is difficult to break.

Anticipating hunger and keeping nutrient-rich snacks readily available can help you avoid this negative cycle. By being mindful of your eating habits and focusing on self-care at every meal, rather than adhering strictly to a diet, you can achieve results more quickly and sustainably. This approach encourages a balanced relationship with food, where the focus is on nourishing your body and enjoying the process rather than solely on restriction.

Ideally, frame your mindset to seek out diverse meals that fuel the metabolism and bolster overall health. It's important to identify genuine hunger by paying close attention to the body's signals, like the tightening of the stomach and the secretion of ghrelin, among others.

Choosing what to eat carefully, especially when hunger isn't yet overwhelming, can avert poor dietary decisions and contribute to a healthy metabolism.

Preparedness and foresight are essential; keeping snacks and hydrating drinks handy gives you a constructive attitude toward eating and can substantially revamp your dietary habits. Be conscious of your desires for food and prepare meals to ensure your eating habits meet your body's legitimate physiological requirements. Favor foods rich in nutrients as substitutes to quench cravings and emphasize small yet positive modifications that enhance a gratifying connection with your food cravings.

Understanding the requirements of actual hunger is a process that should be approached with a degree of focus. This becomes clearer after dedicating effort toward familiarizing oneself with its indicators. Routinely indulging in accessible sustenance, succumbing to the convenience of pre-packaged snacks, or deferring meals until hunger fades can lead to a diminished capacity to perceive true hunger cues. For example, under time constraints and faced with hunger, an individual may turn to a caffeinated drink for a swift uptick in energy, which offers only a temporary solution to hunger. This method postpones the necessary engagement with nutritional requirements.

If you ignore your body's signals to eat, a mild reminder can turn into a strong urge, leading you to choose "unhealthy" foods. The motivation for a calorie-rich meal is rooted in the body's dwindling energy reserves and instinct to preserve its metabolic operations. When in dire need of calories, you might find yourself at the closest fast-food outlet, confronted with an indulgent meal, scarce in vegetables and abundant in carbohydrates and fats – not the ideal nutritional choice. The body's demand for calories is insistent, as it's impossible to outwit your system's physiological requirements.

It might seem counterintuitive, but increasing the number of times you eat each day is beneficial to lose weight effectively. Aim for six small meals. This consistent eating schedule plays a crucial role in controlling your weight and is particularly important at the start of switching to a nutritious diet. If you're accustomed to eating once or twice a day and struggle to lose weight, it's critical to recognize that this eating pattern may contribute to your weight challenges. By establishing a routine of six smaller meals, you will avoid constant hunger, eliminate the sensation of being on a restrictive diet, and distribute your nutrient intake more evenly throughout the day.

Managing hunger and maintaining a healthy diet involves a combination of understanding macronutrients, addressing psychological factors, planning and preparing meals, practicing self-care, and cultivating a positive relationship with food. By taking a holistic approach to nutrition and self-care, you can create a sustainable, balanced, and enjoyable way of eating that supports your long-term health and well-being.

EATING LESSONS

Common Cravings and Their Nutrient Dense Alternatives:

1. **Chocolate**: Indicates magnesium deficiency. Replace with dark leafy greens, nuts, seeds, or a high-quality dark chocolate rich in cacao.
2. **Cheese**: Could signal a need for fatty acids. Substitute with avocados, nuts, seeds, or a plant-based cheese made from cashews or almonds.
3. **Sweets**: Often a sign of blood sugar imbalances. Opt for fruit, dates, or a smoothie with natural sweetness from bananas and berries.
4. **Ice Cream**: Could be craving for comfort and fats. Opt for banana-based nice cream, blended with berries and a dash of almond milk.
5. **Salty Snacks**: Could point to a chloride deficiency. Choose seaweed snacks, celery sticks with almond butter, or a handful of salted nuts.
6. **Soda**: Often a craving for sugar or caffeine. Replace with sparkling water flavored with fresh citrus or herbal teas like peppermint or hibiscus.
7. **Pasta**: Can be a sign of chromium deficiency. Opt for whole-grain pasta or zoodles (zucchini noodles) topped with tomato sauce and nutritional yeast.
8. **Red Meat**: Often indicates an iron deficiency. Substitute with iron-rich foods like lentils, spinach, and tofu, paired with vitamin C-rich foods to enhance absorption.
9. **Potato Chips**: A sign of needing salt or fat. Replace with baked sweet potato fries or kale chips seasoned with sea salt.
10. **Fried Foods**: Could indicate a craving for fats. Replace with baked or air-fried veggies, such as zucchini fries or roasted chickpeas.

Know Your Cravings

11. **Candy**: Often linked to a sugar craving. Substitute with fresh fruit, dates, or a homemade energy ball made with nuts and dried fruits.
12. **Coffee**: Could indicate a need for a stimulant or a comforting habit. Replace with green tea, matcha, or a caffeine-free herbal coffee substitute like chicory root.
13. **Pizza**: A craving for carbs and fats. Replace with a whole grain or cauliflower crust topped with marinara, roasted veggies, and a sprinkle of nutritional yeast.
14. **Sugary Cereals**: Often indicates a need for quick energy. Replace with oatmeal sweetened with fresh fruit and nuts.
15. **Ice**: Chewing ice can signal an iron deficiency. Substitute with iron-rich foods such as beans, lentils, and fortified cereals.
16. **Doughnuts**: A combination of sugar and fat cravings. Replace with a baked vegan doughnut made from almond flour and sweetened with maple syrup.
17. **Alcohol**: Can be a craving for sugar or relaxation. Replace with kombucha, herbal teas, or a mocktail made from sparkling water and fresh juice.
18. **Cookies**: A craving for sugar and fat. Substitute with homemade oatmeal cookies sweetened with banana and studded with nuts and seeds.
19. **Butter**: Could indicate a craving for fats. Replace with avocado, coconut oil, or a drizzle of olive oil on your food.
20. **Creamy Foods**: Often a craving for comfort and fats. Substitute with a cashew-based cream sauce or a rich avocado dressing for your salads.

12
MUSCLE, MOOD, & THE HOPE MOLECULE: HORMONE HEALTH

Within the complex workings of the human body, exercise stands out as a crucial regulator of hormonal balance, generating a series of biochemical reactions that impact the entire system. Regular physical activity fosters this balance, underpinning excellent health and vitality. Every step taken, pedal turned, or weight lifted causes the body to unleash a burst of endorphins—neurotransmitters known as "feel-good" hormones. These endorphins lift the spirit, alleviate stress, and rev up the metabolism, making exercise essential to overall well-being.

The benefits of exercise extend beyond the immediate release of endorphins. Engaging in regular physical activity drives long-term hormonal balance, influencing systems from metabolism to reproductive health. Aerobic activities like jogging or cycling stimulate the secretion of growth hormones and adrenaline, which mobilize energy reserves and promote tissue repair. Strength training, on the other hand, triggers the release of testosterone and human growth hormone, essential for muscle growth, strength, and resilience. These hormones play a pivotal role in the body's adaptation to physical challenges.

In women, testosterone is primarily produced in the ovaries and adrenal glands and plays a critical role in health. It contributes

Muscle, Mood, & the Hope Molecule: Hormone Health

to the growth, maintenance, and repair of reproductive tissues, including the ovaries and uterus, while also influencing bone density and muscle mass. A balanced level of testosterone in women supports physical performance, metabolic health, and overall well-being, yet this hormone is often overlooked in discussions about female health.

Exercise's impact on the endocrine system, which regulates hormone production, is profound. Regular physical activity enhances the release of insulin-like growth factor 1 (IGF-1), a hormone that works with growth hormone to promote tissue development. IGF-1 is crucial for muscle repair and regeneration, making it key in achieving and maintaining muscle mass. Exercise also improves insulin sensitivity, reducing the risk of type 2 diabetes and promoting better metabolic health.

Exercise serves as a potent modulator of stress hormones, buffering against modern-day stressors. When the body is subjected to physical exertion, it activates its stress response, releasing cortisol and adrenaline. While cortisol, the "stress hormone," plays a vital role in managing stress by increasing blood sugar levels and enhancing brain function, chronic stress can lead to elevated cortisol levels linked to weight gain, high blood pressure, and impaired immune function.

Regular exercise helps the body manage stress more efficiently, reducing cortisol production over time and promoting relaxation and recovery. This ability to tame the stress hormone cascade endows individuals with resilience, balance, and mental clarity while mitigating the negative effects of chronic stress, including metabolic syndrome—a cluster of conditions that increase the risk of heart disease, stroke, and type 2 diabetes.

Regular physical activity also enhances mood by increasing levels of dopamine, serotonin, and norepinephrine. Dopamine, the "feel-good" neurotransmitter, is released during workouts, regardless of intensity. This neurotransmitter not only lifts mood but also plays a crucial role in the body's reward system, motivating individuals to continue exercising. Serotonin and norepinephrine regulate sleep patterns, appetite, and mood, reducing anxiety and depression. As exercise intensity increases, so does oxygen intake, leading to feelings of euphoria during and after exercise—a phenomenon often referred to as the "runner's high." This metabolic boost is why exercise is so effective for weight management and overall health.

Achieving a lean, toned physique involves maintaining a low body fat percentage relative to muscle mass. This requires regular physical activity, including aerobic exercise and strength training, alongside a balanced diet that supports muscle growth and fat loss. Understanding how different types of exercise impact the body helps individuals tailor fitness routines to meet specific goals. Strength training exercises like weightlifting lead to muscular adaptations that increase muscle mass and strength. Over time, these adaptations improve the body's ability to burn calories at rest, which is essential for maintaining a healthy body composition.

The physical and psychological benefits of exercise are intertwined, making it a powerful tool for improving overall health. After just one session, the heart rate increases, blood flow to muscles is enhanced, and endorphins are released, fostering well-being. Committing to regular aerobic activities like running, swimming, or cycling gradually improves cardiovascular efficiency. Strength training prompts muscular adaptations, leading to increased muscle strength, endurance, and resilience. As the body adapts to regular exercise, these benefits become more pronounced, contributing to long-term health and vitality.

Recognizing that humans are designed for movement is key to treating your body with care. Anyone can incorporate more physical activity into their routine, regardless of current fitness levels. Setting an intention each morning to connect with your body can help you become more attuned to its needs. This practice not only enhances physical health but also aids in recognizing and addressing emotional eating patterns, particularly for those who suffer from anxiety and depression.

Emotional eating often links to the brain's reward system, where dopamine plays a central role. Dopamine, associated with feelings of pleasure and satisfaction, is released in response to rewarding stimuli, including food. This is how people develop emotional eating habits, seeking to alleviate negative emotions through temporary comfort. Cacao, known for its mood-boosting effects, can be beneficial, but when combined with fillers, processed sugar, and additives, its effects diminish, leading to overconsumption and a cycle of emotional eating.

Exercise, however, provides a healthy way to regulate mood and emotions. Physical activity increases serotonin and norepinephrine, boosting mood, regulating sleep patterns, and reducing anxiety and depression. Low serotonin levels have been linked to increased appetite and cravings for sugars and carbohydrates, often used as a quick fix for emotional distress. Regular physical activity harnesses these neurotransmitters' power, improving mood and reducing reliance on unhealthy coping mechanisms.

Endorphins, often called the body's natural painkillers, are released during physical exercise and help alleviate discomfort. This trait likely evolved as a survival mechanism, enabling humans to endure prolonged physical activity, such as running or climbing away from danger. By reducing pain perception and promoting well-being, endorphins help individuals push through challenging workouts and recover more quickly.

Cortisol, released in response to stress, also plays a significant role in metabolism. It increases blood sugar levels and promotes gluconeogenesis, the conversion of proteins and fats into glucose. This provides a quick energy source during stressful situations. However, chronically elevated cortisol levels can disrupt blood sugar regulation and hinder fat loss.

Prolonged exposure to high cortisol levels can lead to muscle breakdown as the body tries to convert muscle proteins into glucose to meet increased energy demands. This muscle loss can negatively impact metabolic rate, making it harder to burn calories efficiently. Promoting healthy fat loss and regulating cortisol levels require stress management techniques, regular exercise, sufficient sleep, mindfulness practices, and a balanced diet. Managing overall calorie intake and engaging in aerobic and strength-training exercises help maintain a healthy body composition. Hormonal adaptations to exercise may take weeks to months to become noticeable, but the long-term benefits are worth the effort.

Incorporating regular movement into your daily routine requires making time for it, which might mean replacing other activities with exercise. Setting aside 30 minutes in the morning and 30 minutes in the evening for activities like stretching, running, or lifting weights can be effective. Consistent physical activity not only taps into the body's natural reward system but also helps regulate hunger and energy levels, making it easier to make healthy food choices.

Exercise releases hunger-related hormones like ghrelin and leptin. Ghrelin stimulates hunger, while leptin suppresses it. Regular physical activity helps regulate these hormones, fostering a balanced relationship with food. After a single session, the body undergoes immediate changes, including increased heart rate, improved blood flow to muscles, and the release of endorphins. Regular aerobic exercise gradually improves cardiovascular efficiency, leading to a stronger heart and more flexible blood vessels.

Strength training leads to muscular adaptations that increase muscle strength and endurance. Initially, muscle soreness may occur as the body adapts, but consistent practice strengthens muscles and makes them more resistant to fatigue. These physical adaptations not only improve overall health but also enhance the body's ability to manage stress and maintain hormonal balance.

Regular exercise positively affects hormone function, particularly those involved in metabolism, mood, and stress response. Exercise increases the release of endorphins and other "feel-good" hormones while reducing cortisol levels. These hormonal adaptations can vary, taking weeks to months to become noticeable, but regular exercise taps into the body's natural reward system and supports overall health and well-being.

Cognitive Behavioral Therapy (CBT) is another effective tool for improving mental health. CBT is a practical psychological approach that involves self-awareness, understanding cognitive distortions, setting clear goals, and using self-help tools like thought records and journaling. Research shows that combining CBT with regular exercise enhances the benefits of both, leading to improved mood, reduced symptoms of depression and anxiety, and better appetite regulation.

Exercise-induced myokines, such as brain-derived neurotrophic factor (BDNF), play a crucial role in supporting mental health. BDNF promotes the growth and maintenance of neurons in the brain, supporting learning, memory, and cognitive function. Exercise increases the release of BDNF and other myokines, which cross the blood-brain barrier and exert antidepressant effects. Although more research is needed to fully understand the mechanisms by which exercise-induced myokines affect the brain, evidence suggests that regular physical activity reduces symptoms of depression and anxiety.

For menopausal women, diet plays a significant role in managing symptoms and maintaining overall health. A plant-based diet rich in whole foods like fruits, vegetables, whole grains, legumes, nuts, and seeds can alleviate menopausal symptoms such as hot flashes, night sweats, and mood swings. Plant foods contain phytoestrogens, which have mild estrogenic effects and may help balance hormonal fluctuations during menopause. Additionally, a plant-based diet benefits heart health, as it is low in saturated fats and cholesterol—risk factors for cardiovascular disease.

Calcium and vitamin D are essential for bone health, particularly for menopausal women at increased risk of osteoporosis due to reduced estrogen levels. Plant-based sources of these nutrients include fortified plant milk, leafy greens, nuts, and seeds. While dairy products are often promoted as primary sources of calcium, recent research challenges the notion that dairy consumption is essential for bone health. Studies have found no strong evidence that drinking milk prevents bone fractures or osteoporosis. In fact, high dairy consumption during adolescence may not provide the bone-strengthening benefits once believed.

Meat-based diets, typically higher in saturated fats and cholesterol, contain heme iron, a known carcinogen, as well as natural animal hormones and potential hormone amplifiers used in farming. These factors can increase inflammation in the body, potentially worsening menopausal symptoms and increasing the risk of chronic diseases. Supplements like ashwagandha, Evening Primrose oil, L-theanine, and Chasteberry extract can be helpful in alleviating hormonal symptoms and imbalances. These supplements support hormonal balance and mood regulation.

Managing cortisol levels is crucial for fat loss and overall health. Chronic elevation of cortisol hinders fat loss, disrupts blood sugar regulation, and contributes to muscle breakdown. Stress management techniques, a balanced diet, and regular exercise help regulate cortisol levels and support a healthy body composition. Incorporating regular physical activity into your routine and making mindful dietary choices harness the body's natural systems, improving both physical and mental health.

The interconnectedness of physical activity, nutrition, and mental health underscores the importance of a holistic approach to well-being. Exercise and diet are not just tools for achieving a desired physique; they are essential components of a healthy lifestyle that supports both physical and mental health. The synergy between these factors can lead to profound changes in how we feel, function, and perceive the world around us.

Maintaining an exercise routine is a cornerstone of overall health and well-being, yet many people face challenges that make consistency difficult. Motivation can wane, especially when results are not immediately visible, and psychological barriers can deter individuals from sticking to a regular exercise regimen. Lack of motivation often stems from viewing exercise as a chore rather than an enjoyable activity. Time constraints, such as busy work schedules or family obligations, can also make it challenging to prioritize physical activity. Additionally, negative associations with exercise—perhaps due to past injuries, feelings of inadequacy, or discomfort with physical exertion—can further discourage consistency.

Overcoming these barriers requires a multi-faceted approach addressing both psychological and practical aspects of exercise. Setting realistic goals is a fundamental strategy. Instead of aiming for drastic changes, breaking down fitness goals into manageable steps can sustain motivation. Rather than setting an initial goal to lose a significant amount of weight, one might focus on attainable objectives like improving endurance, increasing strength or committing to a certain number of workouts per week. Achieving these smaller goals builds confidence and creates momentum, making it easier to stay motivated over time.

Another effective strategy is finding forms of exercise that are genuinely enjoyable. Experimenting with different activities helps discover what feels most engaging, whether it's dancing, swimming, hiking, or practicing yoga. Enjoyment is key to adherence; people are more likely to stick with activities they find pleasurable. Incorporating variety into an exercise routine prevents boredom and keeps the experience fresh and exciting.

Building a supportive community is also crucial for consistency. Group exercise, whether in fitness classes, team sports, or outdoor activities with friends, offers not only physical benefits but also significant social and emotional rewards. Exercising with others provides motivation, accountability, and a sense of camaraderie. Social interaction and shared experiences in group exercise settings improve mental health by reducing feelings of isolation and boosting mood through social connection. For many, the communal aspect of exercise is a powerful motivator that enhances enjoyment and commitment.

The importance of hydration in physical performance and recovery can't be overstated. Proper hydration is critical for maintaining optimal body function, particularly during exercise. Dehydration impairs performance by reducing endurance, increasing the risk of heat-related illnesses, and hindering the body's ability to recover after workouts. Water regulates body temperature, lubricates joints, and maintains the balance of electrolytes necessary for muscle contractions and nerve function.

During exercise, the body loses water through sweat, and this fluid loss needs to be replenished to prevent dehydration. Even a small percentage of body water loss can significantly decline physical performance. A 2% body weight loss through dehydration can decrease endurance, strength, and cognitive function. Therefore, drinking water before, during, and after exercise is essential to maintain hydration levels. Consuming beverages with electrolytes can also help replace the sodium, potassium, and other minerals lost through sweat, particularly during prolonged or intense exercise.

Hydration plays a critical role in recovery. Adequate fluid intake flushes out toxins produced during exercise, reduces muscle soreness, and facilitates nutrient delivery to muscles for repair. Drinking sufficient water after a workout supports the body's recovery processes, preparing it for the next session.

The long-term benefits of consistent physical activity are profound and far-reaching. Regular exercise reduces the risk of chronic diseases such as heart disease, stroke, type 2 diabetes, and certain cancers. Physical activity lowers blood pressure, improves cholesterol levels, and enhances insulin sensitivity, contributing to cardiovascular health. Exercise also supports healthy aging by preserving muscle mass, maintaining bone density, and reducing the risk of cognitive decline. These benefits underscore the importance of making exercise a lifelong habit, not just a short-term endeavor. The long-term benefits of exercise are especially significant for women, particularly those going through menopause. Menopause is a natural aging phase that brings about hormonal changes, including a decline in estrogen levels. This hormonal shift can lead to symptoms such as hot flashes, night sweats, mood swings, and an increased risk of osteoporosis and cardiovascular disease. Regular exercise mitigates these symptoms and promotes overall health during menopause.

Weight-bearing exercises like walking, jogging, and resistance training are particularly beneficial for maintaining bone density and reducing osteoporosis risk—a major concern for postmenopausal women due to the loss of protective estrogen. Strength training also preserves muscle mass, which tends to decline with age, leading to a slower metabolism and increased fat accumulation. Regular physical activity helps women maintain a healthier body composition and reduces the risk of weight gain during menopause.

Exercise plays a crucial role in managing mood and mental health during menopause. The decline in estrogen levels affects neurotransmitter function, leading to symptoms of depression and anxiety. Physical activity increases endorphins, serotonin, and dopamine production, elevating mood and reducing stress. The social aspects of group exercise provide emotional support and a sense of community, which is particularly beneficial during this transitional period.

Individuals may respond differently to exercise and dietary interventions due to factors such as genetics, age, gender, and pre-existing health conditions. Personalized approaches to fitness and nutrition are often more effective in achieving desired outcomes. For example, some women may find that high-intensity interval training (HIIT) is highly effective for weight loss and cardiovascular health, while others benefit more from low-impact activities like yoga or swimming. Similarly, dietary needs vary widely; some individuals thrive on a plant-based diet, while others require more protein to support muscle maintenance and recovery.

Tailoring exercise and dietary plans to individual needs involves understanding one's unique physiology and preferences. Working with a healthcare provider, nutritionist, or personal trainer helps develop a customized plan that aligns with goals and lifestyle. This personalized approach enhances the effectiveness of the intervention and increases the likelihood of long-term adherence.

Maintaining motivation and consistency in an exercise routine involves overcoming psychological barriers, setting realistic goals, finding enjoyable activities, and building a supportive community.

Proper hydration is essential for optimal performance and recovery, and the long-term benefits of regular physical activity include a reduced risk of chronic diseases and support for healthy aging. For menopausal women, exercise offers additional benefits in managing symptoms and promoting overall health. Recognizing the individual variability in response to exercise and diet allows for personalized approaches that are more likely to lead to success. Addressing these factors enables individuals to create a sustainable and effective exercise regimen supporting their overall well-being.

Understanding the body's complex interplay of hormones, neurotransmitters, and metabolic processes allows us to make informed decisions about how we live. By embracing regular physical activity, making mindful dietary choices, and managing stress effectively, we can achieve a state of balance that supports long-term health and vitality.

Moreover, the benefits of this holistic approach extend beyond the individual. When we take care of ourselves, we are better equipped to care for others, contribute to our communities, and lead fulfilling lives. The ripple effects of good health can be felt in every aspect of our lives, from our relationships to our professional endeavors.

In conclusion, the integration of exercise, diet, and stress management is essential for achieving and maintaining optimal health. By understanding and leveraging the intricate connections between the body and mind, we can create a balanced, healthy lifestyle that supports long-term well-being. Whether you are just starting your fitness journey or looking to deepen your understanding of how to support your health, the principles outlined here provide a foundation for making informed, effective choices that will benefit you for years.

13
TRUST YOUR GUT

The intricate bond between our gut microbiome and our desires for certain foods can be traced to elaborate exchanges between our intestinal flora and the brain. Please think of the gut microbiome as an extensive ecosystem of microorganisms, including a rich diversity of bacteria, fungi, viruses, and many other tiny life forms, all nestled in the confines of our gastrointestinal tract. These microbial inhabitants are power players in a host of bodily functions, from breaking down nutrients to safeguarding our immune system, and they even stretch their influence to dictate our dietary preferences.

Within this microscopic biosphere, certain microbes are adept at concocting chemical messengers and brain-modulating substances that can sway the brain's pleasure-seeking and hunger-regulating realms. This messaging occurs via the gut-brain axis, a two-way communication network that intimately links the happenings in our gut to the intricate workings of our central nervous system. The microbiome can steer our cravings and inclinations for certain types of food by tinkering with the levels of specific chemicals that trigger cravings.

Moreover, gut bacteria have a toe in the digestive ballet, orchestrating the dance of the breakdown and assimilation of nutrients, such as fibers and complex sugars. When particular bacterial populations flourish in the digestive system, they can subtly push us toward a preference for sustenance that nourishes them, often items high in fibrous content, thereby weaving a direct connection between their presence and our food cravings.

Once we have embraced the idea that we are host to microscopic organisms necessary for our well-being, more questions arise. Should everyone take a supplemented pro and prebiotic, and are you eating the right foods to feed them?

Prebiotics are non-digestible fibers or carbohydrates that serve as food for beneficial bacteria in the gut. Stomach acid or digestive enzymes do not affect them; they reach the colon intact. Once in the colon, prebiotics are fermented by gut bacteria, promoting the growth and activity of beneficial bacteria. Examples of prebiotic-rich foods include garlic, onions, bananas, oats, asparagus, sunchokes (Jerusalem artichokes), and chicory.

Garlic and onions make our dishes deliciously aromatic, but they are also sending an invite to the beneficial bacteria in our gut, thanks to their fructooligosaccharides.

Then you've got plantains, Maduros, and bananas. When they're still a tad green, they're chock-full of something called resistant starch, which, would you believe, resists digestion? It's like a playground for those microbes; now, imagine the fiber in oats and its buddy, beta-glucan. They're just like cheerleaders for our gut health. And then there's chicory root and Jerusalem artichokes. They're crammed with inulin, a name that might not sound delicious, but trust me, the beneficial bacteria in your gut are big fans.

Just picture your gut's microscopic residents throwing a little party every time you crunch into these fibrous delights. Dandelion greens are the unsung heroes, brimming with various fiber types, including inulin and FOS.

A very common apple with its soluble fiber known as pectin, which has prebiotic powers. And finally, for all you oatmeal lovers out there, those oats are doing more than just filling you up. They're rich in beta-glucan, another prebiotic champion that helps keep the good vibes rolling in your digestive tract.

When you munch on these foods, you're not just eating; you're cultivating a diverse microbiome party in your gut, essential for your overall health.

Remember that many other foods have fiber, but not all are high in the specific prebiotics mentioned. A food like spaghetti squash has a lot of fiber in its noodle-shaped meat, but while it's not as high in prebiotic fiber as other foods, spaghetti squash contains fiber, including soluble and insoluble types, which can contribute to overall gut health.

The fiber in spaghetti squash can help support regularity and digestive function by promoting healthy bowel movements. While it may not be a significant source of prebiotic fibers like inulin or resistant starch, incorporating spaghetti squash into your meals can still provide valuable dietary fiber and micronutrients.

The Recommended Dietary Allowance (RDA) for fiber varies depending on factors such as age, sex, and life stage. However, the general guideline for adults is around 25 grams of fiber per day for women and 38 grams for men, based on a 2,000-calorie diet. This recommendation is set by health organizations such as the Institute of Medicine and aims to promote digestive health, regularity, and overall well-being.

It's important to note that individual fiber needs may vary based on factors such as activity level, dietary preferences, and health conditions. Some people may require more or less fiber depending on their unique circumstances. Additionally, it's recommended to obtain fiber from various sources, including fruits, vegetables, whole grains, legumes, nuts, and seeds, to ensure a balanced dietary fiber intake and other nutrients.

To add spaghetti squash to your diet, you can roast or steam it and then use a fork to scrape out the flesh, which separates into strands resembling spaghetti noodles. It can be used as a nutritious alternative to pasta in dishes like spaghetti squash "pasta" with marinara sauce, stir-fries, or baked casseroles. Roast with a maple syrup glaze and drizzle with a tahini vinaigrette after stuffing with apples, raisins, pepitas, or walnuts. Spaghetti squash is a nutritious vegetable that provides a range of health benefits, including being a source of dietary fiber.

However, when it comes to prebiotic fiber specifically, spaghetti squash is not considered a significant source. Prebiotic fibers are types of dietary fiber that feed beneficial gut bacteria, promoting a healthy gut microbiome. They are found in foods like garlic, onions, leeks, asparagus, bananas, chicory root, Jerusalem artichokes, and whole grains such as oats and barley.

While spaghetti squash does contain fiber, helping with digestion and contributing to satiety, it does not have the high levels of inulin, oligofructose, or other specific types of prebiotic fibers found in the more potent prebiotic foods listed above. Spaghetti squash can still be a valuable part of a balanced diet, offering vitamins like vitamin C, vitamin B6, and potassium and being low in calories, but for targeted prebiotic benefits, incorporating other foods known for their prebiotic content would be more effective.

To support gut health and promote the growth of beneficial bacteria, consider combining spaghetti squash with prebiotic-rich foods. For example, you could prepare a dish that includes garlic, onions, or leeks alongside spaghetti squash, which would provide both fiber and prebiotic benefits.

While spaghetti squash may not be a primary source of prebiotic fiber, combined with other prebiotic-rich foods, it can still contribute to a well-rounded and diverse diet supporting overall gut health; adding lentils to a marinara making a vegan bolognese is an incredibly delicious combination full of nutrients and fiber and relatively low in calories compared to a traditional bolognese.

Beans, lentils, and peas are excellent sources of fiber. For example, cooked black beans contain about 15 grams of fiber per cup, cooked lentils around 15-18 grams per cup, and cooked chickpeas (garbanzo beans) approximately 12-14 grams per cup.

Whole grains such as oats, barley, quinoa, and brown rice are fiber-rich. For instance, one cup of cooked oatmeal provides roughly 4 grams of fiber, while one cup of cooked barley offers about 6 grams. Many vegetables are high in fiber. Others like artichokes, broccoli, Brussels sprouts, kale, and spinach.

For instance, one medium artichoke contains around 7 grams of fiber, and one cup of cooked broccoli provides approximately 5 grams. Fruits like raspberries, pears, apples, and bananas are known for their fiber content. One cup of raspberries contains about 8 grams of fiber, one medium pear provides roughly 6 grams, and one medium apple offers approximately 4 grams.

Nuts and seeds are good sources of fiber. For example, one ounce (about a handful) of almonds contains around 3.5 grams of fiber, and one ounce of chia seeds provides about 10 grams. Avocado is a unique fruit that is high in fiber. One medium avocado contains approximately 10 grams of fiber, making guacamole the healthiest option on some restaurant menus.

Prebiotics are not to be confused with probiotics, which are the live microorganisms that, when taken orally, can improve the colonization of the adequate strains required for optimal health. They are bacteria or yeast that provide health benefits when consumed adequately. They help maintain a balanced gut microbiota by adding beneficial bacteria to the population. Probiotics can be found in certain foods like yogurt, kefir, sauerkraut, kimchi, and in supplement form. Different strains of probiotics may offer different benefits, so it's important to choose specific strains based on individual needs.

The specific probiotics that individuals may lack can vary

significantly based on factors such as childhood exposure to certain strains, diet, lifestyle, health status, and geographic location. Despite these variations, certain probiotic strains have been widely studied for their health benefits and are commonly available as supplements.

Probiotics found in yogurt and those in probiotic pills can differ depending on the specific strains used in their production. Both yogurt and probiotic supplements contain beneficial bacteria that promote gut health and support digestion, but the types and concentrations of probiotics can vary.

Yogurt is a popular source of probiotics, often containing strains like Lactobacillus bulgaricus, which is crucial in yogurt fermentation and contributes to its texture and flavor. This strain also supports digestive health by producing lactic acid, creating an acidic environment that inhibits the growth of harmful bacteria in the gut. Another strain frequently found in yogurt is Lactobacillus acidophilus, which is known for promoting digestive health and supporting immune function. This bacterium helps maintain the balance of beneficial bacteria in the gut and aids in the digestion of lactose, making it particularly beneficial for those with lactose intolerance. Additionally, some yogurt products include Bifidobacterium lactis. This strain promotes digestive health and regularity and has been shown to alleviate symptoms of irritable bowel syndrome (IBS) and contribute to a healthy gut microbiome.

However, it is important to note that not all yogurt provides the full probiotic benefits one might expect. Most commercially available dairy yogurt undergoes pasteurization, a process where the yogurt is heated to kill harmful bacteria and extend shelf life. While pasteurization is essential for ensuring the safety of the product, it also kills a large portion of the beneficial probiotics naturally present in the yogurt.

This means that many of the live cultures initially added to the yogurt may be inactive by the time it reaches consumers.

To counteract this, some manufacturers add live probiotics back into the yogurt after pasteurization, but the effectiveness of these probiotics can vary. The strains added post-pasteurization might not be as resilient as those naturally occurring, and their concentration may not be sufficient to provide the desired health benefits. As a result, consumers looking to obtain probiotics from dairy yogurt should carefully check labels to ensure that the product contains "live and active cultures" and that these cultures are added after pasteurization.

In contrast, probiotic pills typically offer a wider variety of strains in higher concentrations than yogurt.

These supplements are designed to target various aspects of health by delivering specific strains that may not be present in yogurt. For instance, Lactobacillus acidophilus, commonly found in both yogurt and probiotic pills, plays a critical role in maintaining a balanced gut microbiome and is found in many fermented foods.

Another strain, Bifidobacterium bifidum, is often included in probiotic supplements for its ability to enhance gut health by strengthening the gut's barrier function and promoting the growth of other beneficial bacteria. Lactobacillus rhamnosus, also found in many probiotic supplements, is recognized for supporting immune function and digestive health. This strain has been studied for its potential to reduce the severity of gastrointestinal infections and improve overall gut health. Lactobacillus plantarum is another versatile strain frequently included in probiotic pills, known for supporting the gut's natural flora and contributing to overall well-being.

As awareness of the implications of the dairy industry grows, non-dairy yogurts have become increasingly available. These alternatives often contain similar probiotic strains, making them a viable option for those who are lactose intolerant or choose to avoid dairy for other reasons.

Probiotics, particularly those found in both yogurt and supplements, have been extensively studied for their potential benefits in supporting digestive health, immune function, and overall cellular well-being. Some research suggests that certain probiotic strains can even induce a sense of well-being on a cellular level, contributing to feelings of euphoria, although not in a psychoactive way.

Incorporating probiotics into your diet, whether through yogurt or supplements, can be a valuable way to support gut health and overall wellness. However, when choosing yogurt as your source, it is vital to be aware of the effects of pasteurization and to select products that ensure the presence of live and active cultures. The decision between yogurt and supplements ultimately depends on individual preferences, dietary needs, and health goals.

Another common probiotic strain found in the human gut, Bifidobacterium bifidum, has been associated with various health benefits. It has been shown to contribute to a healthy gut microbiota, support digestion, and promote immune function. It may help promote gastrointestinal health, support immune function, and alleviate symptoms of diarrhea and constipation.

Lactobacillus rhamnosus is a probiotic strain that has been extensively studied and is known for its ability to survive the harsh, acidic environment of the stomach. Lactobacillus rhamnosus has been researched for its potential benefits in supporting gut health and immune function and reducing the risk of certain gastrointestinal conditions. This probiotic strain has been studied for its potential benefits in promoting digestive health, supporting immune function, and reducing the risk of respiratory infections.

Lactobacillus plantarum is a versatile probiotic strain that has been investigated for its potential health benefits. It is known for its ability to survive in the gastrointestinal tract and has been studied for its role in digestive health, immune support, and promoting a balanced gut microbiota. Lactobacillus plantarum is a versatile probiotic strain known for its ability to survive in harsh conditions in the gastrointestinal tract. It may help support digestive health, reduce inflammation, and strengthen the immune system. Both yogurt and probiotic pills can be beneficial sources of probiotics, but the specific strains and concentrations may vary.

Saccharomyces boulardii, while technically a yeast and not a bacterium, is a well-known probiotic that has been extensively studied for its potential benefits in supporting gut health. It has been researched for its role in managing diarrhea, including antibiotic-associated diarrhea and certain gastrointestinal infections.

Sauerkraut and kimchi are both fermented foods that are known for their probiotic content. The specific strains and quantities of probiotics can vary depending on factors such as the fermentation process, ingredients used, and preparation methods. They are typically rich in lactic acid bacteria, including species such as Lactobacillus plantarum, Lactobacillus brevis, and Lactobacillus mesenteroides. These strains contribute to the fermentation process and produce lactic acid, which gives these foods their tangy flavor. This genus of bacteria is commonly found in fermented foods and can play a role in the fermentation of sauerkraut and kimchi. Leuconostoc mesenteroides and Leuconostoc citreum are examples of Leuconostoc strains that may be present. Pediococcus species, such as Pediococcus pentosaceus, are lactic acid bacteria that can contribute to the fermentation of sauerkraut and kimchi.

Weissella species, including Weissella koreensis and Weissella cibaria, are commonly found in fermented vegetables like kimchi and can have probiotic potential. Lactic acid production: The beneficial bacteria, primarily lactic acid bacteria (LAB), convert the sugars present in the food into lactic acid through lactic acid fermentation. This acidifies the environment, creating an inhospitable condition for harmful bacteria and pathogens. Fermentation breaks down complex molecules into simpler forms, making nutrients more easily absorbed by the body. For example, the breakdown of proteins during fermentation can form more bioavailable amino acids.

Fermented foods become rich in live beneficial microorganisms, including lactic acid bacteria and yeast strains. These microorganisms can survive the acidic environment of the digestive system and reach the gut, where they may confer health benefits by supporting a balanced gut microbiota and promoting gut health.

Fermentation activates and increases the activity of enzymes naturally present in food. Enzymes help break down food components and aid in digestion. Fermentation leads to the production of various bioactive compounds such as short-chain fatty acids, antioxidants, vitamins (e.g., B vitamins), and other metabolites. These compounds may have anti-inflammatory, antioxidant, and immune-modulating properties, providing potential health benefits.

Gut flora diversity refers to the variety and abundance of different microbial species in the gut. A diverse gut microbiome is associated with better health outcomes. A diet rich in fiber, prebiotics (food for beneficial bacteria), and fermented foods (probiotics) can promote a diversified gut flora.

The time it takes to cultivate a more diverse gut flora can vary from person to person. Changes in the gut microbiome can occur relatively quickly, often within days to weeks, in response to dietary changes. However, achieving long-lasting changes and a stable, diverse gut microbiome may take several weeks to months.

A diet supporting beneficial bacteria growth is the best way to get a diversified gut flora. Here are some dietary practices that can promote a healthy gut microbiome. Consume fiber-rich foods like fruits, vegetables, whole grains, legumes, and nuts. Fiber is an essential source of nutrition for beneficial gut bacteria.

Incorporate fermented foods like yogurt, kefir, sauerkraut, kimchi, and tempeh into your diet. These foods contain live beneficial bacteria that can help support gut health.

Include prebiotic-rich foods like garlic, onions, leeks, asparagus, and bananas. Prebiotics are non-digestible fibers that feed beneficial bacteria in the gut. High consumption of added sugars and highly processed foods can negatively affect the gut microbiome and promote the growth of less beneficial bacteria. Alcohol consumption can disrupt the gut microbiome. Limit alcohol intake to support gut health.

Chronic stress can also influence the gut microbiome. Practicing stress-reduction techniques, such as meditation, yoga, and regular exercise, can be beneficial.

Kombucha is a fermented tea drink made by fermenting sweetened black or green tea with a symbiotic culture of bacteria and yeast (SCOBY). The fermentation process results in the production of organic acids, probiotics, and other bioactive compounds. Kombucha contains live probiotic bacteria, beneficial microorganisms that can support gut health. These probiotics can colonize the gut and promote a balanced and diverse microbiome.

During fermentation, kombucha produces organic acids like acetic, gluconic, and lactic acid. These acids can create an acidic environment in the gut, which may inhibit the growth of harmful bacteria and promote the development of beneficial bacteria. Tea, the primary ingredient in kombucha, contains polyphenols and antioxidants that can have various health benefits. These compounds can have prebiotic effects, meaning they can act as food for beneficial gut bacteria. Some proponents claim that kombucha aids in detoxification, helping to remove toxins from the body. However, there is limited scientific evidence to support this claim.

Some individuals report that consuming kombucha can improve digestion and alleviate gastrointestinal issues. The probiotics and organic acids in kombucha may contribute to these effects.

Probiotics do not differ by the source from which the yogurt is fermented. Dairy does not create yogurt; the bacteria create the yogurt as long as the base is habitable. The same way that coconut cream whips the same way that dairy cream does, not because it has magical powers and was meant to be whipped up for human consumption, but because it has copious amounts of fat, which is required molecularly for emulsification.

On the other hand, sourdough bread is made using a sourdough starter, a mixture of flour and water that naturally captures wild yeast and bacteria from the environment. The starter captures and grows a diverse community of microorganisms, including various yeast strains and lactobacilli. These wild yeast and bacteria produce carbon dioxide and lactic acid during fermentation, giving sourdough bread its unique flavor, texture, and rise.

While yogurt and sourdough involve fermentation and the use of microorganisms, the specific strains of bacteria and yeast involved in each process differ. The starter cultures for yogurt are carefully selected and controlled, while the sourdough starter captures naturally occurring microorganisms from the environment.

It's important to note that yogurt and sourdough bread can have probiotic properties, but the types of probiotics and their concentrations may vary between the two products. Not all commercial yogurt or sourdough bread may contain live and active probiotics, as some processing methods can affect their viability. For the highest probiotic benefit, look for yogurt labeled with live and active cultures and consider making sourdough bread with a well-maintained sourdough starter.

During the baking process of sourdough bread, high temperatures usually eliminate most bacteria, including those essential for fermentation. Although a few heat-resistant spores may persist, lactobacilli and most other beneficial bacteria don't withstand the heat. As a result, it's rare for these bacteria to remain active post-baking. Yet, fermentation prior to baking is vital for sourdough's distinctive flavors, textures, and characteristics.

Potential health benefits might stem from organic acids and enzymes developed during fermentation. Lactic acid bacteria, which are significant during fermentation, create lactic acid from flour sugars, imparting the sour flavor and aiding in preservation. Despite the heat's impact, some of these bacteria might endure, particularly in the crust or near the bread's surface. Still, the primary benefit of fermentation in sourdough is the enhancement of organic acids and texture rather than providing live probiotics.

For individuals with gluten sensitivity or celiac disease, gluten-free sourdough offers a delicious and nourishing alternative. However, to prevent cross-contamination with gluten-containing products, it's imperative to ensure the use of certified gluten-free components and adhere to strict gluten-free methods during preparation. Consulting a healthcare professional or a dietitian is advisable before introducing gluten-free sourdough or similar products into one's diet.

Gluten is a protein in wheat and related grains like barley and rye. It is essential for the structure and elasticity of bread dough, giving it a characteristic chewy texture. Traditional sourdough bread is made using wheat flour, which contains gluten. However, making gluten-free sourdough using alternative flours that do not contain gluten is possible. Gluten-free sourdough is typically made using gluten-free grains and flour, such as rice flour, buckwheat flour, sorghum flour, quinoa flour, or a combination.

These flours can still ferment and produce a sourdough-like

bread with a tangy flavor and improved digestibility compared to conventionally leavened gluten-free bread. In gluten-free sourdough, the rise and structure of the bread are achieved through the fermentation process, similar to traditional sourdough. Wild yeast and lactobacilli from the environment or from a gluten-free sourdough starter (made with gluten-free flour) help break down the carbohydrates and proteins in the dough, producing carbon dioxide and lactic acid. This fermentation process creates air pockets and gives the bread its characteristic texture and flavor.

The relationship between consuming yeasted bread and candida overgrowth is a topic of debate and not fully understood. Candida is a type of yeast naturally present in the body, particularly in the digestive tract, and typically exists in a balanced state with other microorganisms. However, certain conditions, such as a weakened immune system, prolonged antibiotic use, or a high-sugar diet, can disrupt this balance and lead to candida overgrowth.

Scientific evidence does not support the idea that consuming yeasted bread (or other foods containing yeast) can directly cause candida overgrowth. The yeast used in bread-making, such as Saccharomyces cerevisiae (baker's yeast), differs from the Candida species that can cause infections in the body.

However, it is essential to note that consuming a diet high in refined carbohydrates, sugars, and processed foods can create an environment that promotes candida overgrowth. Yeasted bread, especially those made with refined flour and added sugars, may contribute to an imbalanced diet that can favor the growth of candida and other harmful microorganisms in the gut.

If someone suspects they have candida overgrowth or other digestive issues, it is essential to consult with a healthcare professional, such as a gastroenterologist or a registered dietitian, for an accurate diagnosis and appropriate management. Making dietary changes, such as reducing sugar intake, increasing fiber-rich foods, and supporting beneficial gut bacteria with a balanced diet, can help promote a healthy gut microbiome and overall digestive health.

Kimchi is a nutritious Korean fermented dish made with seasoned vegetables like Napa cabbage and Korean radishes. Its probiotics, vitamins, and antioxidants offer health benefits. It promotes gut health, aids digestion, boosts immunity, and enhances nutrient uptake. Its low calories, high fiber, and anti-inflammatory ingredients also support weight management and reduce inflammation.

Regular kimchi intake may regulate blood sugar and improve heart health by managing cholesterol levels. While probiotic supplements are an option, their effectiveness can vary; refrigeration can help maintain their potency.

Maintaining the health of your gut biome is crucial for your overall wellness; it's important to avoid Western antibiotics where possible and choose nutrient-rich prebiotic fiber instead. Much like how a garden flourishes with adequate sunlight and water, the good bacteria in our intestines flourish on premium nutrition. They consistently crave fiber-rich fruits and vegetables. Bear in mind that if you're taking probiotics without seeing results, suffering discomfort, or dealing with inconsistent bowel movements, you might want to try incorporating a variety of fibers from different sources at every meal.

Digestive processes are quite particular; the breakdown of meat, for instance, is more taxing on the system than carbohydrates or fats. It's a protein-heavy affair; our stomachs need to summon more hydrochloric acid (HCl) to transform these proteins into amino acids. While HCl is crucial in protein digestion and facilitating this acidic environment, its overproduction can have downsides.

An excess of this gastric juice can usher in an array of problems—heartburn, acid reflux, and stomach aches are just the beginning. When our bodies continually produce too much HCl, we may grapple with conditions like hyperchlorhydria or even GERD, the latter characterized by the painful re-entry of stomach acid into the esophagus. The sustained assault of high acid levels can give rise to peptic ulcers, scarring our stomach, intestines, or esophageal linings, in addition to daily discomfort; the ripple effects of excessive acid don't end there; it can corrode the stomach lining over time, leading to gastritis, among other digestive issues. Such a hostile environment can disrupt the assimilation of essential minerals, leaving the door open to calcium, magnesium, and iron deficiencies.

A diet centered around meat can have multiple effects beyond just increasing hydrochloric acid production in the stomach; it can disrupt the body's natural digestive processes and lead to imbalances in the microbiome. High meat consumption alters the composition of bile acids, which are essential for breaking down fats and maintaining a healthy gut environment. This shift can promote harmful bacterial populations while suppressing beneficial ones, disrupting the gut's delicate balance. Additionally, compounds in meat, such as carnitine and choline, are metabolized by gut bacteria into trimethylamine (TMA), which the liver converts into trimethylamine N-oxide (TMAO). Elevated levels of TMAO are associated with an increased risk of heart disease, as it contributes to atherosclerosis, or the buildup of fatty deposits in the arteries, which can lead to heart attacks and strokes.

Furthermore, a diet high in meat proteins can alter the gut's acidity, which influences the balance of gut bacteria. Different bacteria thrive in different pH levels, and a shift towards a more acidic gut can promote the growth of harmful bacteria. This imbalance, known as dysbiosis, can lead to inflammation, compromised immune function, and other health issues. Meat-heavy diets are also typically low in dietary fiber, which is crucial for nourishing beneficial gut bacteria. A lack of fiber can cause beneficial bacteria to diminish, allowing harmful bacteria to flourish. In contrast, gut bacteria ferment dietary fibers from plant-based sources like vegetables, fruits, seeds, and whole grains to produce short-chain fatty acids (SCFAs), which support the growth of beneficial bacteria and contribute to a healthy gut environment.

When dietary fiber is scarce, the fermentation process essential for gut health is curtailed, potentially leading to constipation and other digestive issues. Meat decomposition within the gut can further exacerbate these problems, heightening the risk of various ailments. Therefore, a meat-centric diet not only disrupts the microbiome's balance by altering bile acid composition and increasing levels of harmful compounds like TMAO but also changes gut acidity, impacting overall health.

To maintain a healthy microbiome and promote better digestive health, it is crucial to adopt a balanced diet that includes a variety of plant-based foods. These foods are rich in fiber, which supports the growth of beneficial bacteria and ensures the gut remains a balanced ecosystem. Imagine the gut as a delicate ecosystem, like an aquarium, where even small changes can ripple out and unsettle the entire system. Choosing what you eat with mindfulness can help maintain this balance, supporting overall health and reducing the risk of chronic diseases.

14
SODIUM SUCKS. NAVIGATING FOOD LABELS

In a world where food choices are more important than ever, understanding the hidden dangers of commercial ingredients is crucial. The food industry, driven by profit margins, often prioritizes cheaper fillers and artificial enhancers over the nutritional value and health of consumers. This is why it's imperative that we become vigilant in our food choices. The colorful packaging and strategic product placements in grocery stores might catch our eye, but the truth often lies buried in the fine print of the ingredient list. These lists, which reveal a product's true nature by listing components from most to least prevalent, can empower us to make better choices that nourish our bodies rather than harm them. Even though some harmful additives might be present in trace amounts, their potential impacts accumulate over time and should not be ignored.

Salt, for example, is an essential mineral that our bodies need to function properly. Yet, many people have developed an addiction to it. Contrary to popular belief, salt itself does not deaden taste buds. Instead, salt enhances the perception of flavors, making foods taste more pronounced and enjoyable. However, when consumed in excessive amounts over time, this enhancement can lead to a desensitization of the taste buds to saltiness.

This results in a higher preference for salty flavors and a vicious cycle where more salt is needed to satisfy the same taste sensation. This desensitization is particularly concerning given the link between high salt intake and several health issues. Table salt has a long and storied history that dates back to ancient times when it was a highly prized commodity.

Historically, salt was used not only as a seasoning but also as a preservative, currency, and even in religious rituals. The importance of salt in various cultures led to its nickname, "white gold." The word "salary" even originates from the Latin word *salarium*, which refers to the payments made to Roman soldiers for purchasing salt. For centuries, sea salt was the primary source, obtained by evaporating seawater in large pans under the sun. While effective, this method was limited by geography and climate, leading to the need for alternative methods of salt production.

With the advent of the Industrial Revolution and the need to supply growing urban populations with salt, the focus shifted from traditional methods to mining. Rock salt, or halite, is a mineral form of sodium chloride found in large underground deposits left behind by ancient, evaporated seas. These deposits are mined using traditional mining techniques, providing a more consistent and reliable source of salt compared to the unpredictable yields of sea salt production. Mining salt also became more economically viable with advances in drilling and extraction technologies, making it possible to meet the increasing demand for salt in food, industry, and other applications.

The addition of iodine to table salt began in the early 20th century as a public health measure to combat iodine deficiency disorders (IDD), which were prevalent in regions far from the sea and rich in iodine-containing foods. Iodine deficiency can lead to a range of health issues, including goiter (an enlargement of the thyroid gland), hypothyroidism, and intellectual disabilities in children. In 1924, the United States pioneered the iodization of salt, following the Swiss example, to address the widespread issue of goiter in the Great Lakes, Appalachians, and Northwestern regions. By adding potassium iodide to salt, a common staple in households, public health officials could easily and effectively improve iodine intake among the population. This simple intervention drastically reduced the prevalence of goiter and other iodine-related health problems, making iodized salt a standard in many countries worldwide.

The shift to mined salt for commercial table salt production is largely due to the cost-effectiveness and efficiency of extraction, which allows for the production of large quantities at lower costs. Mined salt can be processed to a high degree of purity, ensuring consistent quality and taste, which is important for both consumers and manufacturers. While sea salt is still valued for its trace minerals and distinct flavor profiles, mined salt remains the primary choice for mass production due to its scalability and economic advantages.

Additionally, the iodization process is more easily controlled and standardized with mined salt, ensuring that each grain of salt carries the necessary iodine content to meet public health guidelines.

In summary, the use of mined salt, combined with the addition of iodine, reflects the evolution of salt production from ancient trade to modern public health initiatives. It showcases how a simple dietary staple can play a crucial role in addressing widespread health issues and how technological advancements have shaped the ways we source and consume this vital mineral.

The importance of iodine in our diet cannot be overstated. Iodine is an essential nutrient required for the production of thyroid hormones, which regulate metabolism, growth, and development. These hormones, primarily triiodothyronine (T3) and thyroxine (T4), are crucial for maintaining the body's energy balance and supporting the function of various organs and tissues. A deficiency in iodine can lead to thyroid-related issues such as goiter, hypothyroidism, and developmental delays in children.

To combat iodine deficiency, which was once prevalent in many regions, iodine was added to table salt, a practice that became widespread in the early 20th century. This public health measure significantly reduced the incidence of iodine deficiency disorders, making iodized salt a primary source of iodine for many people. However, this reliance on iodized salt has led to some confusion, particularly when people are advised to reduce their sodium intake for health reasons. The question arises: How can one maintain adequate iodine levels without consuming excess table salt, especially on a plant-based diet?

Ancient or plant-based populations with iodine-rich soil are somewhat challenging to pinpoint precisely due to the limited historical and archaeological data on dietary iodine content. However, we can infer the presence of iodine-rich soils and the resulting adequate iodine intake based on geographic location, historical agricultural practices, and the use of specific crops. Some ancient populations likely had access to iodine-rich soil, supporting their largely plant-based diets.

Japan, known for its abundant coastline, has been home to numerous ancient civilizations that had a diet rich in seaweed and plant-based foods. The Japanese archipelago is surrounded by iodine-rich seawater, leading to higher natural iodine levels in the coastal soils. Japanese diets have traditionally included a variety of seaweeds, such as kombu, nori, and wakame, which are naturally high in iodine. These seaweeds were commonly used in soups, stews, and seasonings, providing a reliable source of iodine for the population. Additionally, the Japanese diet included vegetables, rice, and other plant-based foods, making it possible for ancient coastal Japanese populations to have adequate iodine intake through their plant-based diets.

The ancient Maya and Aztec civilizations, located in present-day Mexico and Central America, also had access to iodine-rich coastal regions. These civilizations thrived in areas with a mix of coastal and inland territories, allowing them to access iodine from marine sources. Although their primary diet was plant-based, consisting of maize, beans, squash, and chili peppers, they could supplement their iodine intake with seafood and seaweed from the Gulf of Mexico and the Pacific Ocean. The use of coastal resources ensured that even predominantly plant-based diets had sufficient iodine to support thyroid health and overall well-being.

Ancient Celtic populations, particularly those living along the Atlantic coastlines of present-day Britain, Ireland, and northern France, had access to iodine-rich soil due to the influence of seawater and marine sediment deposits. The Celts practiced agriculture but also harvested seaweed, known as dulse and laver, which was rich in iodine. Seaweed was used as food and as fertilizer for crops, further enriching the soil with iodine. The Celtic diet included a variety of grains, vegetables, and seaweed, providing a balanced intake of nutrients, including iodine.

The ancient civilizations of South India, including the Dravidian people, lived in regions where the coastline met the fertile lands of the Deccan Plateau. These populations had access to iodine through the use of coastal and marine resources, including seaweed, fish, and saltwater. Although predominantly plant-based, their diet included a wide range of vegetables, grains, legumes, and fruits, supplemented by occasional use of iodine-rich marine resources. The proximity to the ocean and the use of traditional agricultural practices helped maintain iodine-rich soil, supporting a healthy and balanced diet.

Ancient Greek coastal communities, such as those in Crete and other Aegean islands, had access to iodine through both diet and agricultural practices. These populations relied on a Mediterranean diet, rich in fruits, vegetables, olives, and grains. They also utilized seaweed and seafood as part of their diet, which provided essential iodine. Greek farmers practiced crop rotation and used seaweed as a natural fertilizer, enriching the soil with iodine and other trace minerals. The combination of plant-based foods and marine resources helped ensure adequate iodine intake among ancient Greeks.

Traditional Pacific Islander populations, such as those in Polynesia, Melanesia, and Micronesia, relied heavily on the natural resources of their islands, including the iodine-rich ocean. These populations consumed a diet rich in root vegetables like taro and sweet potatoes, fruits like coconuts and bananas, and various forms of seaweed. Seaweed and fish from the ocean provided essential iodine, while volcanic soils often contributed additional minerals. The combination of iodine from marine sources and plant-based foods ensured that traditional Pacific Islander diets were balanced and nutrient-rich.

These ancient populations, through their geographic location, agricultural practices, and dietary habits, likely had access to iodine-rich soils and marine resources that ensured adequate iodine intake, even within predominantly plant-based diets. By utilizing natural sources of iodine, such as seaweed and marine sediment-enriched soils, these populations were able to maintain thyroid health and overall nutritional balance. Today, these historical practices serve as valuable lessons in understanding the importance of natural nutrient sources and sustainable agricultural practices. Soils near coastlines generally have higher iodine content due to the deposition of iodine from seawater. Iodine is naturally present in the ocean, and it can enter the atmosphere through the volatilization of iodine compounds from seawater. This iodine can then be deposited onto coastal soils through precipitation, leading to higher iodine concentrations. Additionally, coastal areas may benefit from the natural accumulation of seaweed and marine detritus, which are rich in iodine, further contributing to the iodine levels in the soil.

Certain geological formations naturally contain higher levels of iodine. These include areas with sedimentary rocks rich in organic matter, such as shale and coal deposits. As these rocks weather and erode over time, iodine is released into the soil. Regions with volcanic activity can also have soils enriched with iodine, as volcanic ash and gases can contain iodine that becomes part of the soil through natural weathering processes.

Areas that were once submerged under ancient seas or oceans can have iodine-rich soils due to the accumulation of marine sediments. When these areas are uplifted or exposed due to geological changes, the sediments become part of the terrestrial soil, carrying with them the iodine content from marine life and seawater.

Fortunately, there are several plant-based sources of iodine that can help meet your daily needs without the associated risks of overconsuming sodium. Seaweed is one of the richest sources of iodine, with varieties such as kelp, nori, and wakame providing significant amounts of this essential nutrient. A small serving of seaweed can easily fulfill or even exceed the recommended daily intake of iodine, making it a valuable addition to any plant-based diet.

In addition to seaweed, certain fruits and vegetables can contribute to your iodine intake. For instance, potatoes with the skin, cranberries, and strawberries offer smaller but valuable amounts of iodine. Navy beans and other legumes also provide iodine, along with a host of other essential nutrients like fiber and protein, which are important for a balanced plant-based diet.

By incorporating these iodine-rich plant foods into your diet, you can maintain healthy thyroid function without relying on iodized salt or animal products. This approach not only supports your overall health by ensuring adequate iodine intake but also helps you avoid the potential health risks associated with high sodium consumption, such as hypertension and cardiovascular disease.

Moreover, it's important to recognize that while iodized salt can be a convenient source of iodine, it shouldn't be the only source of a balanced plant-based diet. Diversifying your iodine intake through whole plant foods ensures that you're getting a range of nutrients while also minimizing your dependence on processed salt. This holistic approach to nutrition aligns with the broader goal of reducing the intake of harmful additives and chemicals commonly found in processed foods, thereby promoting long-term health and well-being.

In summary, while iodine is a vital nutrient for thyroid health, it's entirely possible to meet your daily requirements on a plant-based diet without over-relying on iodized table salt. By embracing a diet rich in natural, plant-based sources of iodine, you can support your thyroid function, enjoy a variety of nutrient-dense foods, and maintain a healthy balance in your overall diet.

The body's craving for salt can also be a signal of underlying issues. For example, dehydration can lead to an increased need for fluids and an electrolyte balance, prompting a craving for salty foods to replenish sodium levels. Conditions like Addison's disease, which involves adrenal gland dysfunction, can cause electrolyte imbalances, including low sodium levels, leading to salt cravings as the body attempts to restore balance. Hormonal fluctuations, such as those that occur before or during the menstrual cycle, can also trigger salt cravings, likely due to changes in fluid balance and stress responses.

As consumers, we must become more aware of what we eat. Rather than memorizing the names of potentially dangerous additives,

Sodium Sucks. Navigating Food Labels

we should acknowledge the reality of the modern food industry and make informed choices that prioritize our health. For instance, if you enjoy having snacks on hand, it is worth shopping for them in the health food aisle or choosing reputable brands that use cleaner, allergen-friendly ingredients. Many people who live health-conscious lifestyles overlap with those who are sensitive or allergic to certain foods, leading to an increased demand for products made without common allergens or harmful additives. Independent grain mills and small-scale food producers often offer superior natural foods, which can serve as healthier alternatives to the chemical-laden, processed products that dominate the market.

One red flag on food labels is the word "enriched." This term often signals that the product has been stripped of its natural vitamins and minerals during processing and then artificially "enriched" with synthetic nutrients. The bleaching, pasteurizing, and milling processes that many foods undergo strip away their natural nutritional content, leaving them non-nutritive. To mask this, companies re-add vitamins and minerals, but often from sources that are not as bioavailable or beneficial as their natural counterparts. Consuming large amounts of these "enriched" products, which include common items like bread, cereals, milk, cookies, crackers, and pasta, can place an additional burden on the liver and kidneys, particularly when combined with the multivitamins that many people take daily.

In addition to being stripped of nutrients, these processed foods often contain high levels of sodium. The modern American diet is notorious for its overconsumption of sodium, a trend that poses several health hazards. Excessive sodium intake can elevate blood pressure, a condition known as hypertension, which increases the likelihood of heart disease, stroke, and other cardiovascular issues. Sodium's water-retaining properties can also lead to fluid retention, bloating, and swelling, further burdening the kidneys and potentially impairing their function. Research has shown that high sodium intake can even contribute to bone loss, increasing the risk of osteoporosis, and it has been linked to an elevated risk of stomach cancer.

While regular table salt, or iodized salt, is a common household staple, it is not the healthiest option for seasoning food. Sodium is essential for survival, but the form in which it is consumed matters greatly. Iodine, which is added to table salt, is crucial for thyroid gland function and the production of thyroid hormones. These hormones, such as triiodothyronine (T3) and thyroxine (T4), regulate metabolism, growth, development, and the operation of various organs and tissues. The body requires about 150 micrograms of iodine daily, which can be obtained from natural sources like strawberries, cranberries, green beans, corn, leafy greens, watercress, kale, seaweed, and potatoes with the skin. By choosing these foods, you can avoid the need for iodized salt while still supporting thyroid health.

Celtic Sea Salt, harvested from clay-lined shores, is often considered one of the best salts in the world. It is enriched with around 82 minerals, including potassium, magnesium, iron, and calcium, which contribute to its mucus-reducing, electrolyte-boosting, body-healing properties. However, as with all salts, moderation is key. A few flakes in your spring water are enough to enrich it with minerals and provide health benefits without the risks associated with excessive sodium intake.

Pink salt, typically a rock salt with minerals and impurities that give it a pinkish hue, can refer to various types of salt, including Himalayan pink salt, Hawaiian pink salt, or other similar varieties. Himalayan Pink Salt, harvested from the Khewra Salt Mine in Pakistan, is often claimed to be more natural and to contain more minerals than regular table salt. However, consumers should be cautious of sourcing labels to ensure they are purchasing a legitimate product, as this salt is sometimes mined from less desirable locations and still labeled as "Himalayan."

Other salts, like Lava Salt or volcanic salt, are produced by evaporating seawater using volcanic heat. They may contain trace minerals and are often prized for their unique flavor and texture. Dead Sea Salt, derived from the Dead Sea, is known for its high mineral content and is commonly used in spa treatments and skincare products. Kosher salt, a coarse-grained salt often used in kosher cooking, has a texture different from table salt but is not significantly different in sodium content.

The Recommended Dietary Allowance (RDA) for sodium varies based on age, sex, and certain health conditions. For most adults, the Adequate Intake (AI) level set by the National Academies is around 1,500 to 2,300 milligrams per day. However, the average sodium intake in the United States far exceeds these recommendations, with the Centers for Disease Control and Prevention (CDC) reporting that it is approximately 3,400 milligrams daily.

This overconsumption is concerning, particularly when comparing the sodium intake of a typical American diet to that of a raw vegan diet, which contains no added sodium.

Most fruits and vegetables are naturally low in sodium, and even nuts, seeds, and sea vegetables contain only moderate amounts. For example, almonds contain around 1-2 milligrams of sodium per ounce, while sea vegetables like nori or dulse range from 30 to 300 milligrams per serving. These numbers illustrate that a raw vegan diet, devoid of added salt, inherently maintains low sodium levels, making it a healthier option for those looking to reduce their sodium intake.

Certain medications, such as diuretics, which are used to treat conditions like high blood pressure, can increase urinary sodium excretion, leading to sodium depletion and subsequent salt cravings. During intense physical activity or hot weather, the body loses fluids and electrolytes through sweat, creating a need for sodium replacement and leading to salt cravings.

Some individuals may experience increased cravings for salty foods during periods of stress, anxiety, or emotional upheaval, as the body's response to stress hormones can lead to comfort eating. In rare cases, individuals with adrenal insufficiency may experience an Addisonian crisis, a life-threatening condition characterized by severe electrolyte imbalances. During such a crisis, salt cravings may be more pronounced.

When you consume salty foods, the taste buds on your tongue detect the presence of sodium ions, triggering a signal to the brain that results in the perception of saltiness. Salt can enhance the perception of other flavors, heightening the taste of various food components, such as sweetness in desserts or savory notes in dishes. However, regularly consuming high amounts of salt can lead to desensitization, where more salt is needed to achieve the same level of perceived saltiness. This can lead to a preference for saltier foods and a diminished appreciation for the natural flavors of less salty options.

To restore sensitivity to salt, it's important to gradually reduce salt intake, allowing taste buds to readjust and regain their ability to detect lower levels of salt. This process not only helps in appreciating the natural flavors of food but also plays a crucial role in regulating metabolism. Thyroid hormones, for instance, are vital in regulating the body's metabolic rate, energy production, and nutrient utilization. A balanced sodium intake supports the proper functioning of these hormones, which in turn supports overall health.

Understanding food labels is your first line of defense against hidden additives. It's advisable to first look at the calorie content before examining the ingredients. If you can't pronounce an ingredient, it's best to avoid it. Ingredients are listed by volume, so the first few components are crucial in determining the product's overall nutritional value.

The World Health Organization (WHO) has classified processed meat as a Group 1 carcinogen and red meat as a Group 2A probable carcinogen. These classifications are based on evaluations by the International Agency for Research on Cancer (IARC), which found sufficient evidence linking the consumption of these meats to an increased risk of certain types of cancer. However, this classification does not imply that consuming these foods will definitely cause cancer, but rather that there is a potential association that consumers should be aware of when making dietary choices.

Despite these classifications, the WHO's dietary recommendations emphasize a balanced and varied diet, including different food groups. While the WHO suggests including lean meats, poultry, and fish in the diet, they also highlight the importance of consuming various plant-based foods, such as fruits, vegetables, legumes, and whole grains, which have been associated with numerous health benefits and a reduced risk of chronic diseases. The confusion around what we "should" eat for the perfect body, mind, and planet has reached a peak. The answer lies in becoming in tune with the symbiosis we seek, understanding that true change begins when we have the information needed to make the right decisions that will lead us to the manifestation of our perfect body.

In some parts of the world, governments have taken a more proactive approach to food safety by banning certain ingredients that are still allowed in the United States. For instance, "Cheez-It" crackers are banned in Austria and Norway, while Ritz crackers are banned in several other countries due to the presence of partially hydrogenated cottonseed oil, a known health risk.

TBHQ (tert-butylhydroquinone) is yet another example of a

controversial food additive. TBHQ is a synthetic antioxidant derived from petroleum, commonly used as a preservative in processed foods, house paint, and cosmetics. Its primary function is to prevent the oxidation of fats and oils, thereby extending the shelf life of products like cereals, cookies, processed snacks, fast food, fried foods, baked goods, and cooking oils. The FDA has set a maximum allowable limit of 0.02% of a food product's total oil and fat content. However, this seemingly small amount does not mean it is entirely safe. Research has found TBHQ to cause liver enlargement, neurotoxic effects, convulsions, paralysis, and vision impairment in laboratory animals, raising concerns about its long-term safety in the human diet.

Artificial sweeteners like aspartame, saccharin, sucralose, acesulfame potassium (Ace-K), erythritol, and maltose are commonly used as sugar substitutes, but they rarely contribute to long-term weight loss. These artificial sweeteners disrupt the brain's natural processing of food, negatively affecting metabolism and triggering an insulin response that can cause a sudden drop in blood sugar. The side effects of these sweeteners range from gastrointestinal discomfort to potential cancer links, suggesting that the minimal calorie savings they offer may not be worth the potential health risks.

Instead of relying on artificial sweeteners to satisfy sweet cravings, it's healthier to enjoy whole foods like fresh watermelon and black cherries dipped in natural chocolate, tahini chocolate brownies sweetened with dates, maple syrup, or molasses, or coconut yogurt with mango puree. These options satisfy the craving and provide nutritional benefits without the risks associated with artificial additives.

Artificial colors are another area of concern. Commonly found in candy products, artificial colors such as Red 40 (Allura Red AC), Yellow 5 (Tartrazine), Yellow 6 (Sunset Yellow FCF), and Blue 1 (Brilliant Blue FCF) are used to make foods more visually appealing. However, these synthetic dyes are often accompanied by other undesirable ingredients. If you notice artificial colors listed on a food label, it's a strong indication that the product may contain other additives that are best avoided. Natural food dyes, derived from sources like beets, spirulina, and turmeric, are preferable. Ethical food companies committed to cleanliness typically avoid mixing artificial and natural dyes. If numbers identify the dye, it's often synthetic or, in the case of carcinogenic Red dye No. 40 (Cochineal), made from crushed beetles.

The National Archives Code of Regulations lists all permitted colorants legally allowed in the U.S., including Annatto extracts with legal limits on arsenic and lead content. Although these numbers seem small, toxicity can build up over time, especially if someone consumes multiple sports drinks or artificially colored cereal daily.

Preservatives like sodium benzoate, potassium sorbate, BHA (butylated hydroxyanisole), and BHT (butylated hydroxytoluene) are chemical compounds used to stave off food's natural degradation. These preservatives, which are banned in Europe due to their carcinogenic properties, do harm once inside the body. However, natural alternatives exist. Rosemary and oregano, for example, have antimicrobial properties and can serve as natural preservatives in place of chemical ones, offering a safer option for those looking to avoid synthetic additives.

Most people have heard of MSG (Monosodium Glutamate), though its true nature remains a mystery to many. MSG is often used to enhance the flavors of foods, particularly in takeout restaurants. Despite blind studies showing no definitive evidence of allergic reactions, lab mice exposed to MSG demonstrated stunted growth and brain tumors. MSG alters flavors and intensities, sending mixed signals to the brain and potentially leading to overeating. Learning to savor the natural flavors of your meals without resorting to this kind of "hyper-seasoning" will serve you better in the long run.

Emulsifiers and stabilizers, such as xanthan gum, guar gum, and carrageenan, are common thickening agents used in food products. While these ingredients add elasticity and texture to foods, they can be difficult for the human body to break down. Lab studies have shown that xanthan gum can slow tumor growth, but it can also cause gastrointestinal discomfort in some individuals. For those with digestive issues, these gums should be consumed sparingly.

Carrageenan, derived from Irish red moss, is particularly controversial. While it is used widely in the food industry as a thickener and stabilizer, some studies have linked it to colon cancer. A study found that food-grade carrageenan contained degraded carrageenan, a substance used to provoke inflammation in animal studies. This raises concerns about its safety in human consumption despite its widespread use.

Acids like citric acid, lactic acid, phosphoric acid, and tartaric acid are some of the most commonly used additives in food products worldwide. Citric acid, originally from sour fruits like limes and lemons, is now mainly produced by black mold. Scientists discovered that this mold can produce citric acid when it consumes sugar, making it a cheaper alternative for companies. Only about one percent of companies still use natural citric acid, which is clearly indicated on their labels.

The black mold version is detectable in the flavor of the food, in my opinion, so much so that I realized early on that the weird underlying flavor in some jarred salsas, salad dressings, and canned diced tomatoes, although seemingly natural and harmless, my senses honed in on the flavor, realized the common ingredient, and did my research. I have a discerning palate. I don't expect everyone to notice these subtle things until you create the space to enjoy the less tainted ones made from local organic restaurants or meal delivery services. Fresh is always better. Stopping at a Mexican restaurant for a pint of fresh pico de gallo or guacamole is always a preservative-free option compared to the ones on grocery shelves.

Silicon dioxide, or silica, is a naturally occurring mineral used as an anti-caking agent in powdered foods. While small amounts of silica are considered safe for consumption, it's wise to be cautious about cumulative intake. Similarly, calcium silicate, another anti-caking agent, is generally recognized as safe but is best consumed in moderation.

Magnesium stearate, used in supplements, is safe but has been scrutinized for potential contaminants. Sodium aluminosilicate, composed of sodium, aluminum, and silicon, is used as an anti-caking agent in powdered foods. While considered safe in small quantities, the presence of aluminum raises concerns due to its association with neurological issues at high exposure levels.

Understanding food labels is your first line of defense. Look for products with fewer additives and recognizable ingredients. Choosing whole foods, such as fresh fruits, vegetables, whole grains, and lean proteins, naturally reduces your intake of unnecessary additives. Cooking at home and preparing meals from scratch gives you control over what goes into your food.

In conclusion, understanding and sometimes avoiding certain food additives is a key step towards improved health and well-being. By being aware of these common additives and their roles, you can make more informed food choices, contributing to a healthier, more natural diet.

When you begin the habit of reading food labels, you have decided to take some of the regrets out of eating. Memorizing harmful ingredients isn't necessary, but committing to purchasing products without those ingredients will force companies to create cleaner options, get you closer to the healthiest version of yourself, or, hopefully, do both.

15
ORGANIC VS. EVERYTHING ELSE

The cost of organic produce and livestock has transformed what was once a basic expectation of our food into a luxury item. In today's economy, many people rely on store sales when shopping, making the affordability of conventionally grown foods appealing. The widespread belief that if a plant grows bigger and stronger after exposure to chemical sprays, tainted soil, and genetic modification must be safe for consumption is a common misconception. However, this belief is misguided.

Investing in organic foods is worth the extra expense. The primary reason is the invaluable return on money spent on foods that nourish the body. Preserving wellness is priceless; the food you invest in directly shapes who you are. Cutting costs in other areas to make room for the best quality foods is not just an option but a worthwhile investment in your health.

Alternatively, many people could benefit from the knowledge needed to start a small garden at home. Growing your own food allows you to control the quality of what you consume. Seasonally jarring, canning, and freezing homegrown food from local farmers' markets can extend the availability of organic foods throughout the year. Buying in bulk from wholesale clubs, such as frozen organic wild blueberries, can be a cost-effective option that retains much of the nutrition found in fresh produce.

Eating organic versus conventionally grown foods yields a

Organic VS. Everything Else

noticeable difference in taste and nutritional content. Organic farming, which employs natural fertilizers and nutrient-rich, pesticide-free soil, produces more nutritionally dense and flavorful food. Comparing an organic tomato or lettuce with its conventional counterpart reveals a significant difference. For example, hydroponic butter lettuce grown in a greenhouse contrasts sharply in taste with a bag of conventionally grown, ready-to-serve salad. Soaking produce in an alkaline solution with one tablespoon of baking soda per quart of water is highly effective in eliminating most pesticide residues. This simple action can protect you from contaminants that may have been introduced from the farm to your kitchen.

Precut, packaged lettuce and baby carrots, processed in warehouses, typically lose their original flavor due to the various steps involved in their preparation. Baby carrots are not naturally small but are, in fact, misshapen carrots that cannot be sold in stores. After peeling and cutting, they are milled into finger-sized pieces and then soaked in chlorine.

Once lettuce is cut, additional substances are often added to maintain its freshness and crunchiness until sold. This process typically involves using sulfites, which keep the product fresh but can impart a sulfurous, rubbery smell. Some producers also use modified atmospheric packaging with gases like nitrogen, carbon dioxide, or argon. Lettuce stored in these artificially sealed ozone bags can be two to three weeks old but remains more stable than fresh, whole lettuce.

Learning simple regrowth techniques can also reduce the need to repurchase organic foods frequently. Organic foods, not having been genetically manipulated, are generally fresher and more inclined to keep growing. However, for instance, pre-packaged lettuce goes through a three-wash cycle, leading to significant water use and waste. In the United States, the USDA's National Organic Program oversees organic products' production, labeling, and certification. To be labeled as organic, a product must meet specific standards and undergo certification by an accredited certifying agent.

Navigating food labels can be confusing, but understanding the regulations behind organic labeling can help consumers make more informed choices. The USDA sets strict standards for labeling foods as organic, ensuring that consumers receive what they expect when they choose organic products. Agricultural products labeled as organic must be produced using approved organic farming practices. These practices prohibit using synthetic fertilizers, pesticides, genetically modified organisms, and certain other substances. Organic farmers must adhere to guidelines and principles that promote soil and water conservation, biodiversity, and animal welfare. This holistic approach ensures that organic farming is sustainable and environmentally friendly.

To label their products as organic, farms and businesses involved in the production, handling, processing, or labeling of organic products must be certified by a USDA-accredited certifying agent. These certifying agents verify that organic standards and practices are being followed and conduct annual inspections to ensure compliance. Certification guarantees that the products meet all organic requirements from farm to table.

The USDA has established four distinct labeling categories for organic products. The "100% Organic" label is used for products that contain only organic ingredients, ensuring that no synthetic substances or GMOs are present. The "Organic" label is for products that contain at least 95% organic ingredients, with the remaining 5% consisting of non-organic ingredients approved on the USDA's National List of Allowed and Prohibited Substances.

These products still adhere to strict organic standards but allow minimal use of approved non-organic substances. Products with the "Made with Organic Ingredients" label contain at least 70% organic ingredients, with the remaining non-organic ingredients also approved on the USDA's National List.

This category offers more flexibility while still emphasizing the use of organic ingredients. The "Specific Organic Ingredients" label is for products that contain less than 70% organic ingredients. Up to three specific organic ingredients can be listed on the front panel of the packaging. These products do not carry the USDA Organic seal but can highlight the use of specific organic components.

Products that meet the USDA organic standards can display the USDA Organic seal on their packaging. This seal indicates that the product has been certified by an accredited certifying agent, which assures consumers of the product's organic integrity.

If a produce label consists of a four-digit code beginning with a 3 or 4, it indicates that the produce is conventionally grown and may have been exposed to synthetic pesticides.

A label with a five-digit code beginning with an 8 indicates genetically modified produce. A label with a five-digit code beginning with a 9 indicates that the produce has been grown using organic farming practices, ensuring it is free from synthetic pesticides and genetic modification.

To be certified organic, food must meet specific standards set by the governing body responsible for organic regulations in a particular country. Organic farming prohibits the use of synthetic pesticides and chemical fertilizers.

Organic certification is more than just a label; it represents a commitment to standards prioritizing environmental sustainability, animal welfare, and consumer health. Organic farmers follow strict guidelines that prohibit the use of synthetic pesticides, chemical fertilizers, and genetically modified organisms.

When discussing GMO labeling, it's essential to understand

the regulations and verification processes in place. In the United States, the USDA and FDA oversee the regulation of GMOs and non-GMO foods. The USDA implemented the National Bioengineered Food Disclosure Standard, which requires food products containing genetically modified ingredients to be labeled accordingly. This law provides consumers with transparency about GMO content in their food. For those seeking additional assurance about non-GMO status, the Non-GMO Project offers third-party verification and labeling through its Non-GMO Project Verified seal for foods that meet strict standards. Food manufacturers can voluntarily submit their products for evaluation, giving consumers confidence that they are free from GMOs.

It is important to note that organic certification inherently prohibits using GMOs. When you see the USDA organic seal on a product, you can trust that it is also non-GMO. Organic foods are produced according to specific regulations that exclude GMOs from farming practices, ensuring a more natural and transparent food choice. By understanding organic certification and GMO labeling, consumers can make informed decisions about the food they buy. Whether choosing organic for its environmental and health benefits or opting for non-GMO for transparency and personal preference, these labels empower consumers to support a food system that aligns with their values.

Horizontal gene transfer, or the transfer of genetic material between organisms, occurs naturally between certain microorganisms. However, the significance and frequency of horizontal gene transfer from dietary DNA fragments to gut microflora or somatic cells lining the intestines are still subjects of scientific debate and ongoing research. Regulatory bodies and scientific organizations evaluate the safety of genetically modified organisms and their potential impact on human health. Factors such as the stability of DNA fragments in the digestive system, the likelihood of horizontal gene transfer, and the potential consequences if it were to occur are considered in this assessment.

To date, regulatory agencies and scientific bodies, including the World Health Organization and the National Academy of Sciences, have concluded that approved GMOs are safe for human consumption. However, it is essential to note that safety does not necessarily equate to being the best option. Just because something is non-toxic does not mean it is the most suitable choice for consumption. Scientific research continues to investigate the behavior of DNA fragments from genetically modified foods in the gastrointestinal tract, their potential for transfer, and any associated risks. Ongoing surveillance and monitoring of the safety and impact of GMOs are crucial aspects of regulatory oversight. However, concerns have been raised about conflicts of interest, as the entities funding some studies may also stand to profit from the sale of GMO crops.

While many fruits and vegetables have been modified or cultivated by humans, most are still considered natural and safe for consumption. It is important to recognize that access to healthy foods varies across different communities. While the availability of whole foods increases, not everyone has equal access. For instance, choosing conventional broccoli over a prepackaged shelf-stable processed snack reflects the essence of simply selecting upwards of your cravings. Selective breeding and cultivation techniques have allowed us to enhance certain traits for improved taste, size, and other desirable characteristics.

The goal is to learn to understand the feelings associated with healthy foods and how your body and mind react to these changes. Weight loss and muscle tone are side effects of self-care. What you choose to eat is the pinnacle of setting yourself up for success in all areas of your life. Corn, wheat, and soybeans are staple crops that have undergone significant modification and cultivation over the years. Corn, originally a wild grass called teosinte, has been selectively bred by Native American farmers over thousands of years to develop the large, edible kernels we know today. In the United States, corn is a widely cultivated crop; extensive modification and crossbreeding have led to the development of various hybrid corn varieties with improved yield, disease resistance, and other desirable traits.

Similarly, wheat has been modified through selective breeding and hybridization to develop high-yielding varieties. Modern wheat varieties, especially those used in commercial baking, often differ from traditional heirloom strains due to hybridization and breeding programs. Soybeans, another essential crop, have been extensively modified through genetic engineering to develop genetically modified soybean varieties resistant to herbicides and pests. These genetically modified soybeans are commonly used in various food products and as animal feed. However, it is important to note that while most soy products available in health food stores may not be genetically modified, the feed given to livestock often contains genetically modified soybeans.

Eating meat from animals fed genetically modified food sources raises concerns about potential health implications. Animals' health, medicinal treatment, and living conditions can all impact the quality of the meat produced. When an animal consumes genetically modified feed, its body processes these substances, which can then be passed on to consumers through meat consumption. This process introduces layers of complexity and potential toxins into the food chain.

Choosing non-GMO sources, such as whole soybeans or edamame, provides a distinct experience regarding digestion and nutritional benefits. Consuming these whole, unprocessed sources allows the body to more efficiently access and utilize the nutrients they provide without the added burden of processing toxins associated with genetically modified feed. Ultimately, being aware of the origins of our food and making informed choices about what we consume can contribute to better health and well-being. Opting for non-GMO sources and supporting sustainable farming practices can help mitigate potential risks associated with genetically modified crops in our food supply.

Heirloom seeds are cultivated, meaning they are intentionally planted, nurtured, and harvested by farmers or gardeners. Unlike commercially produced hybrid seeds or genetically modified organisms, heirloom seeds are open-pollinated and are not the result of extensive crossbreeding or genetic modification.

Heirloom seeds are known for their genetic stability, meaning that if saved and replanted, they will generally produce plants with similar characteristics as the parent plant. This genetic stability allows heirloom plants to retain their unique flavors, colors, and traits across generations. These seeds often have historical or cultural significance and contribute to preserving genetic diversity in agricultural crops. Many heirloom varieties have unique flavors, appearances, or adaptations to specific climates, making them valued by farmers, gardeners, and culinary enthusiasts.

Apples, for instance, have been cultivated for thousands of years, with hundreds of varieties selectively bred for specific tastes, textures, and uses. Apples have been crossbred and selectively bred to create new varieties with desirable traits such as improved taste, texture, size, and disease resistance. Numerous apple varieties are available today, many resulting from intentional breeding efforts. Depending on where you live, apples grow in many climates, and access to local farms is always the best way to find them, rather than buying mass-marketed ones that often lack flavor.

Tomato breeding programs have concentraed on developing

varieties with enhanced shelf life, disease resistance, and uniformity in size and shape. This has led to the production of numerous hybrid tomato varieties suitable for commercial cultivation. The modifications and crossbreeding of these crops are done through traditional breeding methods, and not all of them involve genetic engineering or manipulation. The aim is often to improve crop yields, disease resistance, taste, and other qualities to meet the demands of mass production and consumption. However, it is still somewhat controversial, and you should strive to get the most naturally produced fruits and vegetables. The popularity of farmers markets has grown, but not everyone has equal access to them due to location, budget, transportation, and climate, which also makes some produce unavailable.

Broccoli, a human-modified form of wild cabbage, has been specifically cultivated for its dense flower heads. It is believed to have originated in the Mediterranean region and has been selectively bred over centuries to develop the desired traits. The bananas we consume today result from centuries of human intervention. The modern banana is a cultivated variety called the Cavendish banana, which replaced the Gros Michel variety due to susceptibility to Panama disease. Wild bananas are smaller and contain large seeds, unlike the seedless bananas we are familiar with today.

Potatoes, native to the Andes region of South America, have been selectively bred by indigenous people over thousands of years to develop larger tubers with improved taste and texture. Today, there are numerous cultivated varieties of potatoes with different colors, shapes, and culinary characteristics. Grapes have a long history of cultivation and domestication. The wild grapevine species Vitis vinifera is believed to be the ancestor of cultivated grapes.

Over time, humans selectively bred grapes for larger, sweeter fruits, and different varieties were developed for wine production or consumption as table grapes.

Organic VS. Everything Else

Watermelons, now cultivated to enhance their sweet, juicy flesh and achieve a larger size, are increasingly difficult to find with the extremely health-beneficial seeds inside. In contrast, wild watermelons possess bitter, pale flesh and yield much smaller fruits. Initially, carrots had a tough, fibrous, and pale root. Through dedicated selective breeding, today's orange-colored carrots, which offer a sweeter taste, evolved from their wild counterparts.

Carrots, as cultivated crops, belong to the Apiaceae family and are scientifically known as Daucus carota subsp. sativus. They boast a rich history, having been farmed for thousands of years. Currently, cultivated carrots thrive in various regions across the globe and are a staple in many diets. Available in an array of shapes, sizes, and colors—including orange, purple, yellow, and white—the orange carrot remains the most widely grown variety.

Selective breeding has refined carrots to exhibit desirable traits such as sweetness, crispness, and uniform shape. Over time, this process has led to the development of numerous carrot cultivars with distinct characteristics suited for fresh consumption, cooking, juicing, and processing. Cultivated carrots typically grow from seeds in well-drained soil. They require careful cultivation, receiving ample water, sunlight, and soil fertility to flourish and yield high-quality roots. Carrots are known for their high beta-carotene content, which the body converts into vitamin A. They also provide other essential nutrients, including dietary fiber, vitamin K, potassium, and antioxidants. Carrots are versatile in the kitchen and can be enjoyed raw, cooked, or used in various culinary applications such as salads, soups, stews, and side dishes.

While cultivated carrots are the most common form of carrots available, wild carrot species also exist. Wild carrots, commonly known as Queen Anne's lace, have smaller, more fibrous roots and are generally not consumed like their cultivated counterparts. Cabbage, derived from the wild mustard plant, has been selectively bred by humans to develop different forms, such as green cabbage, red cabbage, and savoy cabbage, each with its unique characteristics. The wild ancestor of tomatoes is native to South America. Through selective breeding, tomatoes were cultivated to have larger fruits, an assortment of colors, and improved taste.

Regarding fruits and vegetables closest to their original form, certain varieties remarkably resemble their wild ancestors. For example, many wild blueberry species closely resemble the cultivated varieties we consume today, although wild ones typically have smaller berries. Despite the size difference, the flavor profile remains similar, offering a delightful taste of nature. Wild strawberries may have smaller fruits than their cultivated counterparts, but their flavor is often just as intense and delightful. Cultivated strawberries have been bred for larger size and increased productivity, but wild strawberries retain the essence of their natural origins. Unlike many cultivated crops, wild mushrooms have undergone minimal alteration from their original forms. While cultivated mushrooms come in various strains and varieties, the general appearance and characteristics of wild mushrooms remain largely unchanged.

However, it is important to note that caution should be exercised when consuming mushrooms, especially raw or undercooked ones. Even common button mushrooms contain traces of carcinogenic compounds in their raw state. Shiitake mushrooms contain naturally occurring formaldehyde, while portobello mushrooms may contain hydrazine, both of which are heat-sensitive and neutralized through cooking. These fruits and vegetables offer a taste of nature in its purest form, providing both a culinary delight and a connection to our ancestral roots.

Proposition 65, or Prop 65, is a California law known as the Safe Drinking Water and Toxic Enforcement Act of 1986. Enacted as a ballot initiative, it requires businesses to warn Californians about significant exposures to chemicals that may cause cancer, birth defects, or other reproductive harm. For the average consumer in California, Prop 65 means encountering warning labels on various products and in specific locations. These warnings are typically found on a wide range of items, including but not limited to consumer products such as household cleaners, electronics, toys, and even food items.

Certain public locations or areas where consumers may be exposed to chemicals on-site, such as parking garages, amusement parks, and restaurants, may also have Prop 65 warnings. Websites selling products that are shipped to California may display Prop 65 warnings to comply with the law. It is important to note that the presence of a Prop 65 warning does not necessarily mean that a product is unsafe or that using it will cause harm. The law requires warnings if a product or location contains even trace amounts of chemicals on the Prop 65 list, which includes hundreds of chemicals, some of which may be naturally occurring or present in very small quantities. Consequently, products with warning labels may still be legally sold in California.

For the average consumer, Prop 65 alerts them to potential exposures to certain chemicals in products and locations, allowing them to make informed choices about their purchases and activities. Suppose a product has a Prop 65 warning label. In that case, consumers may wish to review the provided information and decide whether they are comfortable using the product or seek alternatives if they have concerns. It is important to remember that Prop 65 is specific to California and its residents. It does not apply to other states or countries, though some manufacturers may choose to apply Prop 65 warnings to products sold nationwide to avoid the need for separate labeling.

Another controversial topic in the world of vegetables is lectins. Lectins are a type of protein found in many plant-based foods, including legumes such as beans, grains, and certain vegetables. They serve various plant functions, such as defense against predators and pests. In the context of human nutrition, lectins have received some attention because they can interact with certain cells in the body, potentially affecting nutrient absorption and causing digestive issues in some individuals. It is important to note that not all lectins are harmful, and their effects can vary based on individual sensitivity and the amount consumed.

Lectins are present in beans, but they are generally considered safe to eat when properly prepared. Lectins in raw or undercooked beans can be more challenging to digest and may cause gastrointestinal discomfort in some people. However, cooking beans thoroughly can significantly reduce their lectin content and help make them safe to consume. Soaking beans overnight or for several hours before cooking can help reduce lectin levels and improve their digestibility. Boiling beans at high temperatures for an extended period can further break down lectins, making beans safer to eat. Pressure-cooking beans can be an effective way to reduce lectin content and improve digestibility.

Canned beans have undergone cooking during the canning process, which helps reduce lectin levels. Rinsing canned beans before consumption can also help remove some of the remaining lectins. As with any food, it is essential to have a diverse diet that includes a variety of plant-based foods. This can help minimize potential issues related to lectins or other naturally occurring compounds.

Lectins found abundantly in many plant-based foods, can be particularly concentrated in certain legumes, grains, and nightshade vegetables. For example, red kidney beans, when not cooked thoroughly, are packed with lectins, which can cause issues. Therefore, it is crucial to cook them well to reduce their lectin content and make them safe to eat. Soybeans and soy products are another example. They contain quite a bit of lectin, but the levels are lower in fermented products like tempeh and miso. Lentils, chickpeas, wheat, barley, and rice, especially brown rice, also contain lectins. Proper cooking methods, such as soaking and cooking with excess water, can help reduce the lectin levels in these foods.

While lectins can be a concern, it is important to remember that they serve various functions in plants and are generally well-tolerated by the body when foods are properly prepared. Cooking, soaking, or fermenting these foods can significantly reduce lectin levels, making them safe and nutritious components of a balanced diet. It is also crucial to remember that most people can consume lectin-containing foods as part of a balanced and diverse diet without any issues. However, if you have specific concerns or suspect you are sensitive to lectins, consider discussing it with a healthcare professional or a registered dietitian for personalized guidance. They can help you navigate your diet and make suitable food choices based on your individual needs.

Moreover, an article by Harvard University states that, regarding the negative impact of lectins, "These theories have fueled the profitable anti-lectin movement, spawning bestselling books and enzyme supplements to prevent lectin activity in the body. However, there is extremely limited human research on the number of active lectins consumed in the diet and their long-term health effects. Antinutrients, including lectins, are most often studied in the diets of developing countries where malnutrition is prevalent, or where food variety is minimal and whole grains and legumes are important daily staples."

Meat labels can also be confusing and often obscure the issue of pharmaceuticals in their production. Truly recognizing what these labels mean is essential for making informed choices. For instance, the "100% Grass-fed" label suggests that the cow ate grass, but it does not guarantee that it was free from hormones, antibiotics, or inhumane treatment. The term "Natural" merely indicates that minimal additives, like marinades, were added after the meat was sourced, but it does not mean that the meat is free from drugs or was humanely raised.

The label "Naturally Raised" originally meant that the meat product checked all the boxes for being hormone-free and humanely raised. However, this label is no longer backed by regulation and is used for marketing purposes, making it highly misleading. The label "Organic Meat" signifies that the cattle farm is on organic land and that the animals have access to this land. However, this can be for as little as an hour a day, and the other 23 hours could be spent confined in a cell. The animals are not required to eat only grass; their food must be organic, but it can include grains.

These animals are expected to have access to clean water and shelter, which indicates the utter negligence of conventional farming practices if this is a significant feature of the label. Additionally, farms selling fewer than 5,000 livestock as food can call themselves organic without submitting paperwork proving so.

When a label states "Raised Without Antibiotics," it means that the animal was not given antibiotics at any point in its life—not in its food, water, or through injections. Similarly, the label "Raised Without Hormones" means that the animal received no added hormones during its life. However, it is crucial to understand that anything living naturally produces hormones.

A significant concern in the meat industry is the widespread use of antibiotics, with 80% of antibiotics produced in the U.S. used in raising livestock. This widespread use of antibiotics in meat production presents various risks, explicitly concerning antibiotic resistance,

Organic VS. Everything Else

which is a growing public health issue. When we consume meat treated with antibiotics, we inadvertently contribute to the development of antibiotic resistance in both humans and livestock. This resistance is carried into the human system on a genetic level, weakening our immune system's ability to combat infections effectively. The impact of antibiotic resistance extends beyond individual health, threatening public health by making common infections harder to treat and increasing the risk of disease spread.

Moreover, meat production often involves using hormones to promote faster growth and increase production efficiency. These hormones, along with heme iron found in red meat and various additives used during processing, pose additional health risks. Heme iron, while essential in small amounts, has been linked to an increased risk of certain cancers when consumed in excess. Additives, used to preserve meat and enhance flavor, can contribute to long-term health issues, including metabolic disorders and cardiovascular diseases.

Another concerning aspect of modern meat consumption is the use of plastic packaging. The safety of plastic packaging, especially when it comes into contact with food, has been questioned due to the potential leaching of harmful chemicals. These chemicals can disrupt endocrine function and have been associated with a variety of health problems, including reproductive issues and developmental problems in children.

Given these risks, one might question the necessity of meat in our diets. Childhood conditioning and cultural norms often perpetuate meat consumption as a staple of daily meals. However, with growing awareness of the health implications and the availability of diverse and nutritious plant-based alternatives, there's little justification for continuing this practice if our goal is long-term wellness.

Opting for a diet rich in fruits, vegetables, whole grains, and plant-based proteins can provide all the necessary nutrients without the associated risks of meat consumption. These foods offer numerous health benefits, including reducing the risk of chronic diseases, supporting immune function, and promoting overall well-being. While meat has traditionally been a common component of many diets, the potential health risks associated with its production and consumption suggest that reconsidering our dietary choices is prudent. By reducing or eliminating meat from our diets, we can avoid the hazards of antibiotics, hormones, heme iron, additives, and plastic packaging.

This shift not only supports individual health but also contributes to broader public health goals, fostering a healthier, more sustainable future for all. Understanding these labeling standards and codes can help you make more informed choices when shopping for organic products. By choosing certified organic foods, you support sustainable farming practices and reduce your exposure to synthetic chemicals and GMOs, contributing to both your health and the health of the environment.

16
DON'T EAT YOUR WHEATIEZ

Wheat, a staple food for over 10,000 years, has played a vital role in human civilization, from ancient agricultural societies to modern industrialized nations. Throughout history, this grain has provided sustenance and served as a symbol of agricultural innovation and economic stability. However, the wheat consumed today, especially in the United States, bears little resemblance to the ancient grains that nourished our ancestors. Over time, extensive modification through selective breeding and genetic engineering has altered wheat to enhance yields, pest resistance, and other traits beneficial to large-scale agriculture. While these changes have contributed to the global food supply, they have also brought unintended consequences, particularly concerning human health.

One of the most significant alterations in modern wheat is its gluten content. Gluten, a protein composite found in wheat, barley, and rye, provides elasticity and structure to baked goods. However, the gluten content in modern wheat varieties has increased, making it more challenging to digest and potentially contributing to the rise in gluten sensitivity and celiac disease, especially in the U.S. population. This increased prevalence of gluten-related disorders raises critical questions about the impact of agricultural practices on human health and the future of food production.

The deliberate modification of wheat began long before modern genetic engineering techniques were developed. Ancient farmers practiced selective breeding, choosing the best grains to replant and gradually developing more resilient and productive wheat varieties. This process laid the foundation for the domesticated wheat varieties we know today, such as einkorn, emmer, and spelt. These ancient grains, often referred to as "heirloom" varieties, had lower gluten content and different protein structures compared to modern wheat, making them potentially less irritating to the digestive system.

The Green Revolution, a period of agricultural transformation that occurred between the 1940s and 1960s, marked a turning point in wheat production. Led by American agronomist Dr. Norman Borlaug, the Green Revolution introduced high-yielding, disease-resistant wheat varieties that could thrive in a range of environmental conditions. These new wheat strains were developed through cross-breeding and, later, genetic modification, resulting in dwarf and semi-dwarf varieties that produced more grain per acre and were less likely to lodge (bend over) under the weight of their own seeds. These advancements helped prevent famines and fed millions of people, earning Borlaug the Nobel Peace Prize in 1970.

However, the push for higher yields also led to changes in the nutritional profile of wheat. Modern wheat varieties were engineered to produce more gluten, as gluten helps dough rise and gives bread its chewy texture, making it appealing to consumers and profitable for bakeries. Unfortunately, the emphasis on gluten content has coincided with a rise in gluten-related health issues, suggesting that these modifications may have unintended health consequences. Some research indicates that the altered protein structures in modern wheat, mainly the gliadin and glutenin proteins that comprise gluten, may be more likely to trigger immune responses in sensitive individuals, leading to conditions such as celiac disease and non-celiac gluten sensitivity.

The United States is not alone in confronting the challenges of modern wheat consumption. However, the prevalence of gluten sensitivity and celiac disease appears to be higher in the U.S. than in many other countries. This discrepancy may be partly due to differences in the types of wheat consumed. In Europe, for example, traditional wheat varieties such as Spelt, Einkorn, and Emmer strains are still commonly grown. These ancient grains have lower gluten content and different protein structures, which may be less likely to cause digestive issues.

Italy, a country known for its pasta and bread, has a relatively high awareness of celiac disease, leading to the widespread availability of gluten-free options and ongoing research into ancient grains that might be safer for those with gluten sensitivities. The European approach to wheat cultivation and consumption highlights the importance of preserving agricultural biodiversity, offering a stark contrast to the monoculture practices common in American farming.

The Green Revolution's focus on high-yielding crop varieties led to the widespread adoption of monoculture practices, where vast land areas are dedicated to a single crop. While this approach maximizes efficiency and output, it also reduces genetic diversity, making crops more vulnerable to pests, diseases, and environmental changes. In addition, monoculture farming relies heavily on chemical inputs, such as synthetic fertilizers and pesticides, to maintain crop health and productivity.

The reliance on chemical inputs has environmental and health consequences. Pesticides designed to protect crops from insects and diseases can leave residues on the harvested grain, which may then be ingested by consumers. These residues can accumulate in the human body over time, potentially leading to health issues such as endocrine disruption, neurological disorders, and even cancer. Moreover, the use of chemical fertilizers can deplete soil nutrients, leading to a decline in soil health and fertility, further compromising the sustainability of agricultural systems.

The loss of biodiversity in agriculture also affects the resilience of food systems. With fewer crop varieties in use, the risk of widespread crop failure increases if a pest or disease targets the dominant variety. This vulnerability underscores the importance of preserving and promoting the use of traditional and locally adapted crop varieties that are naturally resilient and well-suited to their environments.

Gluten, a protein found in wheat, barley, and rye, has become a topic of significant concern and controversy in recent years. While gluten is harmless for most people, it can cause serious health problems for those with celiac disease, wheat allergies, or non-celiac gluten sensitivity. Celiac disease is an autoimmune disorder where the ingestion of gluten triggers an immune response that damages the small intestine's lining, leading to symptoms such as chronic diarrhea, bloating, and nutrient deficiencies. Wheat allergies, on the other hand, involve an allergic reaction to specific proteins found in wheat, causing symptoms that range from mild (skin rashes, hives) to severe (anaphylaxis).

Non-celiac gluten sensitivity (NCGS) is a condition in which individuals experience symptoms similar to those of celiac disease but without the characteristic autoimmune response and intestinal damage. The exact cause of NCGS is still not fully understood, but it is believed to involve an immune reaction to gluten or other components of wheat. Symptoms of NCGS can include gastrointestinal discomfort, headache, fatigue, joint pain, and mood disturbances, making it a complex and challenging condition to diagnose and manage.

The proteins responsible for gluten's problematic nature are gliadins and glutenins. Gliadins contribute to dough's elastic and sticky properties, while glutenins provide strength and structure. Together, these proteins give wheat its desirable baking qualities but can also trigger immune responses in susceptible individuals. In people with celiac disease, certain peptide sequences within gliadins, such as QPQLPY, are recognized by the immune system as harmful, leading to inflammation and damage to the intestinal lining.

Hybridized wheat strains developed during the Green Revolution and beyond have been found to contain higher levels of gliadins compared to older heirloom varieties. This increase in gliadin content, combined with the altered protein structures resulting from selective breeding, may help explain why more people are experiencing gluten-related health issues today. While the exact relationship between modern wheat varieties and gluten sensitivity is still being studied, the evidence suggests that the changes in wheat protein composition are a contributing factor.

For individuals with celiac disease, wheat allergies, or non-celiac gluten sensitivity, strict avoidance of gluten-containing foods is essential to prevent symptoms and manage their condition. This can be challenging, given that wheat is a common ingredient in many processed foods, from bread and pasta to sauces and snacks. Fortunately, awareness of gluten-related disorders has increased, increasing the availability of gluten-free products and alternatives made from grains such as rice, quinoa, and buckwheat.

While gluten-free diets are necessary for those with gluten-related disorders, they are not a one-size-fits-all solution. Some people without diagnosed sensitivities choose to avoid gluten for perceived health benefits, although research on the effects of gluten-free diets in the general population is mixed. Eliminating gluten without a medical reason can lead to nutritional imbalances, as gluten-containing grains are a source of important nutrients such as fiber, B vitamins, and iron. Therefore, it is important for individuals considering a gluten-free diet to consult with a healthcare professional to ensure that their nutritional needs are met.

Diagnosing gluten-related disorders can be complicated, as

symptoms often overlap with other conditions, and not all tests are definitive. Traditional diagnostic methods for celiac disease include blood tests that measure antibodies such as tissue transglutaminase (tTG) and endomysial antibodies (EMA), followed by a biopsy of the small intestine to assess the damage. However, these tests may not detect non-celiac gluten sensitivity, which does not cause the same autoimmune response or intestinal damage.

Emerging diagnostic tools, such as hair bio-resonance and skin reactivity tests, offer alternative ways to assess sensitivities. While these methods are less invasive than traditional blood tests or biopsies, their scientific validity is still debated. Hair bio-resonance tests, for example, analyze electromagnetic frequencies emitted by cells to detect imbalances or sensitivities, but their accuracy and reliability are not widely accepted in the medical community. Despite these limitations, some individuals find these tests helpful as part of a broader approach to identifying and managing food sensitivities.

The evolution of wheat from ancient grains to modern hybrids reflects the broader challenges and opportunities of contemporary agriculture. While the Green Revolution and subsequent advancements have helped feed a growing global population, they have also raised questions about the long-term health and sustainability of our food systems. The rise of gluten-related disorders highlights the need for a more nuanced understanding of the relationship between agricultural practices, food production, and human health.

As we move forward, it is essential to strike a balance between the benefits of technological innovation and the preservation of traditional knowledge and practices. By embracing biodiversity, promoting sustainable farming methods, and supporting research into the health impacts of modern agricultural practices, we can create a food system that nourishes both people and the planet.

This holistic approach will help ensure that future generations can enjoy the benefits of wheat and other staple crops without compromising their health or the environment. The wheat consumed in the United States differs from varieties grown and used in other countries. Wheat has been extensively modified through selective breeding and genetic engineering to enhance yields and resistance to pests. These modifications often result in wheat with higher gluten content and altered protein structures. This increased gluten content and altered protein profiles may contribute to a higher prevalence of gluten sensitivity and celiac disease in the U.S. population.

In contrast, many countries, particularly in Europe, still use traditional wheat varieties that have been less modified over time. These traditional wheat varieties often have lower gluten content and different protein structures, which might be less likely to trigger celiac disease in susceptible individuals. Consequently, countries with a higher consumption of traditional wheat varieties, such as Italy or France, report different celiac disease prevalence rates. Although celiac disease rates have been increasing globally, the variations in wheat types and gluten content may play a role in regional differences in the prevalence of this autoimmune disorder. This highlights the complex interplay between agricultural practices and health outcomes in different parts of the world.

Dr. Norman Borlaug, an American agronomist and Nobel laureate, initiated the Green Revolution. During the Green Revolution, which lasted from the 1940s to the 1960s, there was a significant push to address food scarcity caused by geographic and political factors. To boost food production, scientists focused on engineering hardier strains of wheat that could withstand various challenges, such as weather extremes, droughts, and pests. These modifications aimed to create more resilient and productive crops.

While Borlaug's intentions were revolutionary, the very same improvements that made these crops more robust have led some to believe that they are now too strong for our bodies to digest effectively. For many people, what was once a naturally digestible grain has become associated with various health issues. The advancements during the Green Revolution, which included engineered and naturally modified varieties through cross-breeding techniques, significantly altered staple crops like wheat and rice, impacting global food security and individual health.

The Green Revolution was particularly successful in increasing wheat yields by introducing new wheat varieties, agricultural inputs, and improved farming techniques. However, this grand gesture to fatten up crop yields forged a difficult-to-digest super-grain. During this time of "advancement," new hybridized strains were given to farmers all over the world.

In an effort to boost food availability, the Green Revolution led to the widespread use of higher levels of chemical fertilizers, pesticides, and selective breeding techniques. These practices dramatically altered the cellular digestibility of crops. For instance, if a pest dies upon consuming a particular strain of wheat, it indicates that the chemical defenses within the plant are significantly potent.

The impact of such chemicals extends beyond their intended use on pests. Pesticides, while effective at protecting crops from insects and other threats, can also have significant adverse effects on human health. These chemicals are specifically designed to be toxic to insects by targeting their nervous systems, but their residues often remain on crops and, subsequently, the food that humans consume. Although the doses encountered by humans are much smaller than those that would affect an insect, these residues can still accumulate in the body over time, leading to potential health risks.

Research has shown that prolonged exposure to certain pesticides can disrupt human biological systems, even in small amounts. For example, organophosphates, a standard class of pesticides, have been associated with neurological disorders as they interfere with acetylcholinesterase, an enzyme critical for nerve function. Other studies have linked pesticide exposure to endocrine disruption, which can affect hormone regulation and lead to reproductive and developmental issues. Furthermore, some pesticides have been classified as possible carcinogens, meaning they could contribute to the development of cancer after long-term exposure.

When humans ingest food treated with these chemicals, the residues they consume can trigger various health problems, from digestive disturbances to more serious chronic conditions. The very lethal compounds to insects can also pose risks to human health, particularly when they interfere with critical biological processes. This highlights the importance of stringent regulation, careful management, and ongoing research into the safety of chemicals used in agriculture and the potential benefits of reducing or eliminating pesticide use in food production. By understanding the risks associated with these chemicals, consumers can make more informed choices about their food and health.

The focus on a limited number of high-yielding crop varieties reduced crop diversity, displacing traditional and locally adapted varieties. The widespread adoption of a few high-yielding crop varieties, such as dwarf wheat and semi-dwarf rice, led to monoculture practices, where large areas were planted with the same crop. Monoculture can increase the risk of widespread crop failure if a pest or disease affects the single dominant variety. The extensive use of pesticides during the Green Revolution led to the emergence of pesticide-resistant pests. This required the use of more potent and environmentally harmful chemicals, creating a cycle of escalating pesticide use. These pesticides remain in the soil for decades and seep into the drinking water in these farming communities.

Pesticide runoff can have substantial effects on the quality of drinking water and pose risks to human health and the environment. When pesticides are applied to agricultural fields, lawns, gardens, or other areas, water runoff can carry them away from their intended target. This runoff can occur during rain events or irrigation, and the pesticides can find their way into nearby bodies of water, including rivers, lakes, and groundwater aquifers.

The process of creating heartier wheat strains with higher pesticide resistance did not directly lead to difficulty digesting wheat. However, some changes in wheat varieties and agricultural practices associated with the Green Revolution have been linked to an increased prevalence of wheat-related digestive issues in many individuals in the US.

The Green Revolution focused on developing high-yielding wheat varieties, including semi-dwarf and dwarf wheat, to increase crop productivity. While these new varieties successfully increased wheat yields, they also changed wheat's protein composition, specifically the gluten proteins.

Gluten is a complex mixture of proteins found in wheat, barley, and rye. Two significant gluten protein groups are gliadins and glutenins. The structure and properties of gluten are crucial for wheat dough's elastic and adhesive qualities, which are important in baking.

The changes in wheat varieties and the selective breeding for specific traits may have inadvertently influenced the composition of gluten proteins. Some research suggests that modern wheat varieties may contain higher levels of particular gliadin proteins compared to older wheat varieties. Gluten is a group of proteins found in certain grains, primarily wheat, barley, rye, and their related species. Gliadins are one of the two main components of gluten, with the other being glutenins. Gliadins contribute to the elastic and adhesive properties of gluten, making it essential for the texture and structure of baked goods.

Wheat allergy is an immune system reaction to proteins found in wheat. When a person with a wheat allergy ingests wheat or wheat-derived products, their immune system recognizes these proteins as harmful, triggering an allergic response. Wheat allergy symptoms can range from mild to severe. They may include gastrointestinal symptoms, diarrhea, vomiting, stomach cramps, nausea, skin reactions, Hives, rash, itching, respiratory symptoms, sneezing, runny nose, and asthma.

In severe cases, a life-threatening allergic reaction called anaphylaxis may occur, leading to difficulty breathing, a drop in blood pressure, and loss of consciousness. Anaphylaxis requires immediate medical attention.

Celiac disease is an autoimmune disorder triggered by the ingestion of gluten, a protein found in wheat, barley, rye, and their related grains. In individuals with celiac disease, the immune system reacts to gluten, damaging the small intestine's lining over time. This damage impairs nutrient absorption and can lead to symptoms of chronic diarrhea, bloating, gas, stomach pain, weight loss, fatigue, skin rashes, and nutritional deficiencies due to malabsorption. When individuals with celiac disease consume gluten, it triggers an abnormal immune response in the small intestine. This response involves the activation of certain immune cells, particularly T cells, which are part of the body's defense system. In individuals with celiac disease, these T cells mistakenly recognize gluten as a threat and initiate an immune response.

As a result of the immune response, the T cells release inflammatory cytokines, which are chemical messengers that promote inflammation and attract other immune cells to the site. This immune response causes damage to the lining of the small intestine, specifically the finger-like projections called villi that are responsible for absorbing nutrients from food.

Over time, the inflammation and damage to the small intestine can lead to various symptoms, nutrient deficiencies, and long-term complications. The exact mechanisms behind why gluten triggers this immune response in individuals with celiac disease are still being studied, but it is believed to involve a combination of genetic predisposition and environmental factors.

It's important to note that celiac disease and wheat allergy are distinct conditions, although they may share some gastrointestinal symptoms. The immune mechanisms involved in these conditions are different.

For individuals diagnosed with wheat allergy or celiac disease, strict avoidance of wheat and gluten-containing foods is necessary to prevent symptoms and manage the condition effectively. In such cases, working with a registered dietitian can be beneficial to develop a balanced and nutritious gluten-free diet.

For people with celiac disease or non-celiac gluten sensitivity, gliadins can trigger an immune response in the small intestine, leading to inflammation and damage to the intestinal lining. This immune reaction occurs when susceptible individuals consume gluten-containing foods, and it can cause various gastrointestinal symptoms like nausea, constipation, diarrhea, bloating, and nutrient malabsorption.

It's important to note that gluten sensitivity or intolerance is a different condition from wheat allergy. In wheat allergy, the immune system reacts to specific proteins found in wheat, which can lead to allergic reactions that may be different from the symptoms seen in celiac disease or gluten sensitivity.

Celiac, diverticulitis, gluten intolerance, and non-celiac gluten intolerance are all specifically associated with gluten. Gluten is a gum-like substance in wheat that allows "stretch" in the dough when it rises. But that same gummy gluten, when it gets into our digestive tracts, we simply don't have the mechanisms to break it down.

The molecular composition of gliadins in hybridized wheat strains can vary from that of heirloom strains, although the overall structure and function of these proteins remain similar. Hybridization is a process that involves crossbreeding different wheat varieties to create new hybrid strains with desired traits, such as improved yield or disease resistance. The specific gliadin proteins present in hybridized wheat can differ depending on the parent wheat varieties used in the crossbreeding.

While the molecular differences in gliadins between hybridized and heirloom wheat strains can exist, it's important to note that the immune response triggered in individuals with celiac disease is primarily directed at specific peptide sequences within the gliadins rather than the entire molecular structure of the protein. These peptide sequences, such as those containing toxic epitopes like the amino acid sequence QPQLPY, are recognized by the immune system in individuals with celiac disease, leading to an autoimmune response and damage to the small intestine.

Regardless of the specific molecular differences in gliadins between hybridized and heirloom wheat strains, individuals with celiac disease need to strictly avoid all sources of gluten, including both modern and heirloom wheat varieties, to manage their condition and prevent adverse reactions.

The specific peptide sequence QPQLPY is found in the alpha-gliadins, which are a group of proteins found in gluten-containing grains such as wheat, barley, and rye. These grains are the primary sources of this peptide sequence. It's important to note that the presence of QPQLPY in other foods is unlikely because it is specific to the gliadin proteins in gluten-containing grains. However, other grains and foods may contain similar or related peptide sequences that can also trigger immune responses in individuals with celiac disease or gluten sensitivities.

The toxicity of wheat can indeed vary based on the strain, environmental factors, and historical context. However, studies consistently show that gluten can be problematic for many individuals. Given this, the simplest approach for those who suspect gluten intolerance is to eliminate it from their diet.

If you've experienced symptoms suggestive of gluten intolerance and have continued consuming wheat-containing products, it might be wise to consult a specialist. They can conduct diagnostic tests to assess any potential damage to your gut lining.

Regardless, it's always prudent to eliminate foods that cause adverse reactions. If a particular food makes you feel unwell, it's a clear signal from your body that it may not be benefiting you on a cellular level. Listening to these signals and adjusting your diet accordingly is a key step toward better health.

There are less invasive tests than an endoscopy to check for intolerances, as an endoscopy will diagnose the internal damage more than detect a sensitivity. Blood tests and Bio-resonance tests are a good way to get an overview of how your body reacts to specific foods. Blood allergy tests, hair bio-resonance allergy tests, and skin reactivity allergy tests are different methods used to identify allergies and sensitivities to various substances.

Blood allergy tests measure the levels of specific antibodies called Immunoglobulin E (IgE) in the blood.

The immune system produces IgE in response to allergens. These tests can identify immediate-type allergies, where the body reacts quickly and strongly to an allergen.

Blood tests can be customized to check for specific allergens, such as pollen, mold, pet dander, certain foods, or insect stings. They are relatively noninvasive and can be useful for detecting IgE-mediated allergies. Healthcare providers can order them and perform them in a laboratory setting. Unfortunately, these tests only show reactivity if the allergen has been ingested recently and the antibodies are still in your bloodstream. If you haven't ingested the allergen, you won't be able to measure the blood's cellular reactivity, giving you a false negative to potential allergens.

Hair bio-resonance tests claim to detect allergies and sensitivities by analyzing a sample of the individual's hair. This is based on measuring the reactivity of the hair cells, which have been extracted in a special machine. The allergens reactivity upon contact with the hair cell is relevant to a number on a scale, over a certain level of reactivity is classified as potentially harmful on a cellular level. Proponents of this method assert that hair samples can retain information about a person's health and can be used to identify allergens, from food allergens to environmental ones, and can also potentially detect vitamin and gut bacteria deficiencies as well as levels of heavy metals in the body.

Different bio-resonance devices and methods exist, but they generally involve measuring and analyzing electromagnetic frequencies or energy fields that are purportedly emitted by cells and tissues in the body. Some bio-resonance devices claim to detect imbalances or disturbances in these energy fields, which are then associated with specific allergies or health conditions.

The scientific validity of hair bio-resonance tests is a subject of debate. Many experts in the medical and scientific communities consider these tests to lack scientific evidence and have raised concerns about their reliability and accuracy. But, they can be a helpful and very low-cost way to see what potential foods are triggering you, and when you remove these foods for a period of time from a week to a month and reintroduce them individually, you can have an easier time realizing what foods make you feel a certain way, and or have reactions or symptoms.

In a skin prick test, a small amount of the suspected allergen is pricked into the skin, usually on the forearm or back. The test measures the skin's reaction, such as redness or swelling, to determine whether an allergic reaction occurs.

Intradermal testing involves injecting a small amount of the allergen just under the skin's surface. This test is more sensitive than the skin prick test and is typically used when the skin prick test results are inconclusive.

A patch test is used to diagnose delayed-type allergies, such as contact dermatitis. Small amounts of allergens are applied to patches that are then placed on the skin. The skin's reaction is assessed after a period of time.

Skin reactivity tests are widely used and considered the standard for diagnosing allergic contact dermatitis and certain IgE-mediated allergies. They are relatively quick and straightforward. However, as the skin is being used, only so many items can be tested at once, and they are uncomfortable to administer, especially if there is a reaction.

It's crucial to recognize that the accuracy and reliability of allergy testing can vary, and false positives and false negatives are possible with any testing method. Discussing your symptoms and concerns with a qualified healthcare professional, such as an allergist or immunologist, who can determine the appropriate tests based on your medical history and symptoms is essential. They can help you interpret the test results and develop an appropriate management plan for any identified allergies or sensitivities.

It's important to remember that if you do eat meat, it's almost a guarantee that the animals you are eating high GMO high pesticide feed that once is in their muscle tissue can be passed to you. However, the allergen itself, if eaten by the animal, won't be present in the same form of protein as the initial allergen.

Understand the implications of consuming meat in the context of modern agricultural practices. When animals are fed diets high in genetically modified organisms (GMOs) and exposed to pesticides, these substances can accumulate in their bodies. This accumulation can have a ripple effect, potentially influencing the health of those who consume their meat.

Livestock, particularly in industrial farming systems, are often fed with grains and soy that are genetically modified to resist certain pests and herbicides, such as glyphosate. Glyphosate, the active ingredient in many herbicides, has been found to accumulate in the tissues of animals that consume treated crops. Studies suggest that when humans consume meat from animals exposed to such substances, traces of these chemicals can be ingested, leading to potential health risks, including endocrine disruption, antibiotic resistance, and other chronic conditions.

Bioaccumulation refers to the process by which substances, such as pesticides, accumulate in the tissues of living organisms over time. When animals ingest feed containing GMOs and pesticides, these compounds can build up in their muscle tissues, which are then passed on to humans when the meat is consumed.

Although the levels of these substances may vary, long-term exposure to even small amounts can contribute to health issues. For example, research has shown a potential link between dietary exposure to certain pesticides and increased risks of cancers, neurodevelopmental issues, and reproductive harm.

However, it's also essential to note that not all risks are directly transferred. The proteins within allergens, if consumed by animals, undergo significant metabolic processing. When the animal ingests these allergens, their proteins are broken down and reconfigured during digestion and subsequent muscle formation. This means that the allergenic proteins are not present in the meat in the same form as in the original feed. Thus, while the risk of direct allergen transfer is minimal, other components, such as pesticide residues, can still be a concern.

While the direct risk of allergen transfer from animal feed to meat is low, the broader implications of consuming meat from animals raised on GMO and pesticide-laden diets cannot be ignored. Awareness of these factors can guide more informed dietary choices, potentially reducing exposure to harmful substances and promoting better overall health.

Regardless, it's always prudent to eliminate foods that cause adverse reactions. If a particular food makes you feel unwell, it's a clear signal from your body that it may not benefit you on a cellular level. Listening to these signals and adjusting your diet is a crucial step toward better health and understanding your body.

17
SOMETHING'S FISHY

Imagine the oceans as vast, pristine bodies of water teeming with life, a boundless resource for nourishment and vitality. This vision has long been the narrative surrounding fish consumption, an image of health and abundance that drives millions to incorporate seafood into their diets. Yet, beneath the shimmering surface of this narrative lies a darker truth.

As the world's oceans bear the brunt of industrial pollution, overfishing, and unsustainable farming practices, the once-ideal source of nutrition now raises critical concerns. The hidden dangers of contaminants, environmental degradation, and ethical dilemmas cloud fish consumption's promise of clean eating and health benefits.

Understanding these issues is crucial in an age where dietary choices impact personal health and the planet's well-being. By exploring these complex factors, we can make more informed decisions about what ends up on our plates and find sustainable, plant-based alternatives that promote both health and ecological balance.

While fish is often praised for its nutritional benefits, including omega-3 fatty acids and high-quality protein, significant concerns about the impact of fish consumption on health and the environment persist. One major issue is the contamination of fish with harmful substances. Our oceans are polluted with various toxins, including heavy metals like mercury, PCBs (polychlorinated biphenyls), and pesticides. These pollutants accumulate in the fat of fish and, when consumed, can lead to serious health problems such as neurological damage, reproductive issues, and an increased risk of cancer. Pregnant women and young children are particularly vulnerable to these risks, as the toxins can affect fetal development and childhood growth.

Plant-based sources can provide the same nutritional benefits as fish while avoiding many of the health and environmental concerns associated with seafood. For instance, flaxseeds, chia seeds, and walnuts are rich in alpha-linolenic acid (ALA), a type of omega-3 fatty acid that is essential for heart health and cognitive function. ALA is a plant-based alternative to the eicosapentaenoic acid (EPA) and docosahexaenoic acid (DHA) found in fish. These plant-based sources offer a sustainable and healthful way to obtain omega-3s without the risks of mercury contamination or environmental degradation.

In addition to omega-3s, plant-based proteins can match the high-quality protein found in fish. Legumes, such as lentils, chickpeas, and black beans, are excellent sources of protein and essential amino acids. Quinoa and hemp seeds are also complete proteins, meaning they provide all nine essential amino acids needed by the body. These plant-based proteins not only support muscle growth and repair but also contribute to overall health and wellness.

Furthermore, vegetables like spinach, kale, and seaweed are rich in essential nutrients often associated with fish, such as iron, calcium, and iodine. Sea vegetables, in particular, provide a plant-based source of iodine, which is crucial for thyroid function and is often highlighted as a benefit of consuming fish.

Fishing has been a cornerstone of human nutrition and culture for thousands of years. In ancient civilizations, such as those in Egypt, Greece, and China, fishing was not only a vital source of food but also a key element of trade and economy. The Nile River in Egypt and the Mediterranean Sea in Greece were abundant fishing grounds that sustained large populations and contributed to the development of these early societies. Fishing methods ranged from simple nets and lines to more advanced techniques, reflecting the ingenuity and adaptability of ancient cultures. However, not every culture relied on fish for their dietary needs.

Various populations that thrive on plant-based diets without consuming fish offer valuable insights into the health and nutritional adequacy of such diets. Research has examined bone health in these communities through bone density tests and other indicators, revealing that a well-planned plant-based diet can support strong bones and overall health.

In Loma Linda, California, the Seventh-day Adventists are a notable example. Many in this community follow a primarily plant-based diet, avoiding meat and fish. Studies on this group have utilized bone density testing to assess their skeletal health. The results indicate that despite the absence of fish, which is often praised for its bone-healthy omega-3 fatty acids, the Adventists maintain strong bone density. This is attributed to their consumption of nutrient-rich plant foods, including legumes, nuts, and fortified plant-based alternatives.

Similarly, in various regions of India, particularly among the Jain and Brahmin communities, traditional diets are predominantly plant-based. Research involving bone density tests in these populations has shown that individuals following such diets also maintain good bone health. Their diets are rich in calcium from sources like leafy greens and fortified foods, which are crucial for bone strength. This evidence supports the idea that a plant-based diet can meet calcium needs effectively without the inclusion of fish.

The Hunza people of Northern Pakistan provide another example. Their diet, which consists mainly of plant-based foods such as grains, fruits, and vegetables, with minimal animal products, has been studied for its health benefits. Bone density tests among the Hunza people have demonstrated strong bones and a low incidence of bone-related ailments, suggesting that their diet, rich in plant-based nutrients, supports skeletal health.

EATING LESSONS

While the diet in Okinawa, Japan, includes occasional fish, it is primarily plant-based, featuring a variety of vegetables, legumes, and tofu. Studies of Okinawan longevity and health have shown that their diet contributes to good bone density and overall well-being. The inclusion of plant-based sources of calcium and other vital nutrients in their diet plays a significant role in maintaining bone health.

These examples show that plant-based diets, when thoughtfully designed to include a variety of nutrient-dense foods, can provide the essential nutrients needed for strong bones. Bone density testing and health outcomes in these populations affirm that fish is not a prerequisite for maintaining bone health, and plant-based diets can be both nutritious and supportive of skeletal integrity.

During the medieval period, fishing continued to play a crucial role in food security, particularly in regions with abundant freshwater and marine resources. For example, in Europe, fishing villages thrived along coastlines and riverbanks, providing essential nutrients to communities. The introduction of preservation techniques, such as salting and smoking, allowed fish to be stored and transported over long distances, further integrating fishing into the global food supply.

By the 19th and 20th centuries, advancements in fishing technology, including the development of trawl nets and large-scale commercial fishing fleets, expanded the reach of the fishing industry. This era saw a dramatic increase in fish production and consumption, driving both economic growth and technological innovation. However, these developments also led to overfishing and environmental impacts, highlighting the need for sustainable practices and conservation efforts to balance the benefits of fishing with the preservation of marine ecosystems.

Commercial fishing has a profound impact on our oceans. Pollution and selective farming practices have transformed marine environments, and many fishing routes are heavily trafficked, resulting in waters contaminated with various pollutants. Moreover, overfishing threatens the balance of the aquatic food chain, affecting numerous species. The high demand for seafood has led to the depletion of many fish species, disrupting marine ecosystems and threatening biodiversity. Overfishing not only endangers specific species but also destabilizes the entire aquatic food chain, affecting the health of ocean ecosystems and the survival of other marine life. The practice of bycatch, where non-target species are caught and discarded, further exacerbates this issue, leading to the unnecessary deaths of countless marine animals.

Farm-raised fish, too, present their own set of issues. The practices involved in fish farming often fail to replicate natural conditions, leading to an array of problems. The push to farm specific fish breeds has created an industry that prioritizes profit over ecological balance, resulting in overbreeding and the introduction of unnatural conditions in our grocery stores.

Despite these issues, many people continue to view seafood as a healthy option. However, the nutritional benefits of seafood are often overstated, and the nutrients it provides can be obtained from plant-based sources. As awareness of these environmental and health impacts grows, it's important to reconsider the true value of seafood in our diets.

The association of seafood with the Mediterranean and Okinawa diets has often highlighted fish as a healthy dietary choice. However, the longevity attributed to these diets is more closely linked to their reduced consumption of animal meats and fats rather than the seafood itself. Despite this, the notion of seafood as a healthful option remains prevalent, but significant concerns cloud it.

In intensive aquaculture systems, fish may be raised in high densities to maximize production. This can lead to overcrowding, stress, and increased competition for resources, which may adversely affect the fish's health and well-being. In some fish farms, antibiotics and other chemicals may be used to prevent and treat diseases that can spread rapidly in crowded conditions. The routine use of antibiotics raises concerns about the development of antibiotic-resistant bacteria.

Farmed fish may be fed with formulated diets that may not closely mimic their natural diets. Some fish farms use feed made from ingredients like fishmeal and fish oil, which can contribute to overfishing and depletion of marine resources. Genetic engineering and selective breeding are sometimes used to produce fish with specific desirable traits, such as faster growth or disease resistance. This can raise ethical and environmental concerns about altering the genetic makeup of fish populations.

Farmed fish escaping aquaculture facilities can potentially interbreed with wild fish, leading to genetic dilution and altering natural populations. Waste products and uneaten feed from fish farms can contribute to nutrient pollution in surrounding waters, leading to environmental degradation and potential harm to wild fish and other aquatic organisms. Introducing non-native species for aquaculture purposes can result in unintended consequences, including the potential for invasiveness and the transmission of diseases to wild fish populations.

Heavy Metal isn't just in your headphones; Mercury is a heavy metal that can accumulate in certain fish, particularly more significant predatory species like sharks, swordfish, king mackerel, and tilefish. Mercury is a neurotoxin that can harm the nervous system, especially in pregnant women and young children. This is why doctors tell lactating and expectant mothers not to eat fish because of their potential toxicity.

Some fish, predominately those from polluted waters, may

contain polychlorinated biphenyls (PCBs) and other industrial contaminants. These substances can negatively impact human health and have been linked to various health issues, including developmental delays in children and an increased risk of certain cancers. The ocean seems so large that many people assume that the waters their seafood is coming from are unpolluted, but most of these waters are high traffic, and your food is likely coming from one of these places. Gulf of Mexico: The Gulf of Mexico faces pollution from various sources, including agricultural runoff, oil spills, and industrial discharges. Contamination in this region can impact fish species such as grouper, snapper, and shrimp.

The Great Lakes, which include Lake Superior, Lake Michigan, Lake Huron, Lake Erie, and Lake Ontario, have experienced historical pollution from industrial discharges and agricultural runoff. Some fish species in the Great Lakes, like lake trout and walleye, have been affected by contaminants such as PCBs and mercury.

Industrial and agricultural pollution has impacted the Columbia River and its tributaries. Fish species like salmon and steelhead in the Columbia River have been found to contain elevated levels of contaminants like PCBs and mercury.

Industrial discharges and other sources have polluted the Hudson River in the northeastern United States. Fish species like striped bass and bluefish have been found to contain PCBs and other contaminants.

The Chesapeake Bay, the largest estuary in the United States, is polluted by agricultural runoff and urban development. Some fish species in the Bay, such as striped bass, have been affected by contaminants like polycyclic aromatic hydrocarbons (PAHs) and mercury.

San Francisco Bay and its surrounding waters have been impacted by pollution from industrial activities and urban runoff. Fish species like halibut and sturgeon in the bay have been found to contain contaminants like PCBs and mercury. Overfishing: The demand for specific widespread fish species has led to overfishing and the depletion of fish populations. Overfishing disrupts marine ecosystems and threatens the sustainability of fish stocks.

Destructive Fishing Practices: Some fishing methods, such as bottom trawling, can cause significant damage to marine habitats and result in bycatch—catching unintended species, including endangered marine life.

Unsustainable fishing practices can lead to habitat destruction, disruption of marine ecosystems, and loss of biodiversity. While fish farming (aquaculture) can help meet the growing demand for seafood, poorly managed fish farms can contribute to water pollution, the spread of diseases among farmed fish, and the escape of non-native species into the wild, impacting local ecosystems.

Many people are aware that farmed fish is additionally risky due to human interference, from filling pools with antibiotics to counteract infections. To fish fed from the feces of chicken coops suspended above the water, among other concerns. Farmed fish may be raised in crowded conditions, leading to an increased risk of disease and the use of antibiotics and other chemicals. Some of these substances can accumulate in the fish's flesh and pose potential health risks to consumers.

Farmed fish are often fed a diet that differs significantly from their natural food sources in the wild. For example, some farmed fish are fed a diet high in grains and processed fish meals, which can alter their nutritional profile and omega-3 fatty acid content. Wild-caught fish typically have higher levels of beneficial omega-3 fatty acids than farmed fish. The unnatural diets of farmed fish can lead to an imbalance of omega-6 and omega-3 fatty acids, potentially impacting their nutritional value.

In the wild, fish feed on various natural foods, contributing to their nutrient diversity. Farmed fish often have a limited diet, resulting in lower nutrient content and a less diverse range of beneficial compounds. Fish farms in polluted waters may expose the fish to environmental contaminants, such as heavy metals, pesticides, and industrial chemicals. These pollutants are absorbed by the fish and passed on to consumers.

The close quarters in fish farms can promote the spread of parasites and diseases among the fish. To prevent these issues, farmed fish might be treated with medications and chemicals, which can affect their overall health and quality.

Some farmed fish are given artificial coloring agents to enhance their appearance, as they may need to develop the vibrant colors seen in wild-caught counterparts. Synthetic dyes are sometimes added to the fish feed. And then are absorbed by you.

So why are people eating fish? Under the guise of a Mediterranean and Okinawa diet, eating seafood has gained popularity, but fish do not provide nutrients that can't be obtained from plant sources. The added toxins and cholesterol impact the environment and other species and far outweigh what a filet carries in calories. Some fishing methods, such as bottom trawling, can cause significant damage to marine habitats and result in bycatch—catching unintended species, including endangered marine life. Unsustainable fishing practices can lead to habitat destruction, disruption of marine ecosystems, and loss of biodiversity.

While fish farming (aquaculture) can help meet the growing demand for seafood, poorly managed fish farms can contribute to water pollution, the spread of diseases among farmed fish, and the escape of non-native species into the wild, impacting local ecosystems. Many people are aware that farmed fish is additionally risky due to human interference, from filling pools with antibiotics to counteract infections. To fish fed from the feces of chicken coops suspended above the water, among other concerns. Farmed fish may be raised in crowded conditions, leading to an increased risk of disease and the use of antibiotics and other chemicals. Some of these substances can accumulate in the fish's flesh and pose potential health risks to consumers.

Farmed fish are often fed a diet that differs significantly from their natural food sources in the wild. For example, some farmed fish are fed a diet high in grains and processed fish meals, which can alter their nutritional profile and omega-3 fatty acid content. Wild-caught fish typically have higher levels of beneficial omega-3 fatty acids than farmed fish. The unnatural diets of farmed fish can lead to an imbalance of omega-6 and omega-3 fatty acids, potentially impacting their nutritional value. In the wild, fish can feed on various natural foods, contributing to their nutrient diversity. Farmed fish often have a limited diet, resulting in lower nutrient content and a less diverse range of beneficial compounds. Fish farms in polluted waters may expose the fish to environmental contaminants, such as heavy metals, pesticides, and industrial chemicals.

These pollutants are absorbed by the fish and passed on to consumers. The close quarters in fish farms can promote the spread of parasites and diseases among the fish. Farmed fish might be treated with medications and chemicals to prevent these issues, which can affect their overall health and quality. Some farmed fish are given artificial coloring agents to enhance their appearance, as they may need to develop the vibrant colors seen in wild-caught counterparts. Synthetic dyes are sometimes added to the fish feed, then are absorbed by you.

In addition to these environmental and health concerns, there is also the question of ethics. Industrial fishing practices can result in the suffering of marine life, from fish caught in nets to bycatch species that are discarded, often dead or dying. These practices raise ethical questions about our treatment of aquati animals and our responsibility to preserve the natural world.

Plant-based sources can provide the same nutritional benefits as fish while avoiding many of the health and environmental concerns associated with seafood. For instance, flaxseeds, chia seeds, and walnuts are rich in alpha-linolenic acid (ALA), a type of omega-3 fatty acid that is essential for heart health and cognitive function. ALA is a plant-based alternative to the eicosapentaenoic acid (EPA) and docosahexaenoic acid (DHA) found in fish. These plant-based sources offer a sustainable and healthful way to obtain omega-3s without the risks of mercury contamination or environmental degradation.

In addition to omega-3s, plant-based proteins can match the high-quality protein found in fish. Legumes, such as lentils, chickpeas, and black beans, are excellent sources of protein and essential amino acids. Quinoa and hemp seeds are also complete proteins, meaning they provide all nine essential amino acids needed by the body. These plant-based proteins not only support muscle growth and repair but also contribute to overall health and wellness.

Furthermore, vegetables like spinach, kale, and seaweed are rich in essential nutrients often associated with fish, such as iron, calcium, and iodine. Sea vegetables, in particular, provide a plant-based source of iodine, which is crucial for thyroid function and is often highlighted as a benefit of consuming fish.

Various populations that thrive on plant-based diets without consuming fish offer valuable insights into the health and nutritional adequacy of such diets. Research has examined bone health in these communities through bone density tests and other indicators, revealing that a well-planned plant-based diet can support strong bones and overall health.

In Loma Linda, California, the Seventh-day Adventists are a notable example. Many in this community follow a largely plant-based diet, avoiding meat and fish. Studies on this group have used bone density testing to assess their skeletal health. The results indicate that despite the absence of fish, which is often praised for its bone-healthy omega-3 fatty acids, the Adventists maintain strong bone density. This is attributed to their consumption of nutrient-rich plant foods, including legumes, nuts, and fortified plant-based alternatives.

Similarly, in various regions of India, particularly among the Jain and Brahmin communities, traditional diets are predominantly plant-based. Research involving bone density tests in these populations has shown that individuals following such diets also maintain good bone health. Their diets are rich in calcium from sources like leafy greens and fortified foods, which are crucial for bone strength. This evidence supports the idea that a plant-based diet can meet calcium needs effectively without the inclusion of fish.

The Hunza people of Northern Pakistan provide another example. Their diet, which consists mainly of plant-based foods such as grains, fruits, and vegetables, with minimal animal products, has been studied for its health benefits. Bone density tests among the Hunza people have demonstrated strong bones and a low incidence of bone-related ailments, suggesting that their diet, rich in plant-based nutrients, supports skeletal health.

While the diet in Okinawa, Japan, includes occasional fish, it is primarily plant-based and features a variety of vegetables, legumes, and tofu.

Okinawan longevity and health studies have confirmed that their diet contributes to good bone density and overall well-being. The inclusion of plant-based sources of calcium and other vital nutrients in their diet plays a large role in maintaining bone health.

These examples demonstrate that plant-based diets, when thoughtfully designed to include a variety of nutrient-dense foods, can provide the essential nutrients needed for strong bones. Bone density testing and health outcomes in these populations affirm that fish is not a prerequisite for maintaining bone health, and plant-based diets can be both nutritious and supportive of skeletal integrity.

As awareness of these issues grows, it is crucial to consider the broader implications of our dietary choices. While the consumption of fish offers certain health benefits, it carries significant risks that must be weighed carefully. By exploring plant-based alternatives and adopting more sustainable eating habits, we can support our health and the health of our planet. Reducing our reliance on fish and other animal-based foods can help protect our oceans, preserve biodiversity, and promote a more ethical and sustainable approach to nutrition.

While fish has played a vital role in human history and remains a popular dietary choice, its consumption comes with a range of environmental, health, and ethical concerns. As we strive to make more informed choices about our diets, we must consider the impact of fish consumption on our health and the environment. By embracing plant-based alternatives and adopting a more holistic approach to nutrition, we can support a healthier future for ourselves and our planet.

Many people adhere to the "Paleo" diet, thinking it replicates the way cavemen ate. However, many of our ancestors lived inland and never had access to the types of fish available today. Therefore, the idea that fish was always a part of our original ancestors' diet is a fallacy, and overfishing this planet is doing more harm than good.

18
SOY NICE TO MEET YOU!

The media has long misled the public about soy, perpetuating a range of myths and misconceptions that have persisted for decades. Since my teenage years as a vegan, I've encountered numerous erroneous beliefs: "Soy tastes bland," "Soy causes cancer," "Soy makes men grow breasts," and "Soy is an inferior protein." However, the time has come to set the record straight, particularly as a growing body of scientific evidence continues to dispel these outdated myths.

One of the most common concerns people have about soy is related to its association with genetically modified organisms (GMOs) and cancer risk. Ironically, many individuals who avoid soy due to these concerns still consume animal meat, inadvertently ingesting soy through the livestock they eat. Approximately 80% of the world's soy production is used in animal feed, meaning the protein in your meat likely originates from soy.

This reality exposes a significant paradox: many people who shun soy for fear of GMOs still consume it indirectly through their diet. Recognizing soy as a complete protein with all essential amino acids underscores its potential to combat global hunger if we redirected its use from livestock to direct human consumption. In fact, if more soy were consumed directly by humans rather than being used as animal feed, it could significantly reduce the strain on global food resources, given soy's high protein yield per acre compared to animal farming.

Soy is a crop of incredible efficiency and versatility, capable of yielding far more protein per acre than animal farming. For instance, research shows that soy can produce up to 15 times more protein per hectare than beef, making it a far more resource-efficient food source. This efficiency is not only beneficial from a nutritional standpoint but also has significant environmental implications. By shifting our dietary focus from animal proteins to plant-based options like soy, we can drastically reduce the environmental footprint of our food production.

The cultivation of soy requires significantly less water and land compared to animal farming, and it generates fewer greenhouse gases, which is crucial in the fight against climate change. Studies have shown that transitioning to plant-based diets could reduce global greenhouse gas emissions from food production by up to 70%, with soy playing a key role in this transformation.

The widespread use of GMO soybeans, particularly in cattle feed and soy sauce production, has further fueled concerns about the safety and nutritional value of soy. These genetically modified soybeans are engineered for herbicide tolerance, allowing for more effective and cost-efficient weed control in large-scale farming operations. While this technology has made GMO soybeans prevalent in livestock feed, it has also sparked considerable debate about their long-term environmental and health impacts. Some studies suggest that GMO crops can reduce the need for chemical inputs, thereby lowering the environmental footprint of agriculture. However, other research highlights potential risks, including the development of herbicide-resistant weeds and the potential for GMO genes to spread to wild plant populations.

For example, research has documented the emergence of "superweeds" that have developed resistance to commonly used herbicides like glyphosate, which is often applied to GMO soy crops. These superweeds require even more potent herbicides for control, leading to a cycle of increasing chemical use that contradicts the original intent of reducing agricultural inputs.

There is concern about the potential for GMO genes to transfer to non-GMO crops or wild plants through processes like cross-pollination, which could have unforeseen ecological consequences. These issues highlight the complexity of GMO technology and the need for ongoing research and monitoring to fully understand its long-term effects on both human health and the environment.

In the context of soy sauce production, traditional methods typically involve fermenting whole soybeans or soybean paste. However, some commercial soy sauce brands may use GMO soybeans, raising concerns among consumers who prefer to avoid genetically modified ingredients. For those seeking to avoid GMOs, choosing soy sauce brands labeled as non-GMO or organic provides an assurance that the soybeans used were not genetically modified. The availability of such products has increased in recent years, reflecting growing consumer demand for transparency and sustainability in food production.

For individuals who avoid soy while continuing to consume meat from animals fed on soy, it's crucial to recognize the indirect consumption of GMOs. This paradoxical behavior is emblematic of a broader issue in dietary choices: prioritizing perceived health benefits while neglecting the hidden risks.

For example, many people readily discard a bruised banana despite its richness in antioxidants and essential nutrients while willingly consuming processed foods laden with preservatives, artificial flavors, and other chemicals. This contradiction highlights a significant disconnect between how food is perceived and its actual nutritional value. The same individuals who avoid natural imperfections in fruit may unknowingly expose themselves to greater health risks by consuming processed foods that contain residues from industrial agriculture.

One of the most pervasive myths about soy is that it induces estrogenic effects, such as breast tissue growth in men. This belief is rooted in media misrepresentation and early scientific studies that were either poorly designed or misinterpreted. Soy contains phytoestrogens, such as isoflavones (genistein and daidzein), which are plant-based compounds structurally similar to human estrogen.

Early research raised concerns that these compounds could mimic estrogen's effects in the body, leading to hormonal imbalances. However, subsequent studies have demonstrated that phytoestrogens exert much weaker effects than human estrogen and can even have protective benefits. Critics of the soy industry have argued that the pharmaceutical industry played a role in perpetuating these myths, particularly to undermine soy-based alternatives to hormone replacement therapy (HRT).

The science behind phytoestrogens is complex and nuanced. Phytoestrogens can bind to estrogen receptors in the human body, but their effects are much weaker than those of human estrogen. In fact, phytoestrogens can act as selective estrogen receptor modulators (SERMs), meaning they can have both estrogenic and anti-estrogenic effects depending on the target tissue and the hormonal environment. This dual role allows phytoestrogens to potentially offer protective benefits against certain cancers, particularly those that are hormone-related, such as breast and prostate cancers.

For example, a comprehensive meta-analysis published in the journal Cancer Causes & Control found that soy intake was associated with a significantly reduced risk of breast cancer in both premenopausal and postmenopausal women. This protective effect is thought to be due to the ability of isoflavones to modulate estrogen metabolism and inhibit the growth of cancer cells.

Similarly, another study published in the American Journal of Clinical Nutrition found that men who consumed higher amounts of soy had a reduced risk of developing prostate cancer, further challenging the myth that soy induces harmful estrogenic effects.

Contrary to popular belief, cultures with high soy consumption, such as those in Asia, exhibit no such health concerns related to soy intake. In fact, these populations have some of the lowest rates of hormone-related cancers globally, suggesting that soy's role in the diet is beneficial rather than harmful.

Epidemiological studies have consistently shown that individuals in countries like Japan, where soy is a dietary staple, have significantly lower rates of breast and prostate cancers compared to populations in Western countries. This stark contrast suggests that the issue lies more with media portrayal and cultural biases than with scientific evidence. The current scientific consensus supports the idea that soy can be part of a healthy diet without adverse hormonal effects and may even offer protective benefits.

My personal experience with soy further underscores its nutritional value and versatility. Growing up, soy was a staple in my household, and I have vivid memories of making tofu from fresh soybeans. We would boil the soybeans until they emulsify into a thick, bubbling mixture, then add a splash of vinegar to curdle it. After skimming off the curds, we pressed them into tofu, which we used in a variety of dishes. The process of making tofu is remarkably similar to making cheese from cow's milk, yet tofu has never achieved the same popularity in Western households.

Despite its nutritional benefits and culinary versatility, tofu remained a niche product, often misunderstood or overlooked. In my home, tofu was a key ingredient in everything from savory dishes to desserts like brownies, showcasing its adaptability and potential as a protein source.

The nutritional benefits of tofu and other soy products are

well-documented in scientific literature. Soy is recognized as a complete protein, meaning it contains all essential amino acids necessary for muscle growth and repair. This characteristic makes soy an excellent alternative to animal proteins, which often come with unhealthy fats, cholesterol, and other undesirable components.

Unlike cow's milk, which is lower in protein and frequently contains antibiotics and hormones, soy offers a clean, high-protein alternative that supports muscle health without the associated risks of animal products. The claim that "soy tastes bland" is another misconception, often based on unfair comparisons. Critics typically compare unseasoned tofu to seasoned and cooked meat, but this is not a fair assessment.

When comparing unseasoned tofu to unseasoned chicken breast, the difference in taste is negligible. In fact, tofu's neutrality provides an excellent opportunity to season it according to personal preference, making it an incredibly versatile ingredient.

Modern research continues to shed light on the protective benefits of soy, particularly in relation to cancer prevention. The narrative has shifted dramatically in recent years, with a growing body of evidence supporting soy's role in reducing the risk of breast and prostate cancers. Earlier fears that soy could contribute to cancer development were based on studies that failed to account for the complex interactions between isoflavones and human hormones. Today, it is widely recognized that soy can actually help protect against these cancers. For instance, studies have shown that women who regularly consume soy have a lower risk of breast cancer, particularly when soy is introduced early in life. Similarly, men who include soy in their diet are less likely to develop prostate cancer, a benefit attributed to the anti-inflammatory and antioxidant properties of isoflavones.

A wealth of research supports soy's anti-cancer properties. A study published in the Journal of the National Cancer Institute found that women who consumed soy products regularly had a 30% lower risk of breast cancer recurrence compared to those who consumed little or no soy.

This protective effect was particularly pronounced in women who began consuming soy at a young age, suggesting that early exposure to isoflavones may help modulate estrogen metabolism in a way that reduces cancer risk. Additionally, a study published in the journal Cancer Research found that men who consumed soy protein isolate experienced a significant reduction in prostate-specific antigen (PSA) levels, a marker of prostate cancer risk. These findings underscore the potential of soy as a dietary intervention for cancer prevention and challenge the notion that soy is harmful to hormonal health.

Soy is also recognized as a complete protein, meaning it contains all the essential amino acids necessary for muscle growth and repair. This characteristic makes soy an excellent alternative to animal proteins, which often contain unhealthy fats, cholesterol, and other undesirable components.

Unlike cow's milk, which is lower in protein and frequently contains antibiotics and hormones, soy offers a clean, high-protein alternative that supports muscle health without the associated risks of animal products. The claim that "soy tastes bland" is another misconception, often based on unfair comparisons. Critics typically compare unseasoned tofu to seasoned and cooked meat, but this is not a fair assessment. When comparing unseasoned tofu to unseasoned chicken breast, the difference in taste is negligible. In fact, tofu's neutrality provides an excellent opportunity to season it according to personal preference, making it an incredibly versatile ingredient.

The myth that soy causes men to grow breast tissue is another example of misinformation rooted in a fundamental misunderstanding of how phytoestrogens work. While soy does contain phytoestrogens, these compounds are not the same as mammalian estrogen and do not have the same effects on the body. The estrogen found in cow's milk, for example, is much more potent and has been documented to cause breast tissue growth in prepubescent girls in regions with high dairy consumption.

If soy had a similar effect on men, we would expect to see widespread cases in Asia, where soy is a dietary staple, yet no such phenomenon exists. This myth is not only scientifically unfounded but also reflects a broader misunderstanding of how phytoestrogens interact with the body. Phytoestrogens can bind to estrogen receptors in human cells and elicit weak estrogenic effects, but their potency is much lower than that of endogenous estrogen. Moreover, phytoestrogens can act as selective estrogen receptor modulators (SERMs), meaning they can have both estrogenic and anti-estrogenic effects depending on the target tissue and hormonal environment.

Because of their ability to interact with estrogen receptors, there has been considerable debate about the potential health effects of phytoestrogens, particularly in relation to hormone-related cancers and reproductive health. However, the current scientific consensus suggests that phytoestrogens are unlikely to have significant adverse effects on human health when consumed in moderate amounts as part of a balanced diet. On the contrary, much research suggests that phytoestrogens have health benefits, such as reducing the risk of certain hormone-related cancers, including breast and prostate cancers, and providing cardiovascular protection. Furthermore, phytoestrogens in soy may actually help prevent the absorption of errant estrogen that can enter the body through the consumption of animal products, including dairy and meat.

The consumption of animal products like eggs and chicken meat, which are high in estrogen due to their production in the hormonal epicenter of the animal, has been linked to a range of health issues, including polycystic ovary syndrome (PCOS) in women. Eggs, in particular, are a concentrated source of estrogen, while chicken meat is also extraordinarily high in this hormone. In contrast, the traditional Asian diet, which is rich in soy and other plant-based foods, is celebrated for its health benefits and association with longevity. This diet, which includes leafy greens, legumes, nuts, seeds, and fruits, underscores the long-term benefits of soy consumption and stands in stark contrast to the short-lived dietary fads that often dominate Western culture.

The notion that soy causes cancer is yet another myth that has been thoroughly debunked by modern science. Early studies that suggested a link between soy and cancer were based on flawed methodologies and did not account for the complexities of human metabolism. I remember a wave of people who began telling me that they had heard soy causes cancer, prompting them to cut it out of their diets. For years, there was little media coverage to counter these claims, but more recent research has finally begun to correct the record.

Comprehensive studies now show that soy actually helps prevent cancer, particularly breast and prostate cancer. The protective benefits of soy are largely attributed to its isoflavones, which have been shown to reduce the proliferation of cancer cells, inhibit tumor growth, and modulate the body's hormonal balance in a beneficial way. So, forget the rumors; the truth about soy has been thoroughly documented in scientific literature, readily accessible to anyone willing to look beyond the myths.

The idea that soy is an inferior protein source is similarly outdated and incorrect. Soy is not only a complete protein, but it also offers a unique profile of amino acids that are particularly beneficial for muscle growth and recovery. Unlike some plant-based proteins that need to be combined with other foods to provide all essential amino acids, soy stands alone as a complete protein source.

For example, Eden soy boasts 12 grams of protein per cup with only one ingredient, a stark contrast to cow's milk, which contains just one or two grams of protein per cup and is often laden with added antibiotics and hormones. This comparison highlights the nutritional superiority of soy and underscores the progress we are making as a community in dissolving media-driven, government-subsidized misconceptions, such as those perpetuated by the outdated food pyramid, and embracing more informed and health-conscious dietary choices.

Soy protein is also highly digestible, with a protein digestibility-corrected amino acid score (PDCAAS) comparable to that of animal proteins like eggs and milk.

This score, which measures the quality of a protein based on its amino acid composition and digestibility, indicates that soy protein is just as effective as animal proteins in supporting muscle growth and repair. Furthermore, soy protein has been shown to have additional health benefits, such as reducing cholesterol levels and improving heart health. A study published in the Journal of Nutrition found that individuals who consumed soy protein regularly experienced significant reductions in LDL cholesterol (the "bad" cholesterol) and total cholesterol levels, which are major risk factors for cardiovascular disease.

Progress lies in dismantling media-driven misconceptions and embracing scientifically-backed truths. For too long, soy has been vilified based on misinterpretations and, at times, deliberate misinformation. By reevaluating our understanding of soy, we open the door to its numerous health benefits and its potential as a sustainable food source. This reassessment is not just about clearing soy's name; it's about making informed dietary choices that benefit both our health and the planet.

It's also important to consider the historical and cultural contexts of soy consumption. In many Asian countries, soy has been a dietary staple for centuries, incorporated into daily meals in various forms such as tofu, tempeh, miso, and soy sauce. These populations have not only thrived but also have some of the lowest rates of certain cancers and cardiovascular diseases globally. This stark contrast with Western skepticism towards soy suggests that the fear surrounding soy might be more cultural than factual. The health benefits observed in populations with high soy consumption provide compelling evidence that soy is not only safe but also advantageous as part of a balanced diet.

The introduction of soy-based foods into Western diets has often been met with resistance, driven by unfamiliarity and the powerful influence of the meat and dairy industries. These industries, which have a vested interest in maintaining their market dominance, have been known to fund studies or disseminate information that casts doubt on plant-based alternatives like soy. The claims about soy's estrogenic effects, for example, are a clear case of science being twisted to serve commercial interests. It is crucial to recognize that much of the anti-soy rhetoric is not rooted in solid science but rather in efforts to protect the profits of industries that rely on animal agriculture.

The science supporting soy is robust and continues to grow. Numerous studies have demonstrated that soy can help reduce cholesterol levels, improve heart health, and lower the risk of certain cancers. For instance, research has shown that women who consume soy regularly have a lower risk of breast cancer, and the effect is even more pronounced when soy consumption begins early in life. Similarly, men who include soy in their diet are less likely to develop prostate cancer, a benefit attributed to the anti-inflammatory and antioxidant properties of isoflavones. These findings are supported by a wealth of epidemiological data and clinical trials, making soy one of the most well-researched and evidence-based foods in the human diet.

Moreover, soy's environmental benefits can't be overstated. Producing soy requires significantly less water and land compared to animal farming, and it generates fewer greenhouse gases, making it a more sustainable food source. In a world grappling with climate change and resource scarcity, adopting more plant-based foods like soy is a practical and necessary step toward sustainability. The environmental impact of soy is particularly relevant in the context of global food security, as the efficient use of resources becomes increasingly important in feeding a growing population.

Soy's role in combating climate change is supported by a growing body of research. A study published in the journal Nature Communications found that replacing half of the animal products in the global diet with plant-based alternatives like soy could reduce agricultural greenhouse gas emissions by 35% and free up millions of square kilometers of land currently used for livestock farming. This land could then be repurposed for reforestation or other conservation efforts, further mitigating the impact of climate change. Additionally, soy's nitrogen-fixing properties make it beneficial for soil health, reducing the need for synthetic fertilizers and promoting more sustainable agricultural practices.

It's time to reintroduce soy into our diets and our collective consciousness. The myths that have tarnished its reputation are gradually being debunked by science and by the cultural wisdom of societies that have consumed soy for centuries. By embracing soy, we're making a healthier choice for ourselves and a more sustainable choice for the planet. Let's move beyond the misinformation and start seeing soy for what it truly is: a nutritious, versatile, and environmentally friendly food that deserves a prominent place in our diets. The future of food lies in embracing evidence-based nutrition, and soy is at the forefront of this transformation.

19
NOT MYLK!

Dairy has long held a prominent place in the market, thanks to relentless marketing campaigns, ubiquitous viral dairy commercials, and its integration into countless food products. For decades, the dairy industry has maintained its stronghold. However, recent shifts in consumer behavior are starting to disrupt this longstanding dominance, particularly in how people are changing their coffee habits.

According to a Reuters article by Carey Gilam, the cattle and livestock pharmaceutical industry is a lucrative sector dominated by a few prominent companies. These companies not only control the food supply but also have influence over labeling and government subsidies. They are responsible for enforcing the legal limits on the amount of somatic cells, often referred to as "cow pus," allowed in milk and cheese products. This legal limit underscores a concerning reality about the dairy industry: there is an acceptable level of pus in the milk consumed by the public.

If humans were naturally designed to drink cow's milk, one might expect that infant formula would commonly include dairy milk as a supplement for those not breastfeeding. However, this is not the case, highlighting the notion that cow's milk is primarily intended for the young of the species from which it originates rather than for mass consumption by humans. Using another species' milk as a widespread food ingredient appears increasingly questionable.

The nutritional composition of cow's milk significantly differs from that of human milk. Cow's milk is higher in protein and minerals like sodium and potassium, which can put undue stress on an infant's developing kidneys. The nutritional profile of cow's milk does not meet the specific needs of infants, who require essential nutrients like iron, vitamin C, and certain fats that cow's milk lacks. Furthermore, the proteins in cow's milk, particularly casein, are more challenging for infants to digest compared to the proteins in breast milk or specially formulated infant formulas. This difficulty in digestion can lead to issues such as constipation, colic, and gastrointestinal discomfort. Long-term exposure to casein proteins, known as casomorphins, can lead to an addiction-like effect in humans due to their high concentration in milk compared to human breast milk.

Cow's milk is also a common allergen, affecting about 78 percent of the global population. Allergic reactions can manifest as skin rashes, cystic acne, hives, digestive problems, and respiratory issues. Since the skin is the body's largest organ and often the first to show signs of food intolerance, individuals with skin conditions like eczema or rosacea may find relief by eliminating dairy from their diet. Excessive milk consumption has a long association with increased respiratory tract mucus production and asthma.

Infants, with their developing immune systems, may recognize the proteins in cow's milk as foreign, triggering immune responses that could increase the risk of allergies and autoimmune conditions. This immune response can hinder infants' natural growth and development, mirroring the impact of any immune system disruption during early developmental stages.

Milk contains various growth factors and bioactive compounds specific to the species it is intended for, along with natural hormones. Additionally, dairy production can involve antibiotics and pesticides from genetically modified feed, making dairy a significant endocrine disruptor. The hormones present in dairy products, such as estrogen and progesterone, concern some individuals who choose to avoid dairy to mitigate potential health impacts.

Not Mylk!

Ethical and environmental concerns also drive some people to adopt a plant-based diet. The dairy industry is associated with greenhouse gas emissions, significant land and water use, and animal welfare issues. Consequently, individuals committed to a sustainable and compassionate lifestyle often exclude dairy products from their diets.

Plant-based diets commonly include alternatives to dairy, such as non-dairy milk options like almond, soy, oat, rice, coconut, cashew, hemp, and pea milk. These alternatives vary in their nutritional profiles and ingredients. For example, soy milk, made from soybeans, is rich in protein and often fortified with calcium and vitamins.

Almond milk, derived from ground almonds, is lighter and slightly sweet but can contain added stabilizers and sugars. Homemade almond milk can be made from raw almonds or almond butter blended with water and optionally flavored with ingredients like dates or vanilla extract. It is important to be aware of the potential arsenic content in almonds, which is generally low but present in some cases.

Dairy products can act as endocrine disruptors due to their content of natural hormones and potential contaminants. Cows' milk contains various hormones, such as estrogen and progesterone, which can influence human hormonal balance when consumed regularly. The dairy industry's use of antibiotics and growth hormones in cattle can lead to residues in milk that may further disrupt endocrine function. These hormones and residues, even in small amounts, may interfere with the body's endocrine system, potentially leading to a range of health issues, including hormonal imbalances and increased risk of certain cancers. The concern over endocrine disruption has prompted many individuals to seek dairy-free alternatives or choose organic dairy products to minimize exposure to these potentially harmful substances.

Conventional dairy milk may possibly contain naturally occurring hormones, such as estrogen and progesterone because cows are often treated with synthetic hormones (e.g., bovine growth hormone) to increase milk production. When humans consume dairy products containing these hormones, there is a concern that it may disrupt the body's hormonal balance. These hormones are present because cows are often treated with synthetic hormones (e.g., bovine growth hormone) to increase milk production.

When humans consume dairy products containing these hormones, there is a concern that the. Dairy cows may be exposed to environmental contaminants such as pesticides, industrial chemicals, and pollutants. These contaminants can accumulate in the cows' tissues and milk. When humans consume dairy products from these cows, they may also be exposed to endocrine-disrupting chemicals.

An endocrine disruptor is a chemical substance that interferes with the normal functioning of the endocrine system in humans and animals. The endocrine system is a complex network of glands that produce and secrete hormones, which are chemical messengers that regulate various physiological processes. These processes include growth and development, metabolism, sexual function, reproduction, mood, etc.

Endocrine disruptors can mimic or block the action of natural hormones, leading to hormonal imbalances and disrupting the body's normal hormone signaling pathways. They can bind to hormone receptors, alter hormone production or metabolism, and interfere with hormone transport and signaling. There are various endocrine disruptor sources, including certain manufacturing chemicals, pesticides, plasticizers, and some pharmaceuticals. They can be found in the environment, food, and consumer products, and exposure can occur through ingestion, inhalation, or skin contact.

Oat milk, made from oats, is naturally sweet and creamy, often fortified with calcium and vitamin D. Rice milk, derived from milled rice, has a thinner consistency and a mild taste. Coconut milk,

Not Mylk!

made from coconut flesh, is rich and creamy with a distinct flavor and higher fat content. Cashew milk, made from cashews, has a creamy texture and mild sweetness. Hemp milk from hemp seeds offers a nutty flavor and is a good source of omega-3 fatty acids. Pea milk, made from yellow peas, provides a neutral taste and is fortified with nutrients. However, caution is advised for pea milk due to potential lead contamination in soil.

Protein powders derived from various sources, including dairy and plant-based options, are processed differently. Whey protein, a dairy derivative, is obtained from the liquid remaining after cheese-making. Casein protein, also from dairy, is separated during cheese production and digested more slowly. Soy protein is extracted from soybeans using hexane, a chemical solvent. Though hexane is considered safe within regulatory limits, some concerns exist about its residual presence in food products. Pea protein is extracted from peas using water and centrifugation, while rice protein is derived from brown rice through enzyme treatment. Hemp protein comes from cold-pressed hemp seeds.

In recent years, consumption of cow's milk has declined as more people opt for non-dairy alternatives. The rise in demand for organic milk suggests a growing consumer concern over contaminants associated with conventional dairy production. Tests on milk samples have revealed the presence of antibiotics and pesticides in conventional milk, with some residues exceeding federal limits. On the other hand, organic milk generally shows lower levels of contaminants.

The use of ractopamine, a feed additive that promotes lean muscle growth in livestock, is controversial due to its health impacts on animals and potential effects on humans. Studies show that ractopamine use in pigs results in increased reports of illness and death.

Overall, while plant-based milk and alternative protein sources provide options for those avoiding dairy, it is crucial to be mindful of the ingredients and production processes involved. Homemade versions of plant-based milk can offer a healthier and more customizable alternative to store-bought options.

Understanding the potential risks and benefits of different products can help individuals make informed choices about their diets and health. Some individuals choose to eliminate dairy. You may seek alternative sources of nutrients typically found in dairy, such as calcium, by consuming plant-based foods like leafy greens, fortified non-dairy milk, tofu, and fortified plant-based yogurts or cheeses. That changed in January 2013 when Pfizer Inc. spun off its animal health business Zoetis, raising $2.2 billion. Shares have climbed more than 40 percent since then to around $38.

One of Zoetis' hottest draws is a vaccine for pregnant hogs to ward off a virus that has killed millions of newborn pigs in the United States". This didn't make the news obviously because it would shed light on the fact that the Big Farm industry has its claws deeper in than a lot of people realize; the USDA reports that Cattle production is the most important agricultural industry in the United States, consistently accounting for the largest share of total cash receipts, which is forecast to represent about 17 percent of the $462 billion in total cash receipts for agricultural commodities.

Although many people have opted for nondairy milk in their coffee in the last few years, they still haven't removed cheese, butter, and other products containing milk, and so these contaminants are leaking into many people's diets regardless of their "oat milk Lattes."

Synthetic growth hormones (e.g., rBGH/rBST) are approved for use in dairy cattle in the US. Banned in the European Union, Canada, Japan, Australia, and other countries because (rBGH) is a synthetic hormone used to increase milk production in dairy cows. Due to concerns about potential adverse effects on human health and animal welfare, several countries have chosen to ban its use.

Not Mylk!

The World Health Organization recently called antimicrobial resistance "an increasingly serious threat to global public health that requires action across all government sectors and society." This is why, of all antibiotics sold in the United States, approximately 80% are sold for use in animal agriculture.

About 70% of these are "medically important," meaning the conditions the animals are kept in are breeding grounds for sickness and death. Antibiotics are administered to animals in feed to marginally improve growth rates and prevent infections, a practice projected to increase dramatically worldwide over the next 15 years.

There is growing evidence that the widespread use of non-therapeutic antibiotics in animals promotes antibiotic resistance in humans. Resistant bacteria are transmitted to humans through direct contact with animals, exposure to animal manure, consumption of undercooked meat, and contact with uncooked meat or surfaces meat has touched.

Bovine somatotropin (bST), also known as bovine growth hormone (BGH), is a naturally occurring hormone cows produce. It regulates various physiological processes, including growth and milk production. In the United States, recombinant bovine somatotropin (rbST) is an artificial version of this hormone that was developed for use in dairy cows to increase milk production.

The U.S. Food and Drug Administration (FDA) approved rbST for use in dairy cows in 1993. However, its use has become controversial, and there are varying opinions on its safety and potential impacts on human health and animal welfare. Some concerns include potential effects on milk quality, antibiotic use, and animal well-being. The United States does not require companies to label the use of rBST in their products, although it was banned in the European Union in 1990. The use of rBST in dairy cows has been shown to increase the concentrations of IGF-1, a protein naturally found in milk.

According to contemporary reports, European bans of the product were based on the fear of potential health risks rBST posed to humans, including cancer and animal welfare. However, Monsanto argues that the ban was based on economics and politics.

There is a legally allowed level of contaminants in Dairy products. These contaminants vary depending on environmental factors, the specific conditions of the plant where the cattle are bred and confined, the feed contaminants, pharmaceutical intake, and the process where the product is bottled.

The Somatic Cell Count measures the level of white blood cells in milk and is used as an indicator of udder health in dairy cows. High SCC can indicate the presence of infection or inflammation.

Maximum residue limits (MRLs) for pesticides and veterinary drug residues may be established to prevent unsafe levels of these substances in milk. Regulations often limit the presence of antibiotics in milk due to concerns about antibiotic residues and potential health risks to consumers. Aflatoxins are toxic compounds produced by certain molds. Limits on aflatoxin levels may be set to prevent contamination of milk.

Some standards may include limits for heavy metals, such as lead, cadmium, and mercury, to ensure that milk is not contaminated with these potentially harmful substances. In some areas, regulations may address the presence of radioactive materials in milk, particularly in regions with nuclear facilities. Limits may be established for various chemicals used in agriculture or during milk production, such as cleaning agents and sanitizers.

Consumption of cow's milk has plummeted in the last few years as people embrace non-hormonal, antibiotic-free, and suffering-free options. The simultaneous increase in demand for more costly organic milk suggests consumer concern about exposure to production-related contaminants may be contributing to this decline.

Not Mylk!

While the contaminants in hand-held milk jugs can be blindly tested, all of the hidden dairy in foods, sauces, dressings, and ice creams can not be sussed out and tested as efficiently. However, the ones that were tested showed levels of pharmaceuticals high enough that if you were once a dairy consumer, you probably wouldn't ever look at it the same way again. Volunteers collected half-gallon containers of organic and conventional milk in each of the nine US regions and shipped them on ice for analysis.

Laboratory analysis of retail milk samples showed that current-use pesticides (5/15 tested) and antibiotics (5/13 tested) were detected in several conventional but not in organic samples. Among the conventional samples, residue levels exceeded federal limits for amoxicillin in one sample (3 %) and in multiple samples for sulfamethazine (37 %) and sulfathiazole (26 %). Median bGH and IGF-1 concentrations in conventional milk were 9·8 and 3·5 ng/ml, respectively, twenty and three times that in organic samples.

Current-use antibiotics and pesticides were undetectable in organic but prevalent in conventionally produced milk samples, with multiple samples exceeding federal limits. Higher bGH and IGF-1 levels in conventional milk suggest the presence of synthetic growth hormone.

Ractopamine is a beta-agonist drug used in the United States as a feed additive in livestock production, chiefly for pigs and cattle. It promotes lean muscle growth and improves feed efficiency in animals, leading to increased meat production. Ractopamine works by increasing protein synthesis while reducing fat deposition. The U.S. Food and Drug Administration (FDA) regulates the use of ractopamine in animal agriculture to ensure its safety for animal and human consumption. The FDA has established maximum residue limits (MRLs) for ractopamine in meat products, and meat from animals treated with ractopamine must meet these standards before entering the food supply.

It's worth noting that the use of ractopamine is a topic of debate and has been banned in some countries, including the European Union, China, and Russia, due to concerns about its potential effects on animal welfare and food safety. However, it is still permitted for use in the United States, and meat products from animals raised with ractopamine may be available on the market.

The Center for Food Safety heeds additional warnings on the effect of this one of many pharmaceuticals: Studies on the potential human health effects of ractopamine are extremely limited. The only human study on which the new 2012 "international standard" from Codex is based examined the effects of ractopamine on six young, healthy men, one of whom dropped out after experiencing adverse health effects. Data from the European Food Safety Authority indicates that ractopamine causes elevated heart rates and heart-pounding sensations in humans.

Ractopamine has significant known health impacts on animals. Fed to an estimated 60 to 80 percent of pigs in the U.S. meat industry, ractopamine use has resulted in more reports of sickened or dead pigs than any other livestock drug on the market. According to the FDA's calculations, more pigs have been adversely affected by ractopamine than any other animal. Ractopamine's effects include toxicity and other exposure risks, such as behavioral changes and cardiovascular, musculoskeletal, reproductive, and endocrine problems. It is also associated with high-stress levels in animals, "downer" or lame animals, hyperactivity, broken limbs, and death.

Now, not all plant milks are created equally. The mass production of many things has caused companies to cut corners on many products. Large brands use fillers and stabilizers to stretch products to maintain a creamy texture. Sugar finds its way into some vanilla-flavored milk substitutes but is usually also available unsweetened. This sneaky sugar can add to your daily values without realizing it.

Not Mylk!

Look for brands without carageen on the label because it is a very inflammatory stabilizer. Also, guar gum, sunflower lecithin, and potassium citrate are all ingredients that don't need to be in there. If you like almond milk, the easiest thing to do is make your own; you can do this from organic, raw, unsalted almonds. Or, with a scoop of almond (or any pure nut butter, blend and strain after adding a cup to two cups of water per tablespoon of almond butter. Adding a date, a tablespoon of maple syrup, a splash of real vanilla extract, or even cocoa powder can transform simple almonds into homemade natural milk for pennies on the dollar compared to products sold in stores.

Made from soybeans, soy milk is one of the most widely available and popular plant-based milk options. It has a creamy texture and a mild flavor. Soy milk is a good source of protein and is often fortified with calcium and vitamins.

Made from ground almonds and water, almond milk has a slightly sweet and nutty flavor and a lighter texture than dairy milk. It is often fortified with calcium and vitamin D. While almonds are high in vitamin E, and most almond milk commercially are filled with gums for texture, this is not my first choice for commercial non-dairy milk.

If you are so persuaded to use almond milk on a daily basis versus other types, then it is easier and less costly to make yourself using one to two tablespoons of raw ground almonds and spring water blended in a high-speed food processor and then strained if necessary for a silkier texture, adding a few dates, pure extracts or a dash of maple syrup can customize any homemade nondairy milk to your liking.

Almonds' popularity grew exponentially when dairy milk first lost the spotlight. Almonds were highlighted initially on DR. SEBI's alkaline foods list. Still, then he renounced that after exploring the heightened levels of arsenic that naturally occur in almond milk, he removed it from his list. Although the levels are not high enough to cause issues in everyone, it is important to be aware if you have a diet hefty on almonds, as relying too much on any one food usually doesn't cause enough diversity in the diet, which is very important. Arsenic is a naturally occurring element found in the Earth's crust, and it can be present in varying levels in soil and water. Plants, including almond trees, can absorb arsenic from the soil as they grow. As a result, some almonds may contain trace amounts of arsenic.

There are two primary forms of arsenic: organic and inorganic. Organic arsenic is considered less toxic and is commonly found in plants. Inorganic arsenic, on the other hand, is more harmful and is often associated with potential health risks.

Almonds contain most of the arsenic in the organic form, which is considered less harmful to humans. The levels of inorganic arsenic in almonds are generally low. The U.S. Food and Drug Administration (FDA) has conducted studies on the arsenic content in various foods, including almonds. According to the FDA's data, almonds have been found to contain deficient levels of inorganic arsenic, well below the established safe levels.

It's essential to remember that the overall health benefits of almonds outweigh any potential risks associated with trace amounts of arsenic. Almonds are a nutritious food rich in healthy fats, protein, fiber, vitamins, and minerals. They are known to provide various health benefits, such as supporting heart health, aiding in weight management, and promoting overall well-being.

Made from oats and water, oat milk has a creamy texture and a subtle oat flavor. It is naturally sweet and often fortified with nutrients like calcium and vitamin D. This can also be made at home in a high-speed blender.

Made from milled rice and water, rice milk has a mild, slightly sweet taste. It has a thinner consistency compared to dairy milk. Rice milk is often fortified with nutrients such as calcium and vitamin D.

Made from the flesh of coconuts and water, coconut milk has a rich and creamy texture with a distinct coconut flavor. It is commonly used in cooking, baking, and beverages. Coconut milk is higher in fat compared to other plant-based milks. It can be used alone or blended with other ingredients to make a thicker, creamier-style milk.

Made from ground cashews and water, cashew milk has a creamy texture and a mild, slightly sweet taste. It is often used as a dairy milk substitute in recipes and beverages.

Hemp milk: Made from hemp seeds and water, hemp milk has a slightly nutty flavor and a creamy consistency. It is a good source of omega-3 fatty acids and protein. Hemp seeds are a powerhouse ingredient; the flavor is earthy and nutty.

Made from yellow peas and water, pea milk is a newer addition to the plant-based milk market. It has a creamy texture and a neutral taste. Pea milk is often fortified with nutrients like calcium and vitamin D. This is harder to make at home as the pea protein has been extracted and re-blended. Although a good choice for those with nut allergies, it is also looking for a higher-density amino option. Peas have a warning in California, as they grow in soil that naturally contains lead. This doesn't mean there are necessarily higher doses due to human intervention. Still, in the case of protein powders and processing in general, we need to use this as a general warning that once a food has been processed, the path gets murkier to follow.

Protein powders are derivatives of the above, ranging from dairy-based to plant-based. During processing, some are treated better than others. The process of extracting protein to make protein powders depends on the source of the protein. There are various sources of protein used in protein powders, such as whey protein, casein protein, soy protein, pea protein, rice protein, and hemp protein, among others. Each source requires different extraction methods. Here are some common methods for extracting protein from different sources.

Those who are confused about what whey and casein are are milk derivates, and I advise against them. I have included them here for educational purposes and not as a recommendation, as dairy products do not belong to humans.

Whey protein is derived from milk during the cheese-making process. The liquid that remains after milk is curdled and strained is whey. It undergoes further processing to remove water, fat, and carbohydrates, leaving behind a concentrated form of protein, which is then dried to create whey protein powder.

Like whey, casein protein is also derived from milk. During the cheese-making process, casein is separated and processed into a powdered form. Casein protein is a slower-digesting protein compared to whey and is often used for its sustained release of amino acids.

Soy protein is typically extracted from soybeans using a solvent extraction process. This involves grinding soybeans into a meal, mixing the meal with water, and adding a solvent (usually hexane) to separate the protein from the carbohydrates and fats. After evaporation of the solvent, the remaining protein is dried and turned into powder. Because of this additional processing, it may be simpler for those who want to add soy protein to foods, like smoothies, sauces, etc., by simply using a serving of silken tofu, which is creamy, flavorless, and minimally processed.

Hexane is a chemical compound commonly used as a solvent in various industrial processes, including the extraction of oils from seeds such as soybeans. It is a hydrocarbon of carbon and hydrogen atoms derived from crude oil.

In making protein powder, hexane extracts protein from soybeans while producing soy protein isolate. The process typically involves the following steps:

Soybeans are first cleaned and crushed into a fine powder or meal.

The soybean meal is mixed with water to form a slurry.

Hexane has a high affinity for fats and oils, so it binds to the oil in the soybean, effectively separating it from the protein and other components.

The mixture is allowed to stand or undergo centrifugation, separating the hexane-oil mixture (miscella) from the protein and other solids.

The hexane-oil mixture is then evaporated, leaving behind soybean oil.

The protein-rich solids are further processed through precipitation and filtration to separate the protein from carbohydrates and fiber.

The isolated protein is then dried to remove any remaining moisture, resulting in soy protein isolating in a powdered form.

Hexane effectively extracts oil and separates the protein, but some concerns have been raised about its potential health effects. Hexane is considered a volatile organic compound (VOC) and can release harmful vapors into the air during extraction. As a result, some people are concerned about potential residual hexane in the final product.

To ensure the safety of consumers, regulatory authorities in many countries, including the United States, have set limits on the allowable amount of residual hexane in food products. Reputable manufacturers of soy protein isolate and other food products take measures to minimize the presence of hexane and comply with these safety regulations.

As a consumer, it is essential to choose products from reputable brands that follow good manufacturing practices and safety guidelines. Pea Protein: Pea protein is made from yellow peas. The peas are ground into flour or powder, then the protein is extracted using water and centrifugation. The resulting protein is dried to create pea protein powder.

Rice protein is made from brown rice. Rice is treated with enzymes to break down the carbohydrates and fibers, leaving behind the protein. The protein is then isolated, filtered, and dried to create rice protein powder.

Hemp protein is derived from hemp seeds. The seeds are cold pressed to remove the oil, and the remaining seed cake is ground into a powder. The protein is separated from the remaining carbohydrates and fiber, producing hemp protein powder. You can mimic the benefits of protein powders simply by adding a few tablespoons of sunflower seeds or butter, hemp seeds to your smoothie, cereal, or baked goods to add extra nutrition and amino that have a completely digestible package.

The evolving awareness of "Big Milk's" impact on health, both from a nutritional and environmental perspective, has led many to reconsider their dairy consumption. While milk has been a staple in diets worldwide, increasing evidence highlights the potential drawbacks of dairy, including hormonal and antibiotic residues and its role as an endocrine disruptor. The shift towards plant-based alternatives reflects a growing desire to avoid these concerns and embrace more sustainable and health-conscious choices. As research continues to evolve, individuals are encouraged to make informed decisions based on their health needs and ethical considerations, exploring diverse nutritional options that align with their well-being and values.

20
EAT THE RAINBOW, WHY RAW IS BETTER

Our bodies thrive on the diverse phytonutrients found in raw, living foods. While we all know that carrots are good for our eyes, it's essential to recognize that every edible plant offers its own unique powerhouse of vitality. Incorporating a wide range of fruits and vegetables into your diet ensures you're fueling your body with a variety of essential enzymes, minerals, antioxidants, and vitamins in their most digestible and beneficial form: raw, fresh, and alive.

Phytonutrients are a broad group of natural compounds found in plants. They are responsible for giving plants their color, flavor, and resistance to disease. There are thousands of different phytonutrients, and they can have various effects on human health.

Antioxidants protect cells from damage caused by free radicals, which are unstable molecules that can harm cells. While not all phytonutrients are antioxidants, many of them have antioxidant properties. This means that some phytonutrients can act as antioxidants, helping to neutralize free radicals and prevent cell damage.

In summary, many phytonutrients are antioxidants, but not all antioxidants are phytonutrients.

Natural chemicals found in plants help protect them from harm and give them their color, taste, and smell. Unlike vitamins or minerals, phytonutrients are not essential for our survival, but they can have many health benefits when we eat them.

These compounds can act as antioxidants, helping protect

our cells from damage. They can also reduce inflammation in the body, helping prevent conditions like arthritis and heart disease. Some phytonutrients boost the immune system, helping us fight infections. Others may help protect against cancer by stopping the growth of cancer cells.

Phytonutrients can also help balance hormones in the body, potentially reducing the risk of certain types of cancer. Additionally, they can support heart health by lowering blood pressure and improving blood flow.

A helpful rule of thumb is to eat one fruit or vegetable from every color of the rainbow daily. This simple habit ensures you provide your body with a broad spectrum of nutrients. The concept of "living food" in the Raw Vegan world refers to fruits and vegetables that haven't been heated above 118 degrees Fahrenheit. This is crucial because higher temperatures destroy the enzymes that make these foods special. These enzymes are responsible for digesting the food within our bodies, facilitating chemical exchanges, and converting nutrients into absorbable forms.

The more variety of fruits and vegetables you consume daily, the more you'll support healthy digestion, provide fiber for your microbiome, and promote balance in your skin, hair, mood, and metabolic functions. The real "circle of life" is incorporating fresh, raw foods into every meal. Juice, however, is an exception to the general rule of consuming whole, raw fruits and vegetables. When the fiber is removed from fruit, as in juice, the sugars are absorbed more rapidly into the bloodstream, which can lead to blood sugar spikes.

The decision to eat fruits and vegetables raw or cooked can significantly impact their nutritional value, affecting the availability and retention of vitamins, minerals, and antioxidants. Understanding these differences can help in making dietary choices that maximize nutritional intake.

Eat the Rainbow, Why Raw is Better

Eating fruits and vegetables raw is often recommended for preserving certain vitamins and enzymes sensitive to heat. Raw foods tend to retain more vitamin C and B vitamins, both of which are water-soluble and easily degraded by heat. For instance, red bell peppers and broccoli are excellent sources of vitamin C, which can diminish by up to 50% when cooked. Additionally, raw vegetables like spinach and kale maintain their folate levels better when uncooked, which is crucial for cell growth and DNA synthesis. The natural enzymes in raw foods, such as those found in pineapples (bromelain) and papayas (papain), aid in digestion and may offer anti-inflammatory benefits. These enzymes are often destroyed at high cooking temperatures.

Cooking, on the other hand, can enhance the bioavailability of certain nutrients, making them easier for the body to absorb. For example, cooking carrots and tomatoes helps to release beta-carotene and lycopene, respectively. Lycopene, an antioxidant found in tomatoes, becomes more potent when cooked as the heat breaks down cell walls, making it more accessible.

Similarly, cooking carrots increases the levels of beta-carotene, a precursor of vitamin A, which is essential for vision and immune health. Moreover, cooking can break down fiber, making vegetables like spinach and kale easier to digest and absorb. Some minerals, such as calcium, iron, and magnesium, can also become more readily available when foods are cooked because the cooking process can reduce the presence of oxalates, compounds that inhibit the absorption of these minerals.

Balancing Raw and Cooked Foods: A balanced diet that includes both raw and cooked vegetables and fruits can help ensure that one gets the maximum nutritional benefits. For instance, leafy greens like kale can be consumed raw in salads to benefit from their high vitamin C content, but lightly steaming them can enhance the absorption of calcium and iron. Similarly, while fresh tomatoes in salads are rich in vitamin C, cooked tomato sauces provide a powerful dose of lycopene.

It's also important to consider the type of cooking method. Steaming and microwaving are generally better at preserving nutrients compared to boiling, which can leach water-soluble vitamins into the cooking water. Roasting and grilling can enhance the flavors and increase the nutrient density of vegetables but should be done at moderate temperatures to avoid nutrient loss and the formation of harmful compounds.

Certain foods offer unique benefits when incorporated into your diet. For instance, ginger is incredibly beneficial for the body, and beets, though higher in sugar, are packed with minerals and antioxidants, meaning even a small amount can have a significant impact. Personally, I prefer to consume fruit in its raw, dehydrated, or smoothie form.

Red foods are a powerhouse of nutrients, offering a variety of health benefits through their rich antioxidant content. Tomatoes are a well-known source of lycopene, an antioxidant linked to reduced risk of prostate cancer and heart disease.

Strawberries are packed with vitamin C and manganese, supporting immune health and skin repair. Red bell peppers offer a combination of vitamin C, beta-carotene, and antioxidants, promoting eye health and reducing inflammation.

Cherries contain anthocyanins, which help reduce inflammation and may lower the risk of chronic diseases. Raspberries are rich in dietary fiber, vitamin C, and manganese, supporting digestive health and immune function.

Pomegranates are a superfood packed with polyphenols and flavonoids, which have powerful anti-inflammatory and heart-protective effects. Red grapes, with their resveratrol content, support heart health and have anti-aging properties. Watermelon, a hydrating fruit, provides vitamins A and C, supporting skin health and immune function. Dragon fruit (red variety) is not only visually striking but also rich in vitamin C, fiber, and antioxidants, which aid digestion and boost the immune system.

Goji berries, an ancient superfood, are loaded with antioxidants, vitamins, and minerals that promote eye health, boost immunity, and enhance skin health.

Orange foods are celebrated for their high beta-carotene content, which the body converts into vitamin A, essential for vision and immune function.

Carrots are a classic example, supporting eye health and providing antioxidants that protect against oxidative damage. Sweet potatoes offer a rich source of fiber, vitamins A and C, and potassium, promoting heart health and digestion.

Oranges, known for their high vitamin C content, support immune function and skin health. Mangoes, with their sweet, juicy flesh, provide vitamins A and C, promoting skin health and boosting the immune system.

Cantaloupe is rich in beta-carotene and vitamin C, which are important for eye health and immune support. Papayas offer digestive enzymes, vitamins A and C, and antioxidants, aiding digestion and supporting skin health. Turmeric, a bright orange spice, contains curcumin, known for its anti-inflammatory and antioxidant properties, supporting overall health. Apricots provide vitamins A and C, fiber, and potassium, supporting eye health and heart health.

Papayas are a tropical fruit celebrated for their sweet, vibrant orange flesh and numerous health benefits. They are an excellent source of vitamins A and C, both powerful antioxidants that help protect the body from oxidative stress, boost the immune system, and support healthy skin. Papayas also contain a unique enzyme called papain, which aids digestion by breaking down proteins, making it easier for the body to absorb nutrients.

This enzyme also has anti-inflammatory properties, which can help reduce inflammation in the body and support overall digestive health. Additionally, papayas are rich in folate, fiber, and potassium, which contribute to heart health, help regulate blood pressure, and support the body's overall well-being. Including papayas in your diet can enhance digestion, boost immunity, and provide essential nutrients that promote radiant skin and good health.

Persimmons, with their sweet, honey-like flavor, are rich in beta-carotene, fiber, and vitamin C, promoting heart health and digestion. Sea buckthorn, an exotic orange berry, is a powerhouse of omega-7 fatty acids, vitamins A and C, and antioxidants, supporting skin health, immune function, and reducing inflammation.

Yellow foods bring a burst of sunshine to your diet, packed with nutrients that support overall health. Bananas are a well-known source of potassium, which is vital for heart health and muscle function, as well as vitamin B6, which supports brain health. Yellow bell peppers, rich in vitamin C and beta-carotene, boost the immune system and promote healthy skin.

Lemons, with their high vitamin C content, support the immune system and promote clear skin. Corn, a staple food, provides fiber, B vitamins, and antioxidants, supporting digestive health and energy metabolism.

Yellow squash is rich in vitamins A and C, fiber, and magnesium, supporting eye health and bone health. Golden beets offer similar nutrients to their red counterparts, including folate, manganese, and potassium, which promote heart health and reduce inflammation. Starfruit, a tropical fruit, is low in calories but high in vitamin C, fiber, and antioxidants, supporting immune health and digestion. Yellow dragon fruit, another exotic variety, provides vitamin C, fiber, and antioxidants, aiding in digestion and boosting immunity. Turmeric root, known for its anti-inflammatory and antioxidant properties, is also a vibrant yellow food that supports overall health and well-being.

Green foods are among the most nutrient-dense, providing a variety of vitamins, minerals, and antioxidants. Spinach is rich in vitamins A, C, and K, as well as folate and iron, supporting eye health, immune function, and blood clotting. Kale is another leafy green powerhouse, offering vitamins A, C, and K, along with fiber, calcium, and antioxidants that promote heart health and reduce inflammation.

Broccoli is a cruciferous vegetable that provides vitamins C and K, fiber, and sulforaphane, a compound with potential anti-cancer properties. Avocados are packed with healthy monounsaturated fats, which support heart health, along with vitamin E, an antioxidant that protects the skin. Green peas offer protein, fiber, and vitamins A, C, and K, supporting digestive health and overall wellness.

Green apples provide fiber and vitamin C, helping to regulate blood sugar levels and boost immunity. Kiwi is a small green fruit that packs a punch with its high vitamin C and fiber content, supporting immune function and digestive health. Cucumbers, being mostly water, are excellent for hydration and also provide vitamins K and C, promoting bone health and immune function. Matcha, a powdered form of green tea, is rich in catechins, powerful antioxidants that support brain function, metabolism, and heart health. Moringa, often called the "miracle tree," is a green superfood loaded with vitamins A, C, and E, calcium, protein, and antioxidants, promoting overall health and wellness.

Blue and purple foods are rich in anthocyanins, antioxidants that provide numerous health benefits. Blueberries are a well-known superfood, packed with vitamin C, vitamin K, and antioxidants that support heart health, brain function, and immune health. Blackberries provide fiber, vitamin C, and vitamin K, supporting digestive health and reducing inflammation. Purple cabbage is rich in vitamins C and K, fiber, and anthocyanins, which help reduce inflammation and promote heart health. Eggplant contains Nasunin, an antioxidant that protects cell membranes from damage, as well as fiber and vitamins that support heart health.

Plums are rich in vitamin C, vitamin K, and fiber, promoting bone health and digestion. Acai berries, a popular superfood, are packed with antioxidants, fiber, and healthy fats, promoting heart health and reducing inflammation. Figs offer a good source of dietary fiber, calcium, potassium, and antioxidants, supporting bone health, heart health, and digestion.

Purple grapes contain resveratrol and flavonoids, which have been linked to heart health and longevity. Black currants are rich in vitamin C, anthocyanins, and antioxidants, promoting immune health and reducing inflammation. Purple sweet potatoes are not only visually appealing but also rich in anthocyanins, fiber, and vitamins, supporting gut health and providing powerful antioxidant benefits.

White and brown foods may not be as colorful, but they are still packed with nutrients. Garlic contains allicin, a compound with powerful antimicrobial and anti-inflammatory properties, supporting immune function and heart health. Onions are rich in quercetin, an antioxidant with anti-inflammatory and heart-protective effects.

Cauliflower is a cruciferous vegetable that provides fiber, vitamins C and K, and sulforaphane, a compound that has been shown to have anti-cancer properties. Mushrooms, such as shiitake and maitake, contain beta-glucans, which boost the immune system and have anti-cancer properties.

Potatoes, especially when eaten with the skin, provide fiber, potassium, and vitamin C, supporting heart health and immune function. Turnips offer fiber, vitamin C, and potassium, promoting digestive health and supporting immune function. Ginger, a popular spice, has powerful anti-inflammatory and antioxidant effects, helping to reduce nausea and improve digestion.

Coconut, in its various forms, offers healthy fats, fiber, and minerals like manganese, supporting bone health and heart health. Brown rice is a whole grain that provides fiber, B vitamins, and magnesium, supporting energy metabolism and heart health. Almonds, though technically a seed, offer healthy fats, protein, vitamin E, and antioxidants, supporting heart health and skin health. Maca root, an ancient Peruvian superfood, is rich in vitamins, minerals, and antioxidants, supporting energy, stamina, and hormone balance. Incorporating a variety of these colorful foods into your diet ensures you receive a broad spectrum of nutrients, supporting overall health and well-being. Each color provides unique benefits, making it important to eat a rainbow of fruits and vegetables every day.

By including these foods in your daily diet, you can ensure that you're getting a wide range of nutrients to support your overall health. Each color offers unique benefits, making it essential to eat a diverse array of fruits and vegetables every day.

A common concern is the concentration of sugar in dried fruit. However, I believe dried fruit is an integral part of the Vegan version of the "Paleo" diet. The Paleo diet is based on the idea that we should eat like our ancestors did. While the specifics of prehistoric diets are largely speculative, it's clear that our ancestors relied on dried fruits as part of their winter food stores. When choosing foods, a good rule of thumb is that if it grows from the ground, it's likely a good choice.

Incorporating a variety of fruits and vegetables, whether fresh, dried or in juice form, into your daily routine is essential for maintaining a balanced and healthy diet. By focusing on whole, natural foods, you can nourish your body with the nutrients it needs to thrive.

Before I received professional training, I believed someone who told me that eating bananas and potatoes would make me gain weight, so I cut them out of my diet for years. But as I delved deeper into nutrition, I discovered that no vegetable, including bananas and potatoes, will cause weight gain as much as animal-based foods can. This revelation opened my eyes to the power of plant-based foods, particularly the remarkable compounds they contain.

Take polyphenols, for example. These compounds are abundant in various fruits, vegetables, whole grains, and herbs. Known for their potent antioxidant properties, polyphenols protect the body from oxidative stress, which is linked to chronic diseases like cancer and heart disease. Within this group, you'll find flavonoids, a diverse set of compounds that includes anthocyanins, flavonols, and flavonols. These flavonoids not only contribute to the vibrant colors of fruits and vegetables but also provide anti-inflammatory effects that can help reduce the risk of various illnesses.

Another group of phytochemicals that deserves attention is carotenoids, the pigments responsible for the rich reds, oranges, and yellows in many fruits and vegetables. Carotenoids don't just make your plate more colorful; they act as powerful antioxidants and are converted into vitamin A in the body. This conversion is vital for maintaining healthy vision, supporting immune function, and promoting skin health. Beta-carotene, found in carrots and sweet potatoes, is perhaps the most well-known carotenoid.

Still, others like lycopene, found in tomatoes, and lutein and zeaxanthin, found in leafy greens, are equally important for their roles in protecting against eye diseases and certain types of cancer.

Then glucosinolates are the sulfur-containing compounds

found in cruciferous vegetables like broccoli, kale, cabbage, and cauliflower. These vegetables might not always be the most popular at the dinner table, but they pack a punch regarding health benefits. When you chew or chop these veggies, glucosinolates break down into bioactive compounds called isothiocyanates. These compounds have been extensively studied for their potential anti-cancer properties, as they help the body detoxify harmful substances and may inhibit the growth of cancer cells.

Understanding the variety and potency of these phytochemicals has transformed how I approach food. I now embrace what I once viewed with skepticism as part of a vibrant, nourishing diet. By incorporating a diverse range of raw, living foods into your meals, you're not just eating—you're tapping into a natural pharmacy that has the potential to enhance your health and well-being in profound ways.

Fiber is a type of carbohydrate found in plant foods like fruits, vegetables, whole grains, legumes, and nuts. Though the body doesn't digest it, fiber plays an essential role in maintaining digestive health, regulating blood sugar levels, promoting satiety, and supporting heart health. Incorporating fiber-rich raw living produce into your diet also provides an abundance of vitamins and minerals necessary for optimal health. Fruits and vegetables, in particular, are excellent sources of vitamins C, A, K, and folate, as well as minerals like potassium and magnesium. These nutrients are crucial for supporting immune function, tissue repair, bone health, and overall well-being.

Raw living produce contains enzymes vital for aiding digestion and facilitating various metabolic processes in the body. For example, amylase breaks down carbohydrates, lipase breaks down fats, and protease breaks down proteins. These enzymes are most potent when the foods containing them are consumed raw, as cooking can destroy their activity.

Some colorful foods pack an incredible nutritional punch and are conveniently travel-friendly, making them perfect for preventing extreme hunger and helping you avoid poor food choices on the go.

Fruits like apples, bananas, and oranges are easy to carry, require minimal preparation, and are naturally rich in fiber, vitamins, and antioxidants. Bananas, for instance, are a powerhouse of nutrients, offering vitamin C, vitamin B6, potassium, and magnesium. They are particularly beneficial for heart health due to their potassium content, which helps regulate blood pressure and reduce the risk of cardiovascular diseases. Moreover, the dietary fiber in bananas supports a healthy digestive system. At the same time, carbohydrates provide a quick and easily digestible energy source, making them an excellent choice for athletes and anyone engaging in physical activities.

Nuts and seeds, such as almonds, walnuts, chia seeds, and pumpkin seeds, are nutrient-dense and provide a good source of healthy fats and protein. Creating a custom trail mix with various nuts, seeds, and dried fruits can result in a satisfying, energy-boosting snack that's easy to take. Nut butter packets are another convenient option, offering a perfect pairing with fruits or whole-grain crackers.

Whole-grain crackers or rice cakes make a great base if you want something crunchy. Pair them with avocado or hummus for added flavor and nutrition. Pre-cut veggies like carrot sticks, cucumber slices, or bell pepper strips combined with individual servings of hummus provide a tasty, satisfying snack rich in fiber, vitamins, and minerals.

Dried fruit is often misunderstood due to its concentrated sugar content, but it can be a healthy, natural source of sweetness when consumed in moderation. Portion-controlled packs of dried apricots, raisins, or mangoes are convenient to carry and offer a nutrient boost while satisfying your sweet tooth.

For a more substantial snack or meal, wraps or sandwiches made with gluten-free bread options or collard green/lettuce wraps filled with veggies and plant-based protein sources like tofu, tempeh, or legumes can be incredibly satisfying. A quinoa or grain salad with colorful veggies, herbs, and a simple vinaigrette packed in a portable container is another excellent option for on-the-go nutrition. Energy bars that are vegan, whole-food-based, and low in added sugars can provide a quick nutrient boost when you're short on time.

Roasted chickpeas are a crunchy, protein-packed snack that can be seasoned with various herbs and spices for flavor. Chia pudding, prepared with plant-based milk and left to sit overnight, makes for a nutritious and portable option that's easy to pack in a small container.

Regarding more specific foods, bananas stand out for their nutritional benefits. Beyond their convenience and natural sweetness, they are rich in essential nutrients like vitamin C, vitamin B6, potassium, dietary fiber, and magnesium. These nutrients collectively support heart health, digestion, and even mood regulation, thanks to vitamin B6, which plays a key role in synthesizing serotonin, the "feel-good" hormone.

Apples, whether crab apples or cultivated varieties, contain similar nutrients, including vitamins C and A, dietary fiber, and potassium. While the specific nutrient levels can vary among apple varieties, cultivated apples often have more consistent nutrient profiles.

Phytochemicals like polyphenols and flavonoids contribute to apples' antioxidant properties, supporting overall health and helping to protect the body from oxidative stress.

Beets are another nutrient-rich food belonging to the Chenopodiaceae family and scientifically known as Beta vulgaris.

These root vegetables, valued for their sweet taste, vibrant colors, and nutritional benefits, are rich in folate, manganese, potassium, and dietary fiber. Whether roasted, boiled, steamed, or pickled, beets offer a variety of culinary applications, and their greens can be cooked and enjoyed as a leafy green vegetable. Different varieties of beets, including those with red, golden, or striped flesh, add nutritional value and visual appeal to your meals.

Pineapples, native to South America, are cultivated in tropical and subtropical regions worldwide, including countries like the Philippines, Thailand, Costa Rica, and the United States. These fruits are known for their sweet, tangy flavor and are rich in vitamins A and C, dietary fiber, and antioxidants like beta-carotene and quercetin. Pineapples also offer potassium, which helps regulate blood pressure and fluid balance.

Kale, a leafy green often hailed as a superfood, is an excellent source of vitamins A, C, and K, which promote healthy vision, immune function, and blood clotting. Its high fiber content aids digestion and supports gut health, while minerals like calcium and magnesium contribute to strong bones and muscle function. Kale also contains sulforaphane, a compound with potential anti-cancer properties.

Brussels sprouts, another member of the cruciferous vegetable family, are rich in fiber and vitamins C and K. These nutrients support immune function and bone health, while antioxidants like glucosinolates may offer anti-cancer effects. Additionally, Brussels sprouts provide folate, which is essential for cell division and DNA synthesis, and iron, which is necessary for oxygen transport in the blood.

Canned pumpkin is high in beta-carotene, a precursor to vitamin A, which is crucial for healthy vision and immune function. This versatile ingredient also contains fiber, promoting digestion and satiety, and vitamin C, which acts as an antioxidant to protect cells from damage. The potassium in canned pumpkin supports heart and muscle function, while its antioxidants, like lutein and zeaxanthin, benefit eye health.

Grapes, with their rich antioxidant content, including resveratrol and flavonoids, have been linked to various health benefits, particularly for heart health. These small, hydrating fruits provide dietary fiber to promote digestion and help regulate blood sugar levels. Grapes also contain vitamins C and K, supporting immune function and bone health. Grape seeds are especially rich in antioxidants, including proanthocyanidins, which may offer cardiovascular benefits and contribute to skin health.

Sweet potatoes, cultivated worldwide, with China being the largest producer, are another nutrient-dense food. Whether in the form of traditional cultivars or heirloom varieties, sweet potatoes offer a rich content of vitamins A, C, and some B vitamins, as well as minerals like potassium and manganese. The dietary fiber in sweet potatoes supports digestion, while their antioxidants help protect the body from damage and promote overall health.

Incorporating a variety of these colorful, nutrient-rich foods into your diet can greatly enhance your health and well-being. They provide your body with the vitamins, minerals, fiber, and antioxidants it needs to thrive.

Quinoa is a remarkable grain known for being a complete protein, which means it contains all nine essential amino acids our bodies need. This makes it a standout among plant-based foods, especially for those following vegetarian or vegan diets. Additionally, quinoa is gluten-free and packed with fiber, B vitamins, minerals like magnesium and iron, and a wealth of antioxidants.

These nutrients contribute to various health benefits, including weight management, improved blood sugar control, and enhanced heart health. The amino acid profile of quinoa is impressive, providing balanced amounts of essential amino acids per cooked cup. For instance, quinoa offers approximately 0.72 grams of lysine, an amino acid often lacking in other grains, along with 0.24 grams of methionine and 0.51 grams of phenylalanine. These amino acids are crucial for protein synthesis, muscle repair, and various metabolic processes in the body.

Millet, another gluten-free grain, is celebrated for its rich dietary fiber content, antioxidants, and essential nutrients such as magnesium, phosphorus, and manganese. While millet is not considered a complete protein, it still offers various amino acids, including phenylalanine, leucine, isoleucine, and valine, which support muscle function and overall health. Millet's high fiber content mainly benefits blood sugar management, digestive health, and heart health.

Despite its name, buckwheat is not a grain but a seed. It is gluten-free and highly nutritious, offering a good source of fiber, minerals like manganese and magnesium, and powerful antioxidants. Buckwheat is rich in essential amino acids such as lysine, methionine, and threonine, making it a valuable addition to any diet, especially for those seeking to support heart health, blood sugar control, and digestion.

Forbidden rice, also known as black rice, stands out with its deep purple hue, which indicates a high concentration of anthocyanins—potent antioxidants known for their anti-inflammatory properties. This whole grain is also rich in fiber, vitamins, and minerals, making it an excellent choice for supporting heart health and reducing inflammation in the body.

Teff, a tiny yet mighty grain, is another gluten-free option rich in dietary fiber, iron, calcium, and other essential minerals. Teff is also a good source of protein, containing all the essential amino acids, which is rare for a grain. Its nutrient density supports digestion and bone health and provides sustained daily energy.

Spinach and kale are two leafy greens that are nutritional powerhouses, mainly known for their high content of carotenoids like β-carotene, lutein, and zeaxanthin. These antioxidants are crucial in preventing chronic diseases like cancer and heart disease. Spinach, however, contains oxalates, naturally occurring compounds that can bind with calcium in the urine and potentially form kidney stones in susceptible individuals. While this might sound concerning, it's important to note that not everyone who consumes oxalate-rich foods will develop kidney stones. The overall risk depends on factors like genetics, diet, hydration, and individual health conditions.

Although oxalates can inhibit calcium absorption, the effect is minimal and unlikely to significantly impact overall calcium balance, especially if you maintain a varied and balanced diet. Spinach remains highly nutritious, offering vitamins, minerals, dietary fiber, and antioxidants that contribute to reduced risks of chronic diseases, including heart disease and certain types of cancer. Cooking spinach can help reduce its oxalate levels—boiling or steaming allows some oxalates to leach into the cooking water, which can then be discarded to lower oxalate content further. However, remember that other beneficial nutrients may also be lost during cooking.

For those concerned about oxalate intake, especially if there's a history of kidney stones, it's wise to stay well-hydrated, maintain a balanced diet, and consult a healthcare professional for personalized advice. Ensuring adequate hydration helps dilute the concentration of oxalates in the urine, reducing the likelihood of kidney stone formation.

The body's pH level often comes up in discussions about diet and health. The pH scale ranges from 0 to 14, with 7 being neutral. A pH below 7 is acidic, while a pH above 7 is alkaline. The body, particularly the blood, maintains a slightly alkaline pH between 7.35 and 7.45, which is essential for various physiological processes, enzymes, and chemical reactions within the body to function optimally within this specific pH range.

The idea of eating alkaline foods to maintain or improve the body's pH level has gained popularity, especially in alternative health circles. It's believed that an alkaline environment in the body can help prevent chronic diseases like cancer and cardiovascular issues. While scientific studies specifically proving these claims are limited, the theory aligns with the broader understanding that a diet rich in fruits, vegetables, and whole grains—many of which are considered alkaline—supports overall health and reduces the burden on the body's regulatory systems.

Alkaline foods, which are thought to have an alkalizing effect on the body, include vegetables like spinach, kale, broccoli, and celery; fruits such as lemons, limes, watermelon, and papaya; and a variety of nuts, seeds, legumes, and whole grains like quinoa, amaranth, and millet. Herbal teas, tofu, and seaweeds like nori and kelp are also considered alkaline. These nutrient-dense foods contribute to overall well-being and are believed by some to help the body maintain a slightly alkaline state, which may support various health benefits.

Emphasizing these foods in your diet can improve energy levels, better digestion, and a general sense of well-being. While the body tightly regulates its pH and isn't significantly affected by the pH of the foods we eat, focusing on a diet rich in alkaline foods—largely plant-based and minimally processed—can help you feel more balanced and energized. This dietary shift also reduces the intake of acid-producing foods, which are often linked to inflammation and chronic diseases. By giving your body a break from the onslaught of processed foods, you may notice positive changes in how you feel, making exploring a more alkaline-focused approach to eating worthwhile.

Here are two seven-day meal plans that incorporate all seven colors of the rainbow—red, orange, yellow, green, blue, indigo, and violet—every day. Each day focuses on including a variety of colorful fruits and vegetables to ensure a broad spectrum of nutrients. The beginner version slowly incorporates a full spectrum over the course of the week, while the second encourages that the rainbow of colors of food are incorporated daily for maximum nutritional benefits.

Beginner 7 Days of Eating the Rainbow

DAY 1: RED
- Breakfast: Smoothie with strawberries, raspberries, and pomegranate juice
- Lunch: Red bell pepper slices with hummus, quinoa salad with cherry tomatoes, and beets
- Dinner: Roasted red cabbage, red lentil soup, and a side of steamed red chard
- Nutritional Focus: Red fruits and vegetables are rich in lycopene and anthocyanins, powerful antioxidants known for their role in heart health and cancer prevention.

DAY 2: ORANGE
- Breakfast: Orange and carrot juice, oatmeal topped with dried apricots
- Lunch: Butternut squash soup with a side of roasted sweet potatoes and orange slices
- Dinner: Grilled portobello mushrooms with a side of orange bell peppers and carrots
- Nutritional Focus: Orange foods are high in beta-carotene, which the body converts to vitamin A, supporting vision and immune health.

DAY 3: YELLOW

- <u>Breakfast</u>: Mango and pineapple smoothie with turmeric
- <u>Lunch</u>: Yellow pepper stuffed with brown rice and lentils, corn on the cob
- <u>Dinner</u>: Chickpea curry with yellow squash, served over turmeric-infused rice
- <u>Nutritional Focus</u>: Yellow foods, rich in vitamin C and flavonoids, support immune function and reduce inflammation.

DAY 4: GREEN

- <u>Breakfast</u>: Green smoothie with kale, spinach, green apple, and cucumber
- <u>Lunch</u>: Spinach and avocado salad with green bell pepper, cucumber, and a lemon-tahini dressing
- <u>Dinner</u>: Stir-fry with broccoli, snap peas, and zucchini, served with brown rice
- <u>Nutritional Focus</u>: Green vegetables are packed with chlorophyll, folate, and vitamins K, C, and E, promoting detoxification and cardiovascular health.

DAY 5: BLUE/PURPLE

- <u>Breakfast</u>: Acai bowl with blueberries, blackberries, and chia seeds
- <u>Lunch</u>: Purple cabbage slaw with tahini dressing, side of roasted eggplant
- <u>Dinner</u>: Baked purple sweet potatoes with a side of steamed red kale and black rice
- <u>Nutritional Focus</u>: Blue and purple foods contain anthocyanins, which have been shown to support cognitive function and reduce the risk of heart disease.

DAY 6: WHITE/BROWN
- Breakfast: Banana and almond milk smoothie with flaxseed
- Lunch: Cauliflower and white bean soup with garlic, side of roasted parsnips
- Dinner: Sautéed mushrooms with brown rice and a side of steamed bok choy
- Nutritional Focus: White and brown foods like mushrooms, garlic, and onions contain allicin and other compounds that boost immune function and support bone health.

DAY 7: RAINBOW
- Breakfast: Fruit salad with strawberries, mango, kiwi, blueberries, and pomegranate seeds
- Lunch: Quinoa and mixed vegetable stir-fry (red peppers, carrots, broccoli, purple cabbage)
- Dinner: Stuffed bell peppers (using red, orange, and yellow peppers) with black beans, corn, and kale, served with a side salad of mixed greens and beets
- Nutritional Focus: Combining all colors ensures a wide range of vitamins, minerals, and antioxidants, providing comprehensive support for overall health and vitality.

Advanced 7 Days of Eating the Rainbow (ROYGBIV every day)

DAY 1

Breakfast:
- Smoothie made with strawberries (red), mango (orange),

banana (yellow), spinach (green), blueberries (blue), blackberries (indigo), and chia seeds (violet).

Lunch:
- Mixed salad with red bell pepper (red), shredded carrots (orange), corn (yellow), mixed greens (green), red cabbage (blue), purple cabbage (indigo), and beets (violet).
- Dressing made from lemon juice and olive oil.

Dinner:
- Quinoa bowl with roasted red tomatoes (red), sweet potato (orange), yellow bell pepper (yellow), broccoli (green), black rice (blue/indigo), and roasted eggplant (violet).
- Topped with fresh herbs.

DAY 2

Breakfast:
- Parfait with layers of raspberries (red), apricots (orange), pineapple chunks (yellow), kiwi slices (green), blueberries (blue), figs (indigo), and a drizzle of honey with some chopped nuts.

Lunch:
- Veggie wrap with red hummus (red bell pepper blended with chickpeas), grated carrot (orange), yellow squash (yellow), romaine lettuce (green), pickled red onion (blue), alfalfa sprouts (indigo), and shredded red cabbage (violet).
- Whole grain wrap.

Dinner:
- Stir-fried tofu with diced red chili peppers (red), butternut squash (orange), yellow zucchini (yellow), kale (green), purple potatoes (blue/indigo), and red onions (violet).
- Served over brown rice.

DAY 3

Breakfast:
- Oatmeal topped with cherries (red), dried apricots (orange), banana slices (yellow), kiwi (green), fresh blueberries (blue), and blackberries (indigo), sprinkled with flaxseeds (violet).

Lunch:
- Grain bowl with roasted red beets (red), steamed pumpkin cubes (orange), chickpeas (yellow), green beans (green), cooked wild rice (blue), purple carrots (indigo), and radishes (violet).
- Tahini dressing.

Dinner:
- Pasta salad with cherry tomatoes (red), roasted butternut squash (orange), yellow bell peppers (yellow), arugula (green), kalamata olives (blue), eggplant (indigo), and purple basil (violet).
- Light balsamic vinegar dressing.

DAY 4

Breakfast:
- Smoothie bowl with raspberries (red), papaya (orange),

pineapple (yellow), avocado (green), blueberries (blue), acai (indigo), and passion fruit seeds (violet).
- Topped with coconut flakes.

Lunch:
- Buddha bowl with roasted red peppers (red), carrots (orange), yellow lentils (yellow), edamame (green), sautéed shiitake mushrooms (blue/indigo), and purple kale (violet).
- Lime tahini dressing.

Dinner:
- Vegetable stir-fry with red cabbage (red), orange bell peppers (orange), baby corn (yellow), bok choy (green), purple cauliflower (blue/indigo), and eggplant (violet).
- Served with soba noodles.

DAY 5

Breakfast:
- Fruit salad with watermelon (red), cantaloupe (orange), pineapple (yellow), grapes (green), blueberries (blue), blackberries (indigo), and pomegranate seeds (violet).

Lunch:
- Quinoa salad with roasted red tomatoes (red), diced sweet potato (orange), chickpeas (yellow), spinach (green), red onion (blue), roasted Brussels sprouts (indigo), and beets (violet).
- Lemon olive oil dressing.

Dinner:
- Rainbow vegetable skewers with cherry tomatoes (red), bell

peppers (orange, yellow, and green), red onion (blue), mushrooms (indigo), and purple potatoes (violet).
- Served over a bed of leafy greens.

DAY 6

Breakfast:
- Acai bowl with strawberries (red), goji berries (orange), banana (yellow), kale (green), blueberries (blue), figs (indigo), and edible flowers (violet).
- Topped with granola.

Lunch:
- A veggie platter with red pepper hummus (red), roasted sweet potato (orange), yellow pepper strips (yellow), celery sticks (green), blue corn tortilla chips (blue), purple carrot sticks (indigo), and beetroot hummus (violet).

Dinner:
- Roasted vegetable medley with red beets (red), orange carrots (orange), roasted yellow squash (yellow), green zucchini (green), purple asparagus (blue/indigo), and eggplant (violet).
- Served with a quinoa pilaf.

DAY 7

Breakfast:
- Chia pudding layered with pomegranate seeds (red), pumpkin puree (orange), pineapple (yellow), kiwi (green), blueberries (blue), mulberries (indigo), and blackberries (violet).

Lunch:
- Salad with red lettuce (red), grated carrots (orange), yellow tomatoes (yellow), snap peas (green), radicchio (blue/indigo), and shredded red cabbage (violet).
- Topped with hemp seeds and lemon vinaigrette.

Dinner:
- Ratatouille with red bell peppers (red), orange zucchini (orange), yellow squash (yellow), spinach (green), eggplant (blue/indigo), and tomatoes (violet).
- Served with brown rice.

By incorporating all these colors into your diet daily, you're ensuring a comprehensive intake of essential vitamins, minerals, and antioxidants that support overall health and vitality. This variety makes meals more visually appealing and enjoyable, encouraging more balanced and nutritious eating habits.

21
BOOZE IS MAKING YOU FAT

Alcoholic beverages have been part of human culture for thousands of years, often used in ceremonial and cultural contexts. This historical precedent is frequently cited to justify current drinking habits, arguing that since ancient civilizations engaged in drinking, it must be appropriate or beneficial today.

This reasoning overlooks the significant changes in the nature of alcohol and its consumption over time. Modern alcoholic beverages differ significantly from those consumed by our ancestors regarding their composition, potency, and the cultural contexts in which they are consumed. The reality is that the alcohol we consume today is not the same as what was consumed in ancient times. The nutrient density of ancient foods and the alcohol content of fermented beverages have evolved dramatically.

Modern drinks, such as Cotton Candy vodka, bear little resemblance to the natural, fermented beverages of the past. Today's alcohol, often loaded with added sugars, artificial flavors, and higher potency, has a more immediate and intense effect on the body. The production methods have also changed, with modern processes including additives and techniques that increase the alcohol content and alter the beverage's effects.

Even the source and quality of ingredients have changed.

Ancient wines were made from grapes grown in nutrient-rich soils, and the winemaking process was much simpler without the additives commonly used today. The wood used in barrels, the methods of distillation, and the overall production process have all evolved, resulting in beverages that are far more potent and potentially more harmful than those of the past.

These changes from the soil to the processing and additives mean that alcohol's impact on our bodies today differs from what it was for our ancestors, not just because of the extra calories but also because of how these substances interact with our bodies.

For many people, drinking has become a habit, and for some, it can lead to addiction or serve as a coping mechanism. The idea that alcohol is a normal, healthy part of the diet is often reinforced by media and cultural norms. For example, Superbowl commercials glamorize beer, making it seem like a harmless part of social life. However, it's important to remember that these advertisements are often followed by disclaimers and warnings, prompting us to question what is truly good or bad for our health.

It is essential to examine the role of alcohol in our lives critically. Like any other substance we consume, we should ask ourselves, "How is this serving me?" If answering this question honestly is challenging, it may be because we recognize, deep down, that alcohol is a toxin, one that has been glamorized by the media and normalized by society.

When alcohol is consumed, it is primarily metabolized in the liver, where it takes precedence over other metabolic processes. This can disrupt the body's natural metabolic functions, leading to various health issues. The question isn't just whether alcohol has been part of human culture for thousands of years but whether its role in our lives today is truly beneficial or if it's a habit that needs re-examining in light of modern knowledge and understanding.

Alcohol metabolism involves the liver breaking down ethanol, the active component of alcoholic beverages, into acetic acid,

Booze is Making You Fat

which can be used for energy or stored as fat. However, this process has significant consequences for the body's ability to metabolize other nutrients. When the liver is focused on processing alcohol, its capacity to metabolize fats, carbohydrates, and proteins is reduced, leading to weight gain and hindering weight loss efforts.

The process of metabolizing alcohol can be compared to how a lighter burns fuel. Alcohol, like gasoline, contains calories, but that doesn't make it a beneficial part of your diet. In fact, when you consume alcohol, your body prioritizes burning ethanol over other energy sources. This means that fat loss is essentially put on hold for 24 to 48 hours after drinking, as the body dedicates its energy to metabolizing the alcohol. Any additional calories consumed during this time, whether from food or sugary mixers, are more likely to be stored as fat.

Ethanol provides calories that are different from those derived from carbohydrates, proteins, and fats. Alcohol is a non-essential nutrient, meaning the body cannot store it for later use. When alcohol is consumed, it takes precedence over all other energy sources, disrupting the metabolism of other nutrients, particularly fats, which can remain unprocessed and contribute to weight gain during the 48-hour window following alcohol consumption.

Alcohol is often consumed with additional calories, especially from sugary mixers or high-calorie snacks like chips, wings, and other bar foods. This combination can lead to a positive energy balance, where the body takes in more calories than it burns, storing those extra calories as fat. Additionally, alcohol's interference with muscle recovery exacerbates this issue. It suppresses protein synthesis, the process by which muscle fibers repair and grow after exercise-induced damage, hindering muscle recovery and growth.

Moreover, alcohol disrupts the hormonal balance critical for muscle recovery. It decreases the production of growth hormones, which are vital for muscle repair and growth, and alters the balance of cortisol, a hormone that increases in response to stress, potentially leading to increased muscle protein breakdown. This disruption also affects insulin and glucagon, hormones that regulate blood sugar and fat metabolism, further inhibiting the body's ability to access stored fat for energy.

These effects are particularly detrimental for athletes or anyone engaged in regular physical activity. Alcohol not only delays muscle recovery but also impairs the body's ability to build and maintain muscle mass, undermining the benefits of exercise and making it harder to achieve fitness goals. The celebratory drink that seems harmless can have lasting effects on your metabolism, muscle recovery, and overall health, making it crucial to consider the impact of alcohol on your body beyond just the immediate pleasure it provides.

Alcohol consumption can significantly impact muscle recovery by leading to nutrient deficiencies crucial for the body's repair processes. When alcohol is consumed, it interferes with the absorption and utilization of essential nutrients like vitamin B12, vitamin D, folate, and various minerals. These nutrients are vital for muscle function, tissue repair, and overall health, and deficiencies can severely impede recovery. Without adequate levels of these nutrients, your muscles may not heal properly, leaving you more susceptible to injury and prolonged soreness.

One way alcohol exacerbates these deficiencies is by increasing urine production, which can contribute to dehydration. Dehydration is particularly detrimental to muscle recovery because it impairs blood flow, reducing the delivery of essential nutrients and oxygen to the muscles and hindering the removal of metabolic waste products. This lack of efficient nutrient delivery and waste removal can lead to electrolyte imbalances, further impairing muscle function and delaying recovery.

In addition to nutrient deficiencies and dehydration, alcohol can disrupt sleep patterns, leading to decreased sleep quality and quantity. Quality sleep is crucial for muscle recovery, as during deep sleep, the body secretes growth hormones and repairs exercise-induced muscle damage. Disrupted sleep, therefore, hampers your body's ability to recover and diminishes your overall physical performance and well-being.

Moreover, alcohol affects muscle function and coordination, leading to reduced strength and endurance. It impairs motor skills, balance, and reaction times, all critical components of athletic performance. This can make training harder and increase the risk of injury during physical activity. Excessive alcohol consumption also contributes to poor nutrient absorption, further depleting essential vitamins and minerals necessary for maintaining energy levels, muscle function, and overall health. Over time, these deficiencies can lead to chronic fatigue, reduced athletic performance, and a higher likelihood of injury.

From a personal development perspective, figures like Wayne Dyer, a renowned self-help author and motivational speaker, might have underscored the limitations of alcohol in terms of its impact on motivation, focus, and overall well-being. Dyer's insights likely resonate with those who seek to maximize their potential and maintain a clear, focused mind. However, while his perspectives are valuable, they should be considered alongside the scientific evidence and medical consensus that highlight alcohol's detrimental effects on metabolism, organ function, and athletic performance.

Alcohol might be culturally accepted and even celebrated, but its impact on the body, particularly in the context of muscle recovery and athletic performance, is overwhelmingly negative. It's important to understand these effects and make informed choices about alcohol consumption, especially if your goals include maintaining optimal health, recovering effectively from exercise, and performing at your best.

It's important to recognize that moderate alcohol consumption, defined as up to one drink per day for women and up to two drinks per day for men, may not have significant detrimental effects on health and athletic performance. However, excessive or chronic alcohol consumption can lead to severe consequences. While alcohol has been a part of various cultures throughout history, the way it is consumed and its effects on the body have changed considerably over time.

Historically, many cultures have enjoyed fermented alcoholic beverages with lower alcohol content compared to modern distilled spirits. For example, Pulque is a traditional Mexican drink made from the fermented sap of the maguey or agave plant. Dating back to pre-Columbian times, pulque was considered sacred by indigenous cultures. With its relatively low alcohol content, pulque's effects on the body are milder compared to modern spirits, leading to less intense intoxication.

Sake, a traditional Japanese rice wine, has been produced in Japan for centuries and holds a significant place in Japanese culture. With an alcohol content ranging from 15% to 20%, sake's effects on the body are similar to other fermented beverages, though they can vary depending on the brewing process and specific alcohol content.

Mead, another ancient beverage, is made by fermenting honey with water. Mead has historical significance in cultures like the Norse, Celtic, and Slavic traditions. Its alcohol content can vary, but it is generally lower than distilled spirits. The honey in mead not only provides a distinct flavor but may also contribute additional nutrients, making its impact on the body slightly different from that of other alcoholic beverages.

Chicha, a traditional fermented beverage in various forms

across Latin America, is made from maize (corn), yuca (cassava), quinoa, or fruits. With a low alcohol content similar to that of beer, chicha's effects on the body are comparable to other mild fermented drinks.

These traditional fermented beverages typically had lower alcohol concentrations compared to modern distilled spirits, which can lead to several differences in how they affect the body. Higher alcohol concentrations in modern spirits result in more rapid and intense intoxication, which can place additional strain on the liver and other organs. While the liver metabolizes alcohol at a relatively constant rate regardless of the source, the higher alcohol content in distilled spirits can lead to more significant long-term liver damage, especially with prolonged and excessive consumption.

Moreover, some traditional beverages like pulque or mead may contain additional nutrients or beneficial compounds from their natural ingredients, such as agave or honey. These components might offer some nutritional value or health benefits not found in distilled spirits, which are generally devoid of significant nutrients.

Despite the historical and cultural significance of fermented alcoholic beverages, it's crucial to remember that excessive consumption of alcohol can have detrimental effects on health. Alcohol can harm several organs, including the liver, pancreas, heart, and brain. Prolonged and excessive drinking can lead to serious conditions like cirrhosis, fatty liver, pancreatitis, heart damage, and neurological disorders.

In summary, while moderate consumption of alcohol may be part of a balanced lifestyle for some, it's important to be mindful of the type and amount of alcohol consumed. Understanding the historical context and differences in alcohol content can provide valuable perspectives, but the focus should always be on how these choices impact overall health and well-being.

Beyond the influence of media, some personal relationships likely revolve around alcohol, too. Whether it's nightlife, vacations, celebrations like anniversaries and weddings, sporting events, or even local book clubs, alcohol often plays a central role. This can make it challenging for someone to opt-out, as not partaking can sometimes make you feel like an outsider in these social settings. Self-care is not drinking a glass of wine; often, people associate self-care with using ethanol to numb out reality. If you drink alcohol and call it self-care, it is because you haven't found another way to relax and feel calm. Drinking in lieu of self-care is often masking a deeper need.

The act of pouring yourself a glass of something can be ceremonious. You can pour anything into a beautiful stemware glass, like a calming herbal mocktail, which can signal the beginning of your "you" time. But when you pour alcohol, you often work against your best intentions.

It's natural to want to fit in. As humans, we are wired to seek social acceptance and approval. But sometimes, the need to fit in can pull you away from who you truly are and hinder your pursuit of personal goals. The pressure to conform can lead you to make choices that aren't aligned with your values or long-term aspirations.

Self-actualization, a concept introduced by psychologist Abraham Maslow, is about realizing and fulfilling your potential. It's the process of becoming the best version of yourself, achieving personal growth, and finding true fulfillment. However, the need to fit in and peer pressure can either support or hinder this journey.

On the positive side, fitting in and being accepted by your peers can provide a sense of belonging, which is a fundamental human need. Positive social connections can foster personal growth, offering you emotional support, encouragement, and a network of people who understand you. But it's essential to be mindful of the environments and activities that make up these social connections. If your social life heavily revolves around alcohol, it might be worth exploring activities that aren't centered around drinking.

Consider engaging in hobbies and interests that promote well-being without the influence of alcohol. Activities like bike riding, crochet, video games, dance lessons, and music lessons can offer new avenues for social interaction and personal development. These alternatives not only help you build relationships that aren't based on alcohol but also contribute to your growth and fulfillment.

Ultimately, the decision is yours. Strive to find a balance between blending in and remaining true to yourself. This will help you build a life that aligns with your values and allows you to reach your full potential, even if it means standing out from the crowd.

Filling the time that would otherwise be spent drinking alcohol with activities that enrich your life and nurture your passions can elevate you on the path to self-actualization. Although it may feel lonely at the top, the quality of life and the relationships you build from a healthier foundation will offer long-term rewards that far outweigh the temporary satisfaction of fitting in with unhealthy habits.

Peer groups can expose you to diverse perspectives, ideas, and experiences. Positive peer influences can catalyze personal growth by providing opportunities for learning, skill development, and expanding your horizons. Even peer pressure can sometimes positively impact you when it encourages you to strive for self-improvement. Watching others achieve their goals or engage in positive behaviors can motivate and inspire you to pursue your own personal growth. However, it's essential to choose your friends wisely.

On the flip side, fitting in can sometimes lead to conformity, where you adopt your peer group's values, beliefs, and behaviors, even if they don't align with your true self. This kind of conformity can stifle personal growth by suppressing your individuality, creativity, and the pursuit of unique aspirations. When you rely too heavily on fitting in and adhering to peer pressure, it can limit your personal growth by confining you within the boundaries of group norms and expectations. This can discourage exploration, questioning, and independent thinking, which are crucial for personal development.

While peer pressure might seem like a concept from grade school, the pattern of coaxing others to follow the lead of the "majority" is something that persists into adulthood. This can lead to the adoption of negative or harmful behaviors. When you choose to fit into the "norm" by succumbing to negative peer pressure, whether consciously or not, it can hinder your personal growth and well-being. This might manifest as drinking alcohol simply because it's part of a celebration, eating foods you wouldn't normally choose because you know they aren't good for you, or skipping workouts because you don't feel up to it after engaging in these negative behaviors. All of these actions can impact your mindset, metabolism, and overall sense of well-being.

To truly grow and thrive, it's essential to recognize when the need to fit in is pulling you away from your authentic self and limiting your potential. Focusing on activities that align with your values and goals while surrounding yourself with peers who support and encourage your growth can help you foster a healthier and more fulfilling life. The journey to self-actualization might be challenging, but the rewards are significant—not just in the quality of your life but also in the deep, meaningful connections you build along the way.

Navigating the pressures of fitting in while promoting personal growth requires a delicate balance. It's crucial to learn how to make your own choices about what you put into your body, regardless of what those around you might be doing. Making yourself and your goals the priority is vital. Remember, just because something is offered to you doesn't mean you're obligated to accept it. You have the right to say no to anything that doesn't align with your values or contribute to your well-being.

Embracing your true self, values, and aspirations is key to living a fulfilled life. Strive to fit in on your terms, where your individuality and personal goals are respected. If the people around you create a dissonant or unsupportive environment, stepping back and regaining your footing is okay. Sometimes, the best approach is to allow others to be themselves while expecting the same respect for your own choices.

If your current social circle doesn't align with your values, it might be time to seek out activities and people who resonate more closely with your aspirations. Surround yourself with those who echo your values, or take a break until you feel strong enough that your values become unshakeable. Building a support system within yourself is crucial; becoming the strongest person in the room can lead others to either look up to you or naturally fade out of your life. Positive energy will always outshine negative energy.

It's important to remember that no one else experiences the consequences of what you consume, be it food, drink, or even thoughts, except yourself. Therefore, it's no one's business if you choose to abstain from certain substances or foods. Having a club soda in hand at social events can help keep the focus on the celebration rather than inviting unnecessary questions about why you aren't drinking. Preparing yourself with a decoy beverage can allow you to enjoy social functions without the pressure to conform to the behaviors of others.

By prioritizing your health, values, and goals, you'll find that the right people and opportunities will naturally come into your life, enriching your journey toward self-actualization.

Surround yourself with peers who support and encourage your personal growth. Seek out positive role models and mentors who inspire you to pursue your goals and aspirations. This means if you were to make changes in your diet and drinking, the people around you should support your decision; if they don't, it is a good idea to reevaluate the time you spend with those people as this type of behavior is evident in one-sided and unhealthy relationships, alternatively can be a projection of that person who is too afraid to make changes and wants you to stay on the same paradigm as them.

Considering yourself as an example of strength and perseverance is ideal for maintaining your ground and personal growth, but it creates an opportunity for you to be an example. Having faith in yourself, the core values of a healthy being, and the patience to begin new habits. When you achieve a higher level of self, you "vibrate on a higher frequency. Some people who were a part of your life on lower frequencies will "vibrate right out of your life.

Focus on yourself and be open to the possibilities that elevating your body on a cellular level can foster critical thinking, which becomes clearer when you cease to drink. Alcohol is a depressant to the central nervous system. It dampens functions across the body until you detox, allowing regular functions to reboot. Evaluate the influence of peer pressure and the people you spend your time with and make decisions based on your values and judgments to potentially withdraw from those people and places until you have a solid footing in your new lifestyle.

Develop emotional intelligence skills to navigate social situations effectively; remember that not everyone needs to know what you are doing; sometimes, keeping personal growth changes to yourself or sharing with only your closest people can protect it. Sometimes, friends, family, and coworkers can, intentionally or otherwise, derail the personal growth of others with the injection of their behaviors and influence, like a friend trying to get you to take a shot at a bar, etc.

This includes setting boundaries, asserting yourself and your personal choices, and making decisions aligned with your personal growth, not allowing others to persuade you to do what they are doing in order to validate their own decisions externally.

Remember, personal growth is a unique and individual journey. While connections and peer relationships are meaningful, prioritizing your growth and staying true to yourself is essential for self-actualization and fulfillment.

If you're looking to lower your alcohol intake, several strategies can help guide you through the process. These approaches can also be applied to minimizing any habits in your life that might hinder your growth or well-being.

The first step is to set a clear goal. Define what you want to achieve and commit to it. For example, if your goal is to quit drinking, start by establishing a specific and measurable objective. This could be as simple as reducing the number of alcoholic beverages you consume daily. Negotiating with yourself can also be an effective approach.

You might start by cutting your drinks in half for the first week and then further reducing them in the following weeks. Rewarding yourself for sticking to your plan can make this process more manageable. Developing an "Anything But..." mindset can redirect your brain's reward centers toward healthier alternatives. If you find yourself pouring cocktails out of habit, remember that you don't have to consume them. Instead, replace the alcohol with a mocktail, club soda, or kombucha, which can help satisfy the physical habit of drinking without the negative consequences.

Creating a supportive environment is also crucial. Remove or minimize triggers and temptations in your surroundings. This might mean avoiding alcohol at home and steering clear of situations or social circles that encourage drinking. Surround yourself with friends and family who understand and respect your decision. For some, like myself, this might involve some degree of isolation. I cope best when I work through things independently, focusing on my passions and creative outlets like arts, music, and exercise. There is no right or wrong, as our journeys are individual.

These activities can be a great distraction as you transition from a daily drinker to someone who prioritizes your body and mind. Use this time to explore hobbies you've always wanted to try. Engaging in new interests can help you create the life you've envisioned for your highest self.

Even if you're going through this journey alone, seeking support is essential. Share your intentions with trusted friends or family members who can provide encouragement and hold you accountable. Consider joining support groups like Alcoholics Anonymous (AA) or SMART Recovery, where you can connect with others who are on a similar path.

Education is another powerful tool. Learn about the effects of alcohol on your physical and mental health. Understanding the reasons behind your decision to quit, as well as the benefits it can bring, will strengthen your commitment. It's also important to identify healthier ways to cope with stress, boredom, or emotional triggers that might have led to drinking in the past. Exploring alternative activities such as exercise, hobbies, meditation, or therapy can help manage cravings and improve your overall well-being.

Focusing on self-care is vital. Engage in activities that promote both physical and emotional well-being. This might include getting enough sleep, eating a nutritious diet, practicing relaxation techniques, and participating in activities that bring you joy and fulfillment.

If you've been drinking heavily and experience withdrawal symptoms when you stop, it's recommended to seek medical advice.

Depending on the severity of your symptoms, a healthcare professional may recommend a supervised detox or provide appropriate medications to manage the process safely.

Persistence is everything in this journey. Remember that quitting drinking is a process, and setbacks can happen. Be patient with yourself and stay persistent. Celebrate each milestone, no matter how small, and acknowledge the progress you've made along the way.

Modifying your drinking habits can be challenging, and some people may require professional help or medical support, depending on the severity of their alcohol dependency. If you're struggling or finding it difficult to quit on your own, it's highly recommended to reach out to a healthcare professional, therapist, or addiction specialist who can provide personalized guidance and support throughout the process.

22
SUPP WITH YOU?

The pursuit of optimal health involves more than just eating less or avoiding specific foods. It requires a comprehensive understanding of the nutrients our bodies need and the best ways to obtain them. No single food contains all the nutrients humans need to maintain optimal health. While some foods come close to being nutrient powerhouses, they still cannot provide every essential vitamin, mineral, amino acid, fatty acid, and other compounds required for overall well-being.

Humans require a diverse range of nutrients for various bodily functions, including growth, energy production, immune function, and cellular repair. These nutrients include macronutrients (carbohydrates, proteins, and fats), micronutrients (vitamins and minerals), essential fatty acids, and essential amino acids.

The most reliable sources of vitamins, minerals, and essential fats are the foods we consume daily. However, modern diets, often characterized by calorie restriction or the exclusion of entire food groups, can lead to deficiencies in essential nutrients. When we cut out vegetables, tubers, roots, grains, and other whole foods, we risk more than just reducing our calorie intake; we may also be depriving our bodies of the vital nutrition they need to function optimally.

Despite our best efforts to maintain a balanced diet, there are times when natural supplements can play a crucial role in enhancing our wellness. These supplements can address a variety of health issues, ranging from vitamin deficiencies and allergies to mood swings, hormonal imbalances, anxiety, and even skin and hair health. They can also provide support in preventing infections and promoting overall well-being. However, to harness the benefits of supplements effectively and safely, it is crucial to understand the principles behind their use.

One of the most important considerations when selecting supplements is their bioavailability, which is the degree to which a nutrient is absorbed and utilized by the body. Not all supplements are created equal, and their effectiveness can vary significantly depending on their form. For example, magnesium citrate is known for its high bioavailability, making it a preferred choice over magnesium oxide, which is less efficiently absorbed.

Similarly, natural vitamin E, known as d-alpha-tocopherol, is more readily utilized by the body compared to its synthetic counterpart, dl-alpha-tocopherol. Understanding these differences is crucial for choosing supplements that your body can effectively use. The form in which a supplement is delivered can also impact its bioavailability. For instance, liquid supplements often have higher bioavailability than tablets or capsules because they are more easily absorbed. Liposomal delivery systems, which encapsulate nutrients in lipid spheres, have been shown to enhance the absorption of vitamins like vitamin C and glutathione, making them more effective at lower doses.

While the allure of high-dose supplements may be tempting, more is not always better, especially with fat-soluble vitamins such as A, D, E, and K. These vitamins are stored in the body's fatty tissues and can accumulate over time, potentially leading to toxicity if taken in excessive amounts.

Vitamin D toxicity, for example, can result in hypercalcemia, a condition characterized by elevated calcium levels in the blood, which can cause serious health problems such as kidney stones, heart issues, and bone pain. It is important to follow recommended dosage guidelines, read supplement labels carefully, and understand the recommended daily intake for various nutrients. Dosage needs can vary based on individual factors such as age, sex, health status, and lifestyle. Consulting with a healthcare provider or a registered dietitian can provide personalized guidance on the appropriate dosage for your specific needs.

Timing is another key factor in the effectiveness of supplements. Certain nutrients are better absorbed when taken with food, while others may be more effective on an empty stomach. For example, fat-soluble vitamins like A, D, E, and K should be taken with a meal containing healthy fats to enhance absorption. Calcium supplements are best absorbed in smaller doses throughout the day, rather than all at once. Iron, a mineral essential for oxygen transport and energy production, is better absorbed when taken with vitamin C-rich foods or supplements, such as a glass of orange juice. On the other hand, calcium can interfere with iron absorption, so it is best to take these supplements separately.

Magnesium, a mineral involved in over 300 biochemical reactions in the body, is often recommended to be taken at night, as it can promote relaxation and support a good night's sleep. The timing of B vitamins, which play a crucial role in energy production, should be considered. They are best taken in the morning or early afternoon to avoid interfering with sleep. Understanding these nuances can significantly impact how well your body absorbs and utilizes the nutrients from supplements, maximizing their benefits.

While supplements can offer numerous health benefits, it is important to be aware of potential side effects and interactions. High doses of vitamin C can lead to digestive discomfort, such as diarrhea and stomach cramps. Niacin, or vitamin B3, can cause a temporary redness and warmth of the skin known as the niacin flush. Supplements can also interact with medications, sometimes in ways that are harmful. For example, St. John's Wort, a popular herbal supplement for mood support, can interact with antidepressants, birth control pills, and blood thinners, reducing their effectiveness.

This highlights the importance of consulting with a healthcare provider before starting any new supplement regimen, especially if you are taking prescription medications. A healthcare provider can help identify potential interactions and ensure that supplements are used safely and effectively.

Choosing high-quality supplements is essential for ensuring their safety and efficacy. With so many options on the market, it can be challenging to know which products to trust. Look for supplements that have undergone third-party testing and carry certifications from organizations such as NSF International or the United States Pharmacopeia, USP. These certifications indicate that the product has been tested for quality, potency, and purity, ensuring that it contains what it claims without harmful contaminants.

Be mindful of the sourcing and purity of supplements, especially with herbal products, as the origin of the ingredients can significantly impact their safety and effectiveness. Reputable brands that are transparent about their sourcing and manufacturing practices are more likely to provide high-quality products.

For individuals following a vegan or plant-based diet, selecting vegan-friendly supplements is necessary to ensure alignment with ethical and dietary preferences. Many supplements, especially those in capsule form, may contain animal-derived ingredients such as gelatin. Fortunately, there are plenty of vegan-friendly alternatives available today. Nutrients that are particularly important for vegans, such as vitamin B12, omega-3 fatty acids (DHA and EPA) derived from algae, and vitamin D3 sourced from lichen, should be prioritized. Ensuring that these nutrients are obtained from plant-based sources can support optimal health while adhering to vegan principles.

Numerous myths and misconceptions about supplements need to be addressed. One common misconception is that all supplements are necessary for everyone. Supplement needs are highly individualized and should be tailored to each person's specific health goals, age, sex, and lifestyle.

Not everyone needs to take a multivitamin, and in some cases, taking unnecessary supplements can lead to imbalances or excesses of certain nutrients. Another misconception is that natural supplements are always safe. While natural supplements can offer health benefits, they are not without risks. The term "natural" does not necessarily mean safe, as some natural supplements can have potent effects and may interact with medications or cause side effects. It is important to approach supplementation with a well-informed, personalized strategy.

Ethical considerations and sustainability should also play a role in supplement choices. The production of supplements can have significant environmental impacts, particularly in terms of sourcing ingredients sustainably and minimizing waste. Choosing supplements from environmentally conscious brands that prioritize sustainable practices can help reduce your ecological footprint. Opting for supplements with minimal or recyclable packaging is another way to support sustainability and reduce environmental impact.

Spirulina, a highly regarded superfood, comes in two main varieties: green spirulina (*Spirulina platensis*) and blue spirulina, which is derived from phycocyanin, a pigment present in green spirulina. Green spirulina is renowned for its high protein content, providing all essential amino acids, which makes it a complete protein source.

Rich in vitamins and minerals such as iron, calcium, magnesium, and vitamin B12. However, the B12 found in spirulina is primarily in a form that is not readily absorbed by the human body, making it an unreliable source of this essential vitamin. Green spirulina also offers chlorophyll, a compound known for its detoxifying effects and antioxidant properties.

Blue spirulina is distinguished by its unique blue color, attributed to the presence of phycocyanin, a potent antioxidant with strong anti-inflammatory properties.

Phycocyanin has been shown to protect cells from oxidative stress, enhance liver health, and boost the immune system. Both green and blue spirulina are versatile superfoods that can easily be incorporated into various dietary practices, such as adding them to smoothies, juices, or other recipes, providing a nutritional boost that promotes overall well-being.

Chlorella, a green algae rich in chlorophyll, is a potent detoxifier that helps the body eliminate toxins, including heavy metals like mercury, cadmium, and lead. Its detoxifying properties stem from its unique cell wall structure and high chlorophyll content. Its cell walls contain fibrous materials that bind to heavy metals and toxins in the digestive tract, effectively trapping them and preventing their absorption into the bloodstream. Once bound, these toxins are then safely excreted from the body through regular bowel movements, which aids in reducing the toxic load on vital organs such as the liver and kidneys.

This binding capability is particularly beneficial for individuals exposed to environmental pollutants or those consuming a diet high in processed foods, as it can help cleanse the body and support overall health. Chlorella, particularly in servings ranging from 3 to 5 grams per day, offers a wide range of nutrients that can complement or even substitute for those found in a daily multivitamin. However, chlorella's natural, whole-food composition provides additional phytonutrients and health benefits that are distinct from typical multivitamins.

One of the significant nutrients chlorella offers is vitamin A, which is in the form of beta-carotene. This precursor to vitamin A supports vision, immune function, and skin health. While multivitamins also provide vitamin A, chlorella offers it in a natural form that the body can convert as needed, which may enhance absorption and effectiveness.

Rich in B vitamins, including B1 (thiamine), B2 (riboflavin), B3 (niacin), B6 (pyridoxine), and folate. These vitamins are essential for energy metabolism, nerve function, and red blood cell formation. Unlike synthetic forms found in some multivitamins, chlorella provides these B vitamins in a whole-food matrix, potentially increasing their bioavailability. Notably, chlorella contains bioavailable vitamin B12, making it a valuable source for those on plant-based diets, where B12 can often be deficient.

Although chlorella has some vitamin C content, it is generally lower than the amounts found in a typical multivitamin, which often includes a significant dose of vitamin C to support immune health and provide antioxidant protection. Similarly, chlorella provides vitamin E and vitamin K, which are essential for antioxidant protection and bone health, respectively. However, multivitamins usually offer these vitamins in higher doses.

Chlorella is a good source of iron, offering a bioavailable form that is crucial for oxygen transport and energy production. It also provides magnesium, which supports muscle function, nerve transmission, and energy production. Both minerals are commonly included in multivitamins, but chlorella offers them in a natural, bioavailable form. Calcium is present in chlorella, though not in the high concentrations found in many multivitamins designed to meet daily calcium needs for bone health. Chlorella also contains zinc, which is vital for immune function and wound healing, and potassium, which is essential for maintaining fluid balance, nerve function, and muscle contractions.

One of chlorella's unique features is its high chlorophyll content. Chlorophyll acts as a powerful antioxidant, supports detoxification, and helps reduce body odor. This detoxifying capability is not a feature typically associated with multivitamins, which are primarily designed to provide essential nutrients. Chlorella's chlorophyll content, combined with its ability to bind and eliminate heavy metals and toxins from the body, makes it a valuable detoxifying agent.

Chlorella is also a rich source of antioxidants like phycocyanin, which has strong anti-inflammatory properties. This compound, found in blue-green algae, is not present in most multivitamins. Additionally, chlorella provides carotenoids such as lutein and zeaxanthin, which support eye health. While some multivitamins include these carotenoids, chlorella provides them in their natural, bioactive forms.

Beyond vitamins and minerals, chlorella offers other health benefits that multivitamins do not. It is about 50-60% protein by weight and provides all essential amino acids, making it a complete protein source, which is particularly beneficial for those on plant-based diets. Multivitamins do not provide protein, making chlorella a valuable addition for those seeking to increase their protein intake through natural sources. Furthermore, chlorella contains dietary fiber, which supports digestive health and is generally absent in multivitamin formulations.

Chlorella also includes small amounts of omega-3 fatty acids, which are beneficial for heart and brain health. Although some multivitamins include omega-3s, chlorella offers them naturally, making it an excellent supplement for those looking to enhance their diet with whole-food sources of these essential fats.

While chlorella provides a broad spectrum of essential vitamins, minerals, and additional beneficial compounds, it does not entirely replace the specific and often higher doses of nutrients provided by a daily multivitamin, especially for nutrients like vitamin D and vitamin C. However, chlorella's natural, whole-food composition, combined with its detoxifying properties and complete protein content, makes it a unique and valuable supplement. For those focused on whole foods and natural sources of nutrients, incorporating chlorella into the diet can offer numerous health benefits, complementing a balanced intake of fruits, vegetables, and other nutrient-dense foods. For optimal health, using chlorella alongside other supplements or dietary sources can help ensure all nutritional needs are met, especially for those on vegan or plant-based diets where certain vitamins and minerals might be less abundant.

For detoxification purposes, a daily intake of chlorella can vary depending on individual health goals and needs. For general detoxification and maintenance, a common recommendation is to start with a lower dose, such as 1-2 grams per day, and gradually increase to 3-5 grams per day. This gradual increase allows the body to adjust to the detoxifying effects of chlorella without causing discomfort or digestive upset. For those seeking more intensive detoxification, especially in cases of heavy metal exposure, higher doses ranging from 5-10 grams per day may be used under the guidance of a healthcare professional. It's important to consume chlorella consistently over several weeks or months to allow the body to gradually release and eliminate toxins, leading to improved health and vitality.

The detoxifying effects of chlorella and chlorophyll are not only limited to heavy metal chelation but also extend to supporting the body's natural defense mechanisms. By reducing the toxic burden, these superfoods enhance immune function, support healthy digestion, and improve skin health. As the body detoxifies, many individuals notice a reduction in body odor, clearer skin, and increased energy levels, all signs that the body is functioning more efficiently and effectively. Incorporating chlorella and chlorophyll-rich foods into a balanced diet can be a powerful strategy for promoting long-term health and well-being.

Chlorophyll, the green pigment abundant in chlorella, further enhances its detoxification abilities. Chlorophyll's molecular structure is remarkably similar to hemoglobin, the oxygen-carrying molecule in human blood. This similarity allows chlorophyll to assist in oxygen transport and boost blood purification. By increasing oxygen levels in the bloodstream and promoting the elimination of toxins, chlorophyll helps cleanse the blood, reduce inflammation, and support healthy liver function. Additionally, chlorophyll is known for its alkalizing properties, which help balance the body's pH and create an internal environment less conducive to the growth of harmful bacteria and yeast. This process can significantly impact body odor, as it neutralizes the odor-causing compounds produced by these microorganisms.

Chlorella is often cited for its potential to provide vitamin B12, particularly in its broken cell wall form, which is processed to enhance nutrient bioavailability. However, the bioavailability of B12 in chlorella is a topic of ongoing debate. Some studies suggest that certain strains of chlorella contain bioavailable forms of B12 that can be absorbed and utilized by the body. For instance, research published in the *Journal of Nutritional Science and Vitaminology* by Watanabe et al. (2002) showed that certain strains of chlorella contain significant amounts of bioavailable B12. In their study, rats with vitamin B12 deficiency exhibited improvement when fed chlorella, suggesting that chlorella could serve as a source of bioavailable vitamin B12.

Further research by Miyamoto et al. (2009), published in the *Journal of Medicinal Food*, found that dried powder of *Chlorella pyrenoidosa* contained bioavailable vitamin B12. In trials involving vitamin B12-deficient rats, the chlorella powder was able to restore normal growth, indicating that the B12 in chlorella was indeed bioavailable.

These studies imply that chlorella may be a viable source of vitamin B12, especially in specific strains or preparations. On the other hand, some research challenges these findings, suggesting that much of the B12 present in chlorella is in the form of inactive analogs that humans cannot utilize. A study by Victor Herbert, published in the *American Journal of Clinical Nutrition* in 1992, examined various plant sources, including chlorella, for vitamin B12 content. Herbert found that while chlorella and other algae might contain B12, a significant portion of it was present as B12 analogs. These analogs resemble B12 but are not biologically active and may even interfere with the absorption of true B12, potentially leading to a deficiency.

Additionally, the study by Dagnelie et al. (1991), published in the *Journal of Nutritional Medicine*, focused on the presence of B12 analogs in algal products like chlorella. This study found that these analogs were present in high amounts and were not active in human metabolism. The researchers emphasized the risk of relying solely on chlorella and other algae as sources of vitamin B12, highlighting the need for additional supplementation or consumption of fortified foods to ensure adequate intake of bioavailable vitamin B12.

The study by Dagnelie et al. did not specify its funding sources in the published paper, which is common for research articles from that period. This lack of transparency makes it difficult to ascertain the study's financial backing. However, such studies are typically funded by academic institutions, government research grants, or private foundations. In recent years, research funding sources have been more commonly disclosed due to increased transparency requirements, which helps identify potential conflicts of interest.

The debate over the bioavailability of vitamin B12 in chlorella underscores the importance of using reliable and well-established sources of nutrients to prevent deficiencies. While algae like chlorella and spirulina offer numerous health benefits and contribute valuable nutrients to a diet, they should not be considered complete replacements for all essential vitamins and minerals. For individuals following a plant-based diet, it is particularly crucial to ensure adequate intake of vitamin B12 through more reliable sources.

Vegan B12 supplements, typically derived from synthetic processes or bioengineered through bacterial fermentation, provide bioactive forms of B12, such as methylcobalamin and cyanocobalamin. These supplements are readily absorbed and utilized by the human body, making them essential for those who avoid animal-based foods. Fortified foods, such as plant-based milk alternatives and nutritional yeast, are also recommended to help meet B12 requirements.

While both spirulina and chlorella are nutrient-dense superfoods offering a variety of health benefits, they do not provide every vitamin and mineral essential for life. Whole foods, rich in a diverse array of nutrients, should form the foundation of any diet aimed at achieving optimal health. Where certain nutrients are difficult to obtain from food alone, carefully chosen supplements can support maintaining overall health and well-being.

Individuals should consult healthcare professionals to ensure that their dietary choices and supplement use meet their nutritional needs, preventing deficiencies and promoting long-term health. Ashwagandha, an adaptogenic herb used in Ayurvedic medicine, has gained popularity for its potential to reduce stress and anxiety.

Research suggests that Ashwagandha can lower cortisol levels, the body's main stress hormone, and improve overall well-being. Some studies indicate that it may also have mood-boosting effects and could be beneficial for managing depression and stress-related symptoms. While more research is needed to confirm its effectiveness as a standalone treatment, many people have reported positive experiences with Ashwagandha as part of their wellness regimen.

Reishi mushroom, often referred to as the "mushroom of immortality," is another supplement with a long history of use in traditional Chinese medicine. Reishi is believed to have adaptogenic properties, helping the body manage stress and promote overall health. It is thought to support immune function, reduce inflammation, and provide antioxidant benefits. Some studies suggest that Reishi may also have potential benefits for cardiovascular health, liver function, and even certain types of cancer. While scientific research on Reishi is still evolving, many individuals use it to enhance vitality and support a healthy immune system.

Beet powder is another supplement that has gained attention for its health benefits. Rich in nitrates, beet powder can support cardiovascular health by promoting healthy blood flow and reducing blood pressure. Nitrates in beets are converted to nitric oxide in the body, a molecule that helps relax blood vessels and improve circulation. Beet powder is a good source of vitamins and minerals, including vitamin C, folate, and potassium. It also contains antioxidants that help protect the body from oxidative stress. Athletes and fitness enthusiasts often use beet powder to enhance exercise performance and endurance, as it can improve oxygen delivery to muscles during physical activity.

Supplements like echinacea and goldenseal are often used together to support immune health and overall wellness. Echinacea is known for its ability to stimulate the immune system, helping the body fight off infections. It is commonly used to prevent and treat colds and respiratory infections. Goldenseal, on the other hand, has antimicrobial properties and has been used to address infections of the respiratory and gastrointestinal systems. When combined, echinacea and goldenseal offer synergistic benefits for immune support.

Oil of oregano, derived from the same plant used in cooking, is a potent antimicrobial supplement with a wide range of health benefits. It contains compounds like carvacrol and thymol, which have been shown to have antibacterial, antifungal, and antiviral properties. Oil of oregano can be used to help fight infections caused by bacteria such as E. coli and Salmonella, as well as fungal infections like candidiasis and toenail fungus. It is also believed to have antioxidant and anti-inflammatory effects, making it a valuable addition to a natural wellness regimen.

L-theanine, an amino acid found in green tea leaves, is known for its calming and relaxing effects. It promotes the production of neurotransmitters such as GABA, serotonin, and dopamine, which help regulate mood, emotions, and cognition. L-theanine is often used to reduce anxiety and stress without causing drowsiness, making it a popular supplement for promoting relaxation and mental clarity.

Adaptogenic mushrooms like Chaga, Cordyceps, Lion's Mane, Turkey Tail, Shiitake, and Maitake have been used for centuries in traditional medicine for their health benefits. These mushrooms help the body adapt to stress, boost immune function, and support overall well-being. Chaga is known for its antioxidant properties, Cordyceps for its potential to enhance energy and stamina, Lion's Mane for cognitive support, Turkey Tail for immune health, Shiitake for cardiovascular benefits, and Maitake for its role in supporting blood sugar balance. Incorporating these adaptogenic mushrooms into a supplement routine can provide a wide range of health benefits.

For those interested in collagen supplements, it is worth noting that while traditional collagen is derived from animal sources, plant-based alternatives are available. Ingredients like vitamin C, silica, bamboo extract, and certain plant-based amino acids can support the body's natural collagen production. These plant-based ingredients help maintain skin health, joint function, and overall vitality, offering a vegan-friendly option for those looking to enhance collagen levels without animal-derived products.

Incorporating supplements into your routine can be a powerful way to enhance your health, but it is essential to approach supplementation with a well-informed, personalized strategy. Understanding factors such as bioavailability, timing, dosage, and potential interactions can help you make more effective and safer choices.

Consulting with healthcare professionals can provide valuable guidance, ensuring that your supplement regimen is tailored to your individual needs and health goals. By prioritizing quality, sustainability, and ethical considerations, you can make supplement choices that not only benefit your health but also support a healthier planet. The journey to optimal wellness is unique for each individual, and supplements can play a supportive role in achieving your best health when used wisely and thoughtfully.

23
WORKBOOK

Mindful Eating Prompts

Before giving in to a craving, ask yourself these questions to practice mindful eating:

Am I physically hungry?

What emotions am I feeling?

What time of day is it?

Have I been exposed to food cues?

What have I eaten recently?

Am I craving a specific taste?

How will this food make me feel after eating?

Am I thirsty?

What nutrients might I be lacking?

Is this craving driven by habit?

Can I wait 10 minutes?

What else could satisfy this need?

Personal Growth and Development Prompts

What new skills or abilities do I want to develop?

In what areas do I seek personal growth and improvement?

How do I envision my ideal self in the future?

What is holding me back from achieving my goals?

What motivates me to improve and grow?

Who inspires me, and what can I learn from them?

What habits do I want to cultivate or break?

How can I better manage my time to focus on personal growth?

What does success look like to me, and how can I achieve it?

What challenges have I faced, and what did I learn from them?

How can I step out of my comfort zone to grow?

What small steps can I take daily to reach my long-term goals?

Workbook

Vision Board Prompts

Creating a vision board can help you visualize and achieve your goals. Use these prompts to guide your creation:

"What do I want to achieve in the next year?"

"What would my ideal day look like, from start to finish?"

"Where do I see myself in terms of relationships, career, health, and personal fulfillment in the next five years?"

"Who do I aspire to become, and what qualities define this person?"

"What experiences do I want to attract into my life?"

"What is my ultimate career goal, and what steps will get me there?"

"What personal relationships do I want to nurture and grow?"

"What does financial security mean to me?"

"How can I contribute to my community or causes I care about?"

"What skills or hobbies do I want to develop or improve?"

"What places do I want to visit, and how will I make it happen?"

"What energizes and inspires me, and how can I incorporate more of this into my daily life?"

First Month Lifestyle Transition Prompts

These prompts will help guide you through the first month of transitioning to healthier habits:

What plant-based foods do I enjoy the most?

How can I incorporate a variety of colors in my meals?

What new recipes can I try this week?

How am I feeling physically and mentally after eating more plant-based meals?

What challenges have I faced so far, and how can I overcome them?

What support systems do I have in place to help me on this journey?

What small steps can I take today to stick to my plant-based goals?

What new habits am I forming that contribute to a healthier lifestyle?

How can I make time for meal planning and preparation?

What positive changes have I noticed in my energy levels or mood?

Workbook

Smoothie Recipes

Here are seven nutrient-dense smoothie recipes, perfect for a quick breakfast or post-workout snack:

SMOOTHIE 1: GREEN POWER SMOOTHIE
Ingredients:
- 1 cup almond milk
- 1/2 banana
- 1/2 cup frozen spinach
- 1 tablespoon chia seeds
- 1 tablespoon almond butter
- 1 scoop plant-based protein powder
- 1/4 avocado

Macros: 320 calories, 34g carbs, 12g protein, 14g fat

SMOOTHIE 2: BERRY PROTEIN BLAST
Ingredients:
- 1 cup almond milk
- 1/2 cup frozen mixed berries
- 1/2 cup frozen cauliflower
- 1 tablespoon flaxseeds
- 1 scoop plant-based protein powder
- 1 tablespoon almond butter

Macros: 290 calories, 30g carbs, 15g protein, 13g fat

SMOOTHIE 3: TROPICAL SUNRISE
Ingredients:

1 cup coconut water
1/2 cup frozen pineapple
1/2 cup frozen mango
1/4 cup orange juice
1 tablespoon hemp seeds
1/4 cup silken tofu

Macros: 270 calories, 50g carbs, 10g protein, 5g fat

SMOOTHIE 4: CHOCOLATE PEANUT BUTTER SHAKE

Ingredients:
1 cup almond milk
1 frozen banana
1 tablespoon cacao powder
1 tablespoon peanut butter
1 scoop plant-based protein powder

Macros: 350 calories, 40g carbs, 20g protein, 15g fat

SMOOTHIE 5: MATCHA GREEN TEA SMOOTHIE

Ingredients:
1 cup almond milk
1 teaspoon matcha powder
1/2 banana
1/2 cup frozen spinach
1 tablespoon chia seeds
1 scoop plant-based protein powder

Macros: 290 calories, 32g carbs, 15g protein, 10g fat

SMOOTHIE 6: SPICED APPLE PIE SMOOTHIE

Ingredients:
- 1 cup almond milk
- 1/2 apple, chopped
- 1/2 frozen banana
- 1/2 teaspoon cinnamon
- 1 tablespoon almond butter
- 1/4 cup oats

Macros: 320 calories, 45g carbs, 10g protein, 10g fat

SMOOTHIE 7: CREAMY AVOCADO & LIME

Ingredients:
- 1 cup coconut water
- 1/2 avocado
- Juice of 1 lime
- 1 tablespoon chia seeds
- 1 scoop plant-based protein powder
- 1/2 frozen cucumber

Macros: 310 calories, 28g carbs, 12g protein, 18g fat

7-Day Vegan Meal Plan (High Complete Amino Acid Profiles)

DAY 1

Breakfast:
Quinoa Porridge with Almond Milk, Chia Seeds, and Blueberries
Calories: 400

Protein: 15g
Amino Acids: Complete profile (lysine from quinoa, methionine from chia seeds)

Snack:
Apple slices with almond butter
Calories: 200
Protein: 5g

Lunch:
Lentil Salad with Mixed Greens, Quinoa, and Lemon-Tahini Dressing
Calories: 450
Protein: 20g
Amino Acids: High in lysine, methionine, and cysteine from tahini

Snack:
Edamame beans with a sprinkle of sea salt
Calories: 150
Protein: 12g
Amino Acids: High in lysine, leucine, isoleucine

Dinner:
Stir-fried tofu with Bell Peppers, Snap Peas, and Brown Rice
Calories: 400
Protein: 25g
Amino Acids: High in leucine, valine, threonine

Total Daily Calories: 1,600
Total Daily Protein: 77g

Note: Add a small evening snack like a banana with peanut butter to reach the 2,000-calorie goal.

DAY 2

Breakfast:
Smoothie with Spinach, Chia Seeds, Almond Milk, Banana, and Plant-Based Protein Powder
Calories: 350
Protein: 25g
Amino Acids: High in methionine, lysine, leucine

Snack:
Mixed nuts (almonds, walnuts, cashews)
Calories: 200
Protein: 6g

Lunch:
Chickpea and Avocado Salad Wrap with Lettuce and Tomato
Calories: 450
Protein: 15g
Amino Acids: High in leucine, isoleucine, lysine

Snack:
Sliced cucumber with hummus
Calories: 150
Protein: 5g

Dinner:
Vegan Stuffed Peppers with Quinoa, Black Beans, and Corn
Calories: 450

Protein: 20g
Amino Acids: High in lysine, methionine, threonine

Total Daily Calories: 1,600
Total Daily Protein: 71g
Note: Include a protein-rich evening snack, such as a handful of seeds or nuts, to increase calories and protein intake.

DAY 3

Breakfast:
Oatmeal topped with Pumpkin Seeds, Chopped Nuts, and Fresh Berries
Calories: 350
Protein: 12g
Amino Acids: High in methionine, cysteine, tryptophan

Snack:
Carrot sticks with tahini dip
Calories: 150
Protein: 4g

Lunch:
Quinoa and Lentil Bowl with Roasted Sweet Potatoes and Avocado
Calories: 500
Protein: 22g
Amino Acids: High in lysine, leucine, isoleucine

Snack:
Chia pudding made with almond milk and vanilla extract

Calories: 150
Protein: 8g
Amino Acids: High in methionine, lysine, threonine

Dinner:
Tempeh Stir-Fry with Snap Peas, Carrots, and Jasmine Rice
Calories: 400
Protein: 25g
Amino Acids: Complete profile (tempeh is rich in all essential amino acids)

Total Daily Calories: 1,550
**Total Daily Protein
**: 71g
Note: Add an evening snack like a protein shake or a small portion of mixed nuts to reach the 2,000-calorie goal.

DAY 4

Breakfast:
Chia Seed Pudding with Coconut Milk, Topped with Fresh Mango
Calories: 300
Protein: 10g
Amino Acids: High in methionine, lysine

Snack:
Handful of dried apricots and almonds
Calories: 200
Protein: 5g

Lunch:
Spinach Salad with Tofu, Sunflower Seeds and Lemon Dressing
Calories: 450
Protein: 20g
Amino Acids: High in leucine, isoleucine, methionine

Snack:
Rice cakes with almond butter and sliced bananas
Calories: 200
Protein: 5g

Dinner:
Vegan Chili with Black Beans, Quinoa, and Avocado Slices
Calories: 400
Protein: 20g
Amino Acids: High in lysine, methionine, leucine

Total Daily Calories: 1,550
Total Daily Protein: 60g
Note: A dessert option such as a chia seed pudding or another piece of fruit with nut butter will help reach the 2,000-calorie target.

DAY 5

Breakfast:
Buckwheat Pancakes with Maple Syrup and Fresh Strawberries
Calories: 400
Protein: 10g
Amino Acids: Moderate in lysine, leucine

Snack:
Sliced bell peppers with guacamole
Calories: 150
Protein: 4g

Lunch:
Tempeh Lettuce Wraps with Shredded Carrots, Cucumbers, and Peanut Sauce
Calories: 450
Protein: 25g
Amino Acids: Complete profile from tempeh and peanuts

Snack:
Roasted chickpeas with cumin and paprika
Calories: 150
Protein: 6g

Dinner:
Quinoa-Stuffed Portobello Mushrooms with Spinach and Walnuts
Calories: 400
Protein: 15g
Amino Acids: High in lysine, methionine, leucine

Total Daily Calories: 1,550
Total Daily Protein: 60g
Note: Including a protein smoothie or a protein-rich dessert will help to increase both calorie and protein intake to meet the daily goal.

DAY 6

Breakfast:
Smoothie with Kale, Spirulina, Hemp Seeds, Pineapple, and Coconut Water
Calories: 350
Protein: 18g
Amino Acids: Complete profile from hemp seeds and spirulina

Snack:
Sliced apple with peanut butter
Calories: 200
Protein: 5g

Lunch:
Lentil Soup with Spinach and Quinoa
Calories: 450
Protein: 20g
Amino Acids: High in lysine, methionine, leucine

Snack:
Trail mix with dried fruits and seeds
Calories: 200
Protein: 5g

Dinner:
Vegan Tacos with Black Beans, Quinoa, Avocado, and Salsa
Calories: 400
Protein: 20g
Amino Acids: High in lysine, methionine, isoleucine

Total Daily Calories: 1,600

Total Daily Protein: 68g

Note: Adding a post-dinner snack like a piece of fruit with nuts or a small dessert will help reach the 2,000-calorie goal.

DAY 7

Breakfast:

Vegan Protein Pancakes with Almond Butter and Fresh Berries

Calories: 400

Protein: 20g

Amino Acids: Complete profile from protein powder and almond butter

Snack:

Sliced cucumber and cherry tomatoes with hummus

Calories: 150

Protein: 5g

Lunch:

Roasted Vegetable and Quinoa Bowl with Tahini Dressing

Calories: 450

Protein: 18g

Amino Acids: High in methionine, lysine, leucine

Snack: Rice cakes topped with avocado and a sprinkle of salt

Calories: 150

Protein: 4g

Dinner: Spaghetti Squash with Marinara Sauce and Lentil Meatballs

Calories: 400
Protein: 20g
Amino Acids: High in lysine, methionine, leucine

Total Daily Calories: 1,550
Total Daily Protein: 67g
Note: A bedtime snack such as a bowl of fruit with nuts or a small serving of vegan yogurt will help meet the 2,000-calorie target.

RECIPE 1: VEGAN QUINOA AND BLACK BEAN STUFFED PEPPERS

Macros: 300 calories, 48g carbs, 12g protein, 8g fat

Ingredients:
- 4 large bell peppers, tops removed and seeds cleaned out
- 1 cup cooked quinoa
- 1 can black beans, drained and rinsed
- 1/2 cup corn kernels (fresh or frozen)
- 1/4 cup diced tomatoes
- 1 teaspoon cumin
- 1 teaspoon smoked paprika
- Salt and pepper to taste
- 1/4 cup chopped cilantro
- 1 tablespoon olive oil

Instructions:
1. Preheat oven to 375°F (190°C).
2. In a large bowl, combine quinoa, black beans, corn, tomatoes, cumin, paprika, salt, and pepper. Mix well.

3. Stuff each bell pepper with the quinoa mixture and place them in a baking dish.
4. Drizzle olive oil over the stuffed peppers and cover with foil.
5. Bake for 30-35 minutes until peppers are tender.

RECIPE 2: VEGAN SWEET POTATO AND CHICKPEA CURRY

Macros: 350 calories, 55g carbs, 10g protein, 12g fat

Ingredients:
- 2 medium sweet potatoes, peeled and diced
- 1 can chickpeas, drained and rinsed
- 1 can of coconut milk
- onion, diced
- 2 garlic cloves, minced
- 1 tablespoon curry powder
- 1 teaspoon ground turmeric
- 1 teaspoon cumin
- 1/2 teaspoon cinnamon
- Salt and pepper to taste
- 2 cups spinach
- 1 tablespoon coconut oil

Instructions:
1. In a large pot, heat coconut oil over medium heat.
2. Add onion and garlic, sauté until translucent.
3. Stir in curry powder, turmeric, cumin, and cinnamon. Cook for 1-2 minutes.
4. Add sweet potatoes and chickpeas, stirring to coat with spices.

5. Pour in coconut milk, bring to a boil, then reduce heat to simmer.
6. Cook until sweet potatoes are tender, about 20 minutes.
7. Stir in spinach until wilted. Season with salt and pepper to taste.

RECIPE 3: VEGAN LENTIL AND QUINOA STUFFED PORTOBELLO MUSHROOMS

Macros: 280 calories, 45g carbs, 15g protein, 9g fat

Ingredients:

    4 large Portobello mushrooms, stems removed
    1 cup cooked lentils
    1 cup cooked quinoa
    1/4 cup chopped walnuts
    1 garlic clove, minced
    1/4 cup nutritional yeast
    2 tablespoons olive oil
    1 tablespoon balsamic vinegar
    Salt and pepper to taste
    2 tablespoons fresh parsley, chopped

Instructions:
1. Preheat oven to 375°F (190°C).
2. In a large bowl, combine cooked lentils, quinoa, walnuts, garlic, nutritional yeast, salt, and pepper.
3. Drizzle olive oil and balsamic vinegar over the mixture and toss to coat.
4. Place mushrooms on a baking sheet, gill side up. Spoon the lentil-quinoa mixture into each mushroom cap.

5. Bake for 20-25 minutes until mushrooms are tender and the filling is heated through.
6. Garnish with fresh parsley before serving.

RAW PROTEIN BAR RECIPES

PROTEIN BAR 1: MAPLE ALMOND PROTEIN BARS

Ingredients:
- 1 cup almond butter
- 1/4 cup maple syrup
- 1/4 cup protein powder (plant-based)
- 1/2 cup almond flour
- 1/4 cup chopped almonds
- 1/4 cup shredded coconut
- 1 teaspoon vanilla extract

Instructions:
1. Mix almond butter and maple syrup in a bowl until well combined.
2. Add protein powder, almond flour, chopped almonds, shredded coconut, and vanilla extract. Stir until a thick dough forms.
3. Press the mixture into a lined 8x8 inch baking dish.
4. Refrigerate for at least 2 hours before cutting into bars.

Macros (per bar): 250 calories, 12g carbs, 10g protein, 18g fat

EATING LESSONS

DATE & NUT ENERGY BARS

Ingredients:
- 1 cup pitted dates
- 1/2 cup raw cashews
- 1/2 cup rolled oats
- 1/4 cup protein powder (plant-based)
- 1/4 cup chia seeds
- 1/4 cup almond butter
- 1/2 teaspoon cinnamon

Instructions:
1. Process the dates in a food processor until they form a sticky paste.
2. Add cashews, oats, protein powder, chia seeds, almond butter, and cinnamon. Pulse until well combined.
3. Press the mixture into a lined 8x8 inch baking dish.
4. Refrigerate for at least 2 hours before cutting into bars.

Macros (per bar): 220 calories, 30g carbs, 8g protein, 10g fat

---

CHOCOLATE COOKIES WITH MAPLE SYRUP AND TAHINI

Ingredients:
- 1/2 cup tahini
- 1/4 cup pure maple syrup
- 1/4 cup coconut oil, melted
- 1 teaspoon vanilla extract
- 1 cup almond flour
- 1/4 cup cocoa powder

1/2 teaspoon baking soda
1/4 teaspoon salt
1/2 cup dark chocolate chips (vegan)

Instructions:
1. Preheat your oven to 350°F (175°C). Line a baking sheet with parchment paper.
2. In a large mixing bowl, combine the tahini, maple syrup, melted coconut oil, and vanilla extract. Stir until smooth and well combined.
3. In a separate bowl, whisk together the almond flour, cocoa powder, baking soda, and salt.
4. Gradually add the dry ingredients to the wet mixture, stirring until a dough forms.
5. Fold in the dark chocolate chips until evenly distributed throughout the dough.
6. Scoop tablespoon-sized portions of the dough onto the prepared baking sheet, leaving space between each cookie.
7. Flatten the cookies slightly with the back of a spoon or your fingers.
8. Bake for 10-12 minutes, or until the edges are set and the tops are slightly cracked.
9. Allow the cookies to cool on the baking sheet for a few minutes before transferring them to a wire rack to cool completely.

(Per cookie, assuming the recipe makes 12 cookies)
Calories: 150 kcal Protein: 3g Fat: 11g Saturated Fat: 3.5g
Carbohydrates: 11g Fiber: 2g Sugars: 6g

SPIRULINA BALLS WITH ORANGE

Ingredients:
- 1 cup pitted dates
- 1/2 cup almonds or cashews
- 1/4 cup shredded coconut (unsweetened)
- 1 tablespoon spirulina powder
- Zest of 1 orange
- 2 tablespoons fresh orange juice
- 1 tablespoon chia seeds (optional for extra texture)
- 1/2 teaspoon vanilla extract
- Pinch of salt
- Extra shredded coconut for rolling (optional)

Instructions:
1. In a food processor, pulse the almonds or cashews until they form a coarse meal.
2. Add the pitted dates, shredded coconut, spirulina powder, orange zest, orange juice, chia seeds (if using), vanilla extract, and salt to the food processor.
3. Process until the mixture comes together into a sticky dough. You may need to stop and scrape down the sides a few times to ensure everything is well combined.
4. Once the dough is ready, scoop out tablespoon-sized portions and roll them into balls using your hands.
5. If desired, roll each ball in extra shredded coconut to coat.
6. Place the spirulina balls in an airtight container and refrigerate for at least 30 minutes to firm up.
7. Store the spirulina balls in the refrigerator for up to a week or freeze them for longer storage.Spirulina Balls with Orange

(Per ball, assuming the recipe makes 12 balls)

Calories: 90 kcal Protein: 2g Fat: 4.5g Saturated Fat: 1.5g Carbohydrates: 12g Fiber: 2g Sugars: 8g

Here's a list of twenty creative on-the-go snacks that are nutritious, vegan, and easy to prepare:

1. Apple Slices with Almond Butter: Slice up an apple and add 1 tablespoon of almond butter for a sweet and satisfying snack.
2. Mixed Nuts: A small handful (about 1 ounce) of almonds, walnuts, or cashews provides a boost of healthy fats and protein.
3. Rice Cakes with Avocado: Top a gluten-free rice cake with mashed avocado and a sprinkle of salt for a crunchy, creamy snack.
4. Carrot Sticks with Hummus: 10 baby carrots dipped in 2 tablespoons of hummus for a fiber-rich, savory treat.
5. Energy Balls: Combine oats, dates, almond butter, and chia seeds, then roll into bite-sized balls.
6. Dried Fruit: A small handful of dried apricots, raisins, or dates for a natural sweet treat.
7. Chia Pudding: Mix 2 tablespoons chia seeds with almond milk and a dash of vanilla extract; let it sit overnight for a creamy, pudding-like snack.
8. Edamame Beans: 1/2 cup of steamed edamame, lightly salted, for a protein-packed snack.
9. Vegan Protein Bars: Look for gluten-free brands around 100-200 calories per bar, ideally with simple, whole-food ingredients.

10. Cucumber Slices with Guacamole: Fresh cucumber rounds topped with a dollop of guacamole for a refreshing and creamy snack.
11. Kale Chips: Baked kale leaves with a drizzle of olive oil and a sprinkle of sea salt, for a crunchy, nutrient-dense snack.
12. Banana with Peanut Butter: A banana sliced and spread with 1 tablespoon of peanut butter for a quick energy boost.
13. Homemade Trail Mix: A mix of raw nuts, seeds, dried fruit, and dark chocolate chips for a satisfying and energizing snack.
14. Celery Sticks with Nut Butter: Celery sticks filled with almond or peanut butter, sprinkled with raisins, known as "ants on a log."
15. Seaweed Snacks: Lightly salted nori sheets or seaweed chips, low-calorie and packed with iodine.
16. Olives and Cherry Tomatoes: A small container of mixed olives and cherry tomatoes for a savory, bite-sized snack.
17. Berry and Coconut Yogurt Parfait: A small container of coconut yogurt topped with fresh berries and a sprinkle of granola.
18. Sweet Potato Toasts: Thinly sliced sweet potato rounds, toasted, and topped with almond butter or avocado.
19. Veggie Sticks with Tahini Dip: Sliced bell peppers, cucumber, and zucchini with a side of tahini dip for a creamy and crunchy snack.
20. Pumpkin Seeds (Pepitas): A small handful of roasted pumpkin seeds seasoned with a pinch of salt or spices for a protein-rich, crunchy snack.

Workbook

These snacks offer a range of flavors, textures, and nutrients, making them perfect for staying energized and satisfied on the go.

Websites for Consumer Water Testing

- Environmental Working Group (EWG) Tap Water Database (www.ewg.org/tapwater)
- NSF International: www.nsf.org (www.nsf.org)
- Safe Drinking Water Foundation: (www.safewater.org)
- National Testing Laboratories (www.ntllabs.com)

ROYGBIV Plant-Based Foods Checklist

Eating a variety of colorful foods ensures a range of nutrients. Use this checklist to track your intake:

1. **Red:** Tomatoes, red peppers, strawberries, raspberries, red apples, beets, cherries, watermelon, pomegranate, red cabbage.
2. **Orange:** Carrots, sweet potatoes, oranges, pumpkin, butternut squash, apricots, persimmons, mangoes, papayas, cantaloupe.
3. **Yellow:** Yellow bell peppers, yellow tomatoes, corn, pineapple, bananas, lemons, yellow squash, golden beets, starfruit, yellow watermelon.
4. **Green:** Spinach, kale, broccoli, green beans, zucchini, cucumbers, avocados, kiwi, green apples, green grapes.
5. **Blue:** Blueberries, blackberries, blue potatoes, blue corn,

blue grapes, elderberries, black currants, blue figs, damson plums, blue seaweed.
6. **Indigo:** Blackberries, figs, prunes, purple grapes, purple asparagus, eggplant, purple carrots, purple cabbage, black rice, dark plums.
7. **Violet:** Eggplant, purple cauliflower, purple sweet potatoes, radicchio, purple kale, acai berries, purple figs, purple grapes, purple basil, purple bell peppers.

Glossary of Key Terms

Macronutrients: Nutrients that provide energy—carbohydrates, proteins, and fats. These are required in larger amounts to maintain body functions and energy levels.

Micronutrients: Essential vitamins and minerals required in small amounts. They play a crucial role in metabolism, immune function, and overall health.

Glycemic Index (GI): A measure of how quickly food raises blood sugar levels. High-GI foods cause a rapid increase, while low-GI foods result in a slower, more gradual rise.

GMO (Genetically Modified Organism): Organisms with altered genetic material to enhance certain traits, such as resistance to pests or increased nutritional content.

Antioxidants: Molecules that prevent oxidation and cellular damage by neutralizing free radicals. They help protect the body from diseases and aging.

Phytonutrients: Natural compounds found in plants that provide health benefits, such as anti-inflammatory and antioxidant effects.

Omega-3 Fatty Acids: Essential fats found in foods like flaxseeds, chia seeds, and walnuts. They are crucial for heart health, brain function, and reducing inflammation.

Probiotics: Beneficial bacteria found in fermented foods that support gut health and boost the immune system by maintaining a healthy balance of gut flora.

Prebiotics: Non-digestible ingredients, typically fibers, that promote the growth of beneficial bacteria in the gut, enhancing digestive health.

BPA (Bisphenol A): A chemical used in producing certain plastics, linked to health issues such as hormonal disruptions and developmental problems.

Whole Foods: Foods that are minimally processed and close to their natural form, such as fruits, vegetables, whole grains, and nuts. They are free from artificial additives and preservatives.

Processed Foods: Foods that have been altered from their natural state through methods like canning, freezing, or adding preservatives. Highly processed foods often contain added sugars, unhealthy fats, and artificial ingredients.

Umami: A savory taste found in foods like mushrooms, soy sauce, and aged cheese. It is considered the fifth basic taste, alongside sweet, sour, bitter, and salty.

Gluten: A protein found in wheat, barley, and rye. It gives dough elasticity and can cause adverse reactions in people with celiac disease or gluten sensitivity.

Detoxification: The process of removing toxins from the body, supported by organs like the liver and kidneys. A diet rich in whole foods and adequate hydration can enhance natural detox processes.

Sustainable Agriculture: Farming practices that protect the environment, ensure fair labor practices, and promote animal welfare. This approach focuses on maintaining soil health, reducing chemical use, and conserving resources.

Adaptogens: Natural substances, typically herbs, that help the body adapt to stress and maintain balance. Examples include ashwagandha, rhodiola, and ginseng.

Electrolytes: Minerals in the body, such as sodium, potassium, and magnesium, that are essential for maintaining fluid balance, nerve function, and muscle contractions.

Polyphenols: A category of phytonutrients with antioxidant properties found in foods like tea, red wine, berries, and dark chocolate. They contribute to reduced inflammation and improved heart health.

Flavonoids: A type of polyphenol found in fruits, vegetables, and certain beverages that have antioxidant and anti-inflammatory properties. They are associated with a lower risk of chronic diseases.

Free Radicals: Unstable molecules that can damage cells and lead to oxidative stress. They are neutralized by antioxidants, preventing cellular damage.

Lignans: Plant compounds found in seeds (especially flaxseeds), whole grains, and vegetables. They have antioxidant properties and may help protect against certain cancers.

Nutraceuticals: Products derived from food sources that offer health benefits, often beyond basic nutrition. Examples include fish oil capsules, probiotics, and fortified foods.

Functional Foods: Foods that have a potentially positive effect on health beyond basic nutrition. They may provide benefits such as improving gut health, enhancing immune function, or reducing the risk of chronic diseases.

Isoflavones: A type of phytonutrient found in soy products that have estrogen-like properties. They are studied for their potential role in reducing the risk of hormone-related cancers.

Fermentation: A metabolic process that converts sugar to acids, gases, or alcohol. Fermented foods like yogurt, kimchi, and sauerkraut contain probiotics that support gut health.

Carotenoids: A class of phytonutrients that includes beta-carotene, lutein, and lycopene, found in colorful fruits and vegetables. They are known for their role in eye health and as antioxidants.

Collagen: A protein that provides structure to skin, hair, nails, and connective tissues. Some plant-based foods can help support collagen production in the body.

Ketogenic Diet: A low-carbohydrate, high-fat diet that induces ketosis, a metabolic state where the body burns fat for fuel instead of carbohydrates. It is used for weight loss and managing certain health conditions.

Paleo Diet: A dietary plan based on foods similar to what might have been eaten during the Paleolithic era, focusing on whole foods like lean meats, fish, fruits, vegetables, nuts, and seeds.

Phycocyanin: A pigment-protein complex found in blue-green algae, such as spirulina. It has potent antioxidant and anti-inflammatory properties and is responsible for the blue color in blue spirulina.

Chlorophyll: The green pigment in plants responsible for photosynthesis. It is known for its potential detoxifying properties and is found in green leafy vegetables and algae.

Methylcobalamin: A natural, bioactive form of vitamin B12, essential for nerve function and the production of DNA and red blood cells. Often found in animal products and certain supplements.

Amino Acids: The building blocks of proteins, essential for growth, tissue repair, and various metabolic functions. There are 20 amino acids, 9 of which are essential, meaning the body cannot produce them, and they must be obtained through diet.

Bioavailability: The degree to which a nutrient or supplement is absorbed and utilized by the body. It determines the effectiveness of nutrients and supplements.

Lycopene: A powerful antioxidant found in tomatoes and other red fruits and vegetables. It is linked to reduced risk of certain types of cancer and heart disease.

Sulforaphane: A compound found in cruciferous vegetables like broccoli and kale. It is known for its potential anti-cancer properties and ability to support detoxification processes.

Resveratrol: An antioxidant found in grapes, red wine, and certain berries. It is studied for its potential benefits in heart health, anti-aging, and cancer prevention.

Oxalates: Naturally occurring compounds found in foods like spinach, beets, and nuts. In high amounts, they can bind to minerals and form crystals, potentially contributing to kidney stones in susceptible individuals.

Nutritional Substitution Guide

Cravings can often indicate underlying nutritional deficiencies. Use this guide to address cravings with healthier options:

Chocolate: Magnesium deficiency. Substitute with green leafy vegetables, seeds, raw nuts, beans, and fruits.

Fatty or Oily Foods: Calcium deficiency. Include spinach, collard greens, kale, okra, oranges, almonds, figs, and sesame seeds.

Bread: Nitrogen deficiency. Opt for oatmeal, leafy greens, nuts, and legumes.

Soda and Carbonated Drinks: Calcium deficiency. Eat more mustard greens, kale, and sesame.

Salty Snacks: Chloride deficiency. Eat sea salt, celery, and tomatoes.

Sugary Sweets: Low blood sugar, chromium, or sulfur deficiency. Substitute with quinoa, fruits, legumes, cinnamon, raisins, asparagus, garlic, kale, and onions.

Cheese: Essential fatty acid deficiency. Substitute with flax oil, Omega-3s (EPA and DHA), walnuts, and chia seeds.

Alcohol: Protein, calcium, or potassium deficiency. Substitute with legumes, leafy greens, nuts, seeds, seaweed, tomatoes, citrus fruits, and black olives.

Pasta or Baked Foods: Chromium deficiency. Substitute with cinnamon, grapes, tomatoes, onions, apples, lettuce, and sweet potatoes.

Cheat Sheet for Organic Labeling

Understanding food labels is crucial for making informed choices. Here's a quick guide to common organic labels and symbols:

USDA Organic: Products with this label contain at least 95% organic ingredients and have been certified by the United States Department of Agriculture.

Non-GMO Project Verified: Ensures that the product does not contain genetically modified organisms (GMOs).

Fair Trade Certified: Indicates that the product was made under fair labor conditions with environmentally sustainable practices.

100% Organic: Products contain only organic ingredients with no synthetic additives.

Made with Organic Ingredients: Indicates that the product contains at least 70% organic ingredients.

4-Digit Code (Conventionally Grown): Produce with a 4-digit code (starting with 3 or 4) is conventionally grown using standard agricultural methods, which may include pesticides and synthetic fertilizers.

5-Digit Code Starting with 9 (Organic): Produce with a 5-digit code starting with 9 is organic and grown without synthetic pesticides, fertilizers, or GMOs.

5-Digit Code Starting with 8 (Genetically Modified): Produce with a 5-digit code starting with 8 is genetically modified (GMO).

Additives on Labels to Avoid

To protect your health, avoid certain chemicals commonly found in processed foods. Watch out for:

1. High Fructose Corn Syrup (HFCS)
2. Refined Sugar (Sucrose)
3. Artificial Sweeteners:
   Aspartame
   Saccharin
   Sucralose
   Acesulfame K

Neotame

Cyclamate

4. Trans Fats (Partially Hydrogenated Oils)

5. Vegetable and Seed Oils:

Soybean Oil

Corn Oil

Canola Oil

Sunflower Oil

Safflower Oil

6. Monosodium Glutamate (MSG)

7. Artificial Colors:

Red 40 (Allura Red)

Yellow 5 (Tartrazine)

Yellow 6 (Sunset Yellow)

Blue 1 (Brilliant Blue)

Blue 2 (Indigo Carmine)

Green 3 (Fast Green)

Red 3 (Erythrosine)

8. Preservatives:

Sodium Nitrite and Sodium Nitrate

Butylated Hydroxyanisole (BHA)

Butylated Hydroxytoluene (BHT)

Propyl Gallate

Potassium Sorbate

Calcium Propionate

Sodium Benzoate

9. Flavor Enhancers:

Disodium Inosinate

Disodium Guanylate

Autolyzed Yeast Extract

10. Stabilizers and Emulsifiers:

Carrageenan

Polysorbates (e.g., Polysorbate 80)

Xanthan Gum

Mono and Diglycerides

11. Thickeners:

Modified Corn Starch

Guar Gum

Cellulose Gum

Carboxymethylcellulose

12. Anti-Caking Agents:

Silicon Dioxide

Calcium Silicate

13. Brominated Vegetable Oil (BVO)

14. Potassium Bromate

15. TBHQ (Tertiary Butylhydroquinone)

16. Artificial Flavors

17. Propylene Glycol

18. Sodium Carboxymethyl Cellulose

19. Sodium Erythorbate

20. Aluminum Additives:

Sodium Aluminum Phosphate

Sodium Aluminum Sulfate

Potassium Aluminum Sulfate

21. Phosphates:

Sodium Phosphate

Calcium Phosphate

22. Parabens (Methylparaben, Propylparaben)

23. Sodium Lauryl Sulfate (SLS)

24. Azodicarbonamide (ADA)

25. Ethoxyquin

These ingredients are commonly found in a wide range of processed foods and personal care products. While some are considered safe in low amounts, ongoing consumption, particularly from multiple sources, may lead to health issues over time. To minimize exposure, it's advisable to read food labels carefully and choose whole, minimally processed foods whenever possible.

Justine Bassani

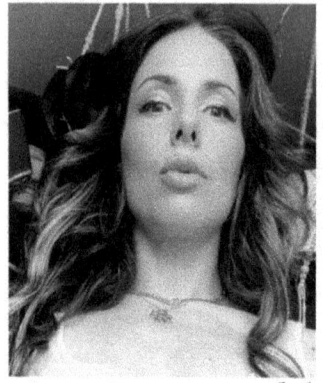

Justine's passion for empowering others with knowledge led her to compile the essential lessons on eating and nutrition into this book, designed for anyone who has ever wanted to take control of their diet and make lasting, positive changes. Her approach is grounded in years of research and a genuine desire to help others live healthier, more fulfilling lives

Justine Bassani is a certified Nutrition Coach and Personal Trainer through the National Academy of Sports Medicine. With a diverse background that uniquely blends her professional training and real-world experience, Justine has dedicated herself to helping others understand the often-confusing world of nutrition and diet. Her journey into the realm of wellness was sparked by her years of experience as a bartender, where she had countless conversations with people from all walks of life. These interactions and learning from her own challenges revealed widespread misconceptions about dieting, inspiring Justine to dive deep into research to uncover the truths about eating habits and nutrition.

Outside of her work in nutrition, Justine is an artist with a deep love for music and classical painting. She is also a member of the Screen Actors Guild, showcasing her multifaceted talents and creative spirit. Despite her work as a bartender, Justine is a proud non-drinker, embodying the principles of self-discipline and health that she advocates.

Looking ahead, Justine is working on new projects, including habit-tracking journals and shadow workbooks designed to create emotional and habitual changes that align with a holistic approach to eating. Her future works aim to encourage readers to respect their bodies, other living beings, and the environment in their daily habits. You can find her on Instagram @JustineBassani and at her website www.weallglowedup.com, where you can find blogs, recommended products, and new release updates. You can also connect with her directly!

Justine's journey is a testament to the power of combining professional knowledge with personal passion, and her work continues to inspire those seeking to make meaningful changes in their lives.

Workbook

www.ingramcontent.com/pod-product-compliance
Lightning Source LLC
Chambersburg PA
CBHW070608030426
42337CB00020B/3711